Endocrine and Metabolic Emergencies

Editors

GEORGE C. WILLIS
M. TYSON PILLOW

EMERGENCY MEDICINE CLINICS OF NORTH AMERICA

www.emed.theclinics.com

Consulting Editor
AMAL MATTU

May 2014 • Volume 32 • Number 2

ELSEVIER

1600 John F. Kennedy Boulevard • Suite 1800 • Philadelphia, Pennsylvania, 19103-2899

http://www.theclinics.com

EMERGENCY MEDICINE CLINICS OF NORTH AMERICA Volume 32, Number 2
May 2014 ISSN 0733-8627, ISBN-13: 978-0-323-29703-5

Editor: Patrick Manley
Developmental Editor: Casey Jackson

Emergency Medicine Clinics of North America (ISSN 0733-8627) is published quarterly by Elsevier Inc., 360 Park Avenue South, New York, NY, 10010-1710. Months of issue are February, May, August, and November. Business and Editorial Offices: 1600 John F. Kennedy Boulevard, Suite 1800, Philadelphia, PA 19103-2899. Customer Service Office: 6277 Sea Harbor Drive, Orlando, FL 32887-4800. Periodicals postage paid at New York, NY, and additional mailing offices. Subscription prices are $155.00 per year (US students), $315.00 per year (US individuals), $523.00 per year (US institutions), $220.00 per year (international students), $450.00 per year (international individuals), $642.00 per year (international institutions), $220.00 per year (Canadian students), $385.00 per year (Canadian individuals), and $642.00 per year (Canadian institutions). International air speed delivery is included in all *Clinics'* subscription prices. All prices are subject to change without notice. **POSTMASTER:** Send address changes to *Emergency Medicine Clinics of North America*, Elsevier Periodicals Customer Service, 11830 Westline Industrial Drive, St. Louis, MO 63146. Customer Service (orders, claims, online, change of address): Elsevier Periodicals Customer Service, 11830 Westline Industrial Drive, St. Louis, MO 63146. Tel: 1-800-654-2452 (U.S. and Canada); 314-453-7041 (outside U.S. and Canada). Fax: 314-453-5170. E-mail: journalscustomerservice-usa@elsevier.com (for print support); journalsonlinesupport-usa@elsevier.com (for online support).

Reprints. For copies of 100 or more of articles in this publication, please contact the Commercial Reprints Department, Elsevier Inc., 360 Park Avenue South, New York, NY 10010-1710. Tel.: 212-633-3874; Fax: 212-633-3820; E-mail: reprints@elsevier.com.

Emergency Medicine Clinics of North America is covered in *MEDLINE/PubMed (Index Medicus), Current Contents/Clinical Medicine, EMBASE/Excerpta Medica, BIOSIS, SciSearch, CINAHL, ISI/BIOMED*, and *Research Alert*.

Contributors

CONSULTING EDITOR

AMAL MATTU, MD
Professor and Vice Chair, Department of Emergency Medicine, University of Maryland School of Medicine, Baltimore, Maryland

EDITORS

GEORGE C. WILLIS, MD
Assistant Professor, Department of Emergency Medicine, University of Maryland School of Medicine, Baltimore, Maryland

M. TYSON PILLOW, MD, MEd
Associate Program Director, Section of Emergency Medicine, Assistant Professor, Undergraduate Medical Education, Baylor College of Medicine; San Antonio Military Medical Center, Houston, Texas

AUTHORS

MICHAEL K. ABRAHAM, MD, MS
Clinical Assistant Professor, Department of Emergency Medicine, University of Maryland School of Medicine, Baltimore, Maryland

OMOYEMI ADEBAYO, MD
Resident, Department of Emergency Medicine, University of Maryland Medical Center, Baltimore, Maryland

MICHAEL G. ALLISON, MD
Division of Pulmonary and Critical Care Medicine, Department of Medicine; Department of Emergency Medicine, University of Maryland School of Medicine, Baltimore, Maryland

WAN-TSU W. CHANG, MD
Assistant Professor, Department of Emergency Medicine, University of Maryland School of Medicine, Baltimore, Maryland

BRIAN CORWELL, MD, FACEP
CAQ Sports Medicine, Assistant Professor, Department of Emergency Medicine, University of Maryland School of Medicine, Baltimore, Maryland

NATHAN S. DEAL, MD
Assistant Professor, Section of Emergency Medicine, Ben Taub General Hospital, Baylor College of Medicine, Houston, Texas

DANIELLE DEVEREAUX, MD
Emergency Medicine and Pediatric Resident, Department of Emergency Medicine, University of Maryland Medical System, University of Maryland, Baltimore, Maryland

SARAH B. DUBBS, MD
Department of Emergency Medicine, University of Maryland School of Medicine, Baltimore, Maryland

THERESA R. HARRING, MD
Section of Emergency Medicine, Ben Taub General Hospital, Baylor College of Medicine, Houston, Texas

BASHAR ISMAIL, MD
Baylor College of Medicine, Houston, Texas

HYUNG T. KIM, MD
Assistant Professor of Clinical Emergency Medicine, Keck School of Medicine of University of Southern California; Medical Director, Department of Emergency Medicine, Los Angeles County + University of Southern California Medical Center, Los Angeles, California

BRANDI KNIGHT, MD
Resident Physician, Department of Emergency Medicine, University of Maryland School of Medicine, Baltimore, Maryland

DICK C. KUO, MD
Associate Professor, Section of Emergency Medicine, Ben Taub General Hospital, Baylor College of Medicine, Houston, Texas

MICHAEL T. MCCURDY, MD
Assistant Professor, Department of Emergency Medicine; Assistant Professor, Division of Pulmonary and Critical Care Medicine, Department of Medicine, University of Maryland School of Medicine, Baltimore, Maryland

LAURA MEDFORD-DAVIS, MD
Division of Emergency Medicine, Baylor College of Medicine; Department of Emergency Medicine, Ben Taub General Hospital, Houston, Texas

LAURA OLIVIERI, MD
Resident Physician, Department of Emergency Medicine, University of Maryland School of Medicine, Baltimore, Maryland

ELIZABETH PARK, MD
Resident Physician, Department of Emergency Medicine, Baylor College of Medicine, Houston, Texas

NADIA M. PEARSON, DO
Department of Emergency Medicine, San Antonio Military Medical Center, San Antonio; Section of Emergency Medicine, Baylor College of Medicine, Houston, Texas

M. TYSON PILLOW, MD, MEd
Associate Program Director, Section of Emergency Medicine, Assistant Professor, Undergraduate Medical Education, Baylor College of Medicine; San Antonio Military Medical Center, Houston, Texas

BETHANY RADIN, DO
Fellow, Division of Pulmonary and Critical Care Medicine, Department of Medicine, University of Maryland School of Medicine, Baltimore, Maryland

ZUBAID RAFIQUE, MD
Division of Emergency Medicine, Baylor College of Medicine; Department of Emergency Medicine, Ben Taub General Hospital, Houston, Texas

MIKE RICE, MD
Baylor College of Medicine, Houston, Texas

JENNIFER T. SOIFER, MD
Assistant Professor of Clinical Emergency Medicine, Keck School of Medicine of University of Southern California; Assistant Medical Director, Department of Emergency Medicine, Los Angeles County + University of Southern California Medical Center, Los Angeles, California

TELEMATÉ SOKARI, MD
Section of Emergency Medicine, Emergency Center, Ben Taub General Hospital, Baylor College of Medicine, Houston, Texas

RYAN SPANGLER, MD
Emergency Medicine Residency Program, University of Maryland Medical Center, Baltimore, Maryland

SEMHAR Z. TEWELDE, MD
Cardiology Fellow/Clinical Instructor, Department of Emergency Medicine, University of Maryland Medical System, University of Maryland, Baltimore, Maryland

ALEXANDER TOLEDO, DO, PharmD
Assistant Professor of Pediatrics and Emergency Medicine, Section of Emergency Medicine, Baylor College of Medicine, Houston, Texas

VERONICA TUCCI, MD, JD
Assistant Professor, Baylor College of Medicine; Section of Emergency Medicine, Emergency Center, Ben Taub General Hospital, Houston, Texas

GEORGE C. WILLIS, MD
Assistant Professor, Department of Emergency Medicine, University of Maryland School of Medicine, Baltimore, Maryland

Contents

epidemic of childhood obesity, causing a paradigm shift in how childhood diabetes is conceptualized. Once thought a consequence of obesity, sedentary lifestyle, and genetics, diabetes with onset in adults has been found to have a variant with autoimmunity. As the lines among adult-onset, child-onset, and type 1 and type 2 diabetes mellitus become more blurred, best practices in management and prevention become more complicated. This article highlights key points regarding 2 variants, juvenile-onset type 2 diabetes mellitus and latent autoimmune diabetes of adults.

Changes in potassium elimination, primarily due to the renal and GI systems, and shifting potassium between the intracellular and extracellular spaces cause potassium derangement. Symptoms are vague, but can be cardiac, musculoskeletal, or gastrointestinal. There are no absolute guidelines for when to treat, but it is generally recommended when the patient is symptomatic or has ECG changes. Treatment of hyperkalemia includes cardiac membrane stabilization with IV calcium, insulin and beta-antagonists to push potassium intracellularly, and dialysis. Neither sodium bicarbonate nor kayexelate are recommended. Treatment of symptomatic hypokalemia consists of PO or IV repletion with potassium chloride and magnesium sulfate.

Derangements of calcium, magnesium, and phosphate are associated with increased morbidity and mortality. These minerals have vital roles in the cellular physiology of the neuromuscular and cardiovascular systems. This article describes the pathophysiology of these mineral disorders. It aims to provide the emergency practitioner with an overview of the diagnosis and management of these disorders.

Although the altered mental status is a common presentation in the emergency department, altered mental status caused by endocrine emergencies is rare. The altered patient could have an endocrine cause that can quickly improve with appropriate diagnosis and interventions. When dealing with limited information and an obtunded patient, it is important to have a broad differential diagnosis, pick up on the physical examination findings, and evaluate laboratory abnormalities that could suggest an underlying endocrine emergency. This article outlines the findings and provides a description of altered patients with endocrine emergencies to facilitate the diagnosis and treatment in the emergency department.

Dysnatremias occur simultaneously with disorders in water balance. The first priority is to correct dehydration; once the patient is euvolemic, the sodium level can be reassessed. In unstable patients with hyponatremia, the clinician should rapidly administer hypertonic saline. In unstable patients with hypernatremia, the clinician should administer isotonic intravenous fluid. In stable patients with either hyponatremia or hypernatremia, the clinician should aim for correction over 24 to 48 hours, with the maximal change in serum sodium between 8 to 12 mEq/L over the first 24 hours. This rate of correction decreases the chances of cerebral edema or osmotic demyelination syndrome.

Acid-base disorders should be considered a process with the goal being to treat the patient and the underlying condition, not the numbers. A good understanding of the normal acid-base regulation in the body, as well as the most common derangements can prepare the emergency physician for this very common disorder that presents on every shift.

The resuscitation principles of securing the airway and stabilizing hemodynamics remain the same in any neonatal emergency. However, stabilizing endocrine disorders may prove especially challenging. Several organ systems are affected simultaneously and the clinical presentation can be subtle. Although not all-inclusive, the implementation of newborn screening tests has significantly reduced morbidity and mortality in neonates. Implementing routine screening tests worldwide and improving the accuracy of present tests remains the challenge for healthcare providers. With further study of these disorders and best treatment practices we can provide neonates presenting to the emergency department with the best possible outcomes.

Diabetic ketoacidosis and hyperosmolar hyperglycemic state are the most feared complications of uncontrolled diabetes seen in emergency medicine. The treatment of both conditions must be tailored to individual patients and relies on aggressive fluid resuscitation, insulin replacement, and electrolyte management. Emergency medicine providers must address the underlying causes and monitor for complications of therapy. Improved understanding of the underlying pathophysiology and application of evidence-based guidelines have significantly improved prognosis and decreased mortality. The purpose of this article is to review the diagnosis, presentation, and emergency department management of diabetic ketoacidosis and hyperosmolar hyperglycemic state with an emphasis on current management and treatment guidelines.

Metabolic alkalosis is a common disorder, accounting for half of all acid-base disturbances in hospitalized patients. It is the result of an increase

EMERGENCY MEDICINE
CLINICS OF NORTH AMERICA

FORTHCOMING ISSUES

August 2014
Hematology/Oncology Emergencies
John C. Perkins, MD, and
Jonathan E. Davis, MD, *Editors*

November 2014
Critical Care in the Emergency Department
Evie Marcolini, MD, and
Haney A. Mallemat, MD, *Editors*

February 2015
Management of Hazardous Material Emergencies
Stephen Borron, MD, and
Ziad Kazzi, MD, *Editors*

RECENT ISSUES

February 2014
Clinical Toxicology
Silas W. Smith, MD, and
Daniel M. Lugassy, MD, *Editors*

November 2013
Dangerous Fever in the Emergency Department
Emilie Calvello, MD, and
Christian Theodosis, MD, *Editors*

August 2013
Pediatric Emergency Medicine
Le N. Lu, MD, Dale Woolridge, MD, and
Ann M. Dietrich, MD, *Editors*

RELATED INTEREST

Endocrinology and Metabolism Clinics of North America, March 2014 (Vol. 43, No. 1)
Diabetes Mellitus: Associated Conditions
Leonid Poretsky, MD, and Emilia Liao, MD, *Editors*

DOWNLOAD
Free App!

Review Articles
THE CLINICS

NOW AVAILABLE FOR YOUR iPhone and iPad

PROGRAM OBJECTIVE

The goal of *Emergency Medicine Clinics of North America* is to keep practicing emergency medicine physicians and emergency medicine residents up to date with current clinical practice in emergency medicine by providing timely articles reviewing the state of the art in patient care.

TARGET AUDIENCE

All practicing physicians and healthcare professionals who provide patient care utilizing findings from *Emergency Medicine Clinics of North America*.

LEARNING OBJECTIVES

Upon completion of this activity, participants will be able to:
1. Discuss approaches to metabolic acidosis and metabolic alkalosis
2. Review treatments for hyperthyroidism and thyrotoxicosis
3. Describe disorders of sodium and water balance

ACCREDITATION

The Elsevier Office of Continuing Medical Education (EOCME) is accredited by the Accreditation Council for Continuing Medical Education (ACCME) to provide continuing medical education for physicians.

The EOCME designates this enduringmaterial for a maximum of 15 *AMA PRA Category 1 Credit*(s)™. Physicians should claim only the credit commensurate with the extent of their participation in the activity.

All other health care professionals requesting continuing education credit for this enduring material will be issued a certificate of participation.

DISCLOSURE OF CONFLICTS OF INTEREST

The EOCME assesses conflict of interest with its instructors, faculty, planners, and other individuals who are in a position to control the content of CME activities. All relevant conflicts of interest that are identified are thoroughly vetted by EOCME for fair balance, scientific objectivity, and patient care recommendations. EOCME is committed to providing its learners with CME activities that promote improvements or quality in healthcare and not a specific proprietary business or a commercial interest.

The planning committee, staff, authors and editors listed below have identified no financial relationships or relationships to products or devices they or their spouse/life partner have with commercial interest related to the content of this CME activity:

Michael K. Abraham, MD, MS; Omoyemi Adebayo, MD; Michael G. Allison, MD; Wan-Tsu W. Chang, MD; Brian Corwell, MD; Nathan S. Deal, MD; Danielle Devereaux, MD; Sarah B. Dubbs, MD; Theresa R. Harring, MD; Kristen Helm; Brynne Hunter; Bashar Ismail, MD; Hyung T. Kim, MD; Brandi Knight, MD; Indu Kumari; Dick C. Kuo, MD; Patrick Manley; Amal Mattu, MD; Michael T. McCurdy, MD; Jill McNair; Laura Medford-Davis, MD; Laura H. Olivieri, MD; Elizabeth Park, MD; Nadia M. Pearson, DO; M. Tyson Pillow, MD, MEd; Bethany Radin, DO; Zubaid Rafique, MD; Mike Rice, MD; Jennifer T. Soifer, MD; Telemate Sokari, MD; Ryan Spangler, MD; Semhar Z. Tewelde, MD; Alex Toledo, DO, PharmD, FAAEM, FAAP; Veronica Tucci, MD; George C. Willis, MD, FAAEM.

The planning committee, staff, authors and editors listed below have identified financial relationships or relationships to products or devices they or their spouse/life partner have with commercial interest related to the content of this CME activity:

UNAPPROVED/OFF-LABEL USE DISCLOSURE

The EOCME requires CME faculty to disclose to the participants:
1. When products or procedures being discussed are off-label, unlabelled, experimental, and/or investigational (not US Food and Drug Administration (FDA) approved); and
2. Any limitations on the information presented, such as data that are preliminary or that represent ongoing research, interim analyses, and/or unsupported opinions. Faculty may discuss information about pharmaceutical agents that is outside of FDA-approved labelling. This information is intended solely for CME and is not intended to promote off-label use of these medications. If you have any questions, contact the medical affairs department of the manufacturer for the most recent prescribing information.

TO ENROLL

To enroll in the *Emergency Medicine Clinics* Continuing Medical Education program, call customer service at 1-800-654-2452 or sign up online at http://www.theclinics.com/home/cme. The CME program is available to subscribers for an additional annual fee of $235 USD.

METHOD OF PARTICIPATION

In order to claim credit, participants must complete the following:
1. Complete enrolment as indicated above.
2. Read the activity.
3. Complete the CME Test and Evaluation. Participants must achieve a score of 70% on the test. All CME Tests and Evaluations must be completed online.

CME INQUIRIES/SPECIAL NEEDS

For all CME inquiries or special needs, please contact elsevierCME@elsevier.com.

Foreword

Endocrine and Metabolic Emergencies in Emergency Medicine

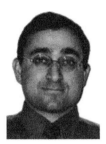

Amal Mattu, MD
Consulting Editor

A junior member of our faculty once approached me for some career advice, inquiring as to what clinical area of emergency medicine in which he should develop an academic niche. I advised him to focus on endocrine and metabolic emergencies. He immediately grimaced as if he had just bitten into a lemon. My reasons for the recommendation were simple: the endocrine system has a direct influence on *every* other organ system in the body; dysfunction of most organ systems produces metabolic derangements that can be life-threatening; endocrine and metabolic emergencies are very common in clinical practice and a not insignificant portion of the emergency medicine core curriculum; and finally, people don't understand these emergencies well. Unfortunately, his visceral reaction was a typical one among emergency physicians when the topic of endocrinology or metabolism arises. These topics are typically taught with poor clinical relevance to emergency medicine, and as a result, they are not enjoyed by most emergency physicians. I explained to this faculty member that, if he could become an expert in these topics and teach them in an interesting and relevant manner, he would find success and opportunities abounding in academic emergency medicine. That junior faculty member was Dr George Willis, one of our guest editors for this issue of *Emergency Medicine Clinics of North America*, who has rapidly become a national expert in endocrine and metabolic emergencies.

Next to enter the scene was Dr Tyson Pillow, another rising academic superstar in emergency medicine with a strong interest in endocrine and metabolic emergencies. Drs Willis and Pillow have combined their talents and similar interests to produce a fantastic issue of *Emergency Medicine Clinics of North America*. In reading through this issue, you will quickly appreciate the tremendous importance of endocrine and

Emerg Med Clin N Am 32 (2014) xv–xvi
http://dx.doi.org/10.1016/j.emc.2014.03.002
0733-8627/14/$ – see front matter © 2014 Elsevier Inc. All rights reserved.

emed.theclinics.com

metabolic issues in the clinical practice of emergency medicine, and you will also appreciate the clinical relevance that they and their authors have brought to topics that are traditionally steeped in basic science minutia.

Articles in this issue discuss core topics such as diabetic, thyroid, and adrenal disorders, sodium and fluid balance, and critical electrolyte emergencies. A separate article is dedicated to simplifying the dizzying array of neonatal endocrine disorders; and a full article is devoted to the influence of the endocrine system on mental status. Finally, a full article is devoted to the all-too-common alcoholic patient in the emergency department, an article that reminds us that these patients are prone to deadly metabolic abnormalities that are easily missed.

For anyone that has ever grimaced at the thought of hearing about or reading about endocrine and metabolic emergencies, I would strongly advise you to take a peek at the articles contained within this issue of *Emergency Medicine Clinics of North America*. You just might be very surprised to discover the clinical relevance of these topics to daily emergency medicine practice, and you'll be pleasantly surprised to see how enjoyable it can be to learn more about these topics from some practical and down-to-earth, stellar clinicians. And for those of you that are starting your careers in academic emergency medicine and are searching for a niche, this issue of *Emergency Medicine Clinics of North America* just might inspire you to choose endocrine and metabolic emergencies as your area of hopeful expertise. Kudos to the authors and guest editors for their contribution to our learning and for their outstanding work!

Amal Mattu, MD
Department of Emergency Medicine
University of Maryland School of Medicine
Baltimore, MD 21201, USA

E-mail address:
amattu@smail.umaryland.edu

Preface

Endocrine and Metabolic Emergencies

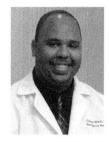 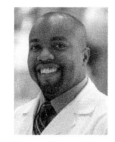

George C. Willis, MD   M. Tyson Pillow, MD, MEd
Editors

Hello everyone and welcome to this issue of the *Emergency Medicine Clinics of North America*. We are excited to have the opportunity to revisit key topics in endocrinology and metabolism.

Often the mention of endocrine and metabolism is met with eye-rolling and sighs, but this continues to be at least a consideration in every patient (you are screening the patient every time you order a basic metabolic panel, for example). As we examined this area of emergency medicine, we tried to incorporate several key themes into the articles. First, endocrine emergencies are a critical part of emergency medicine practice. Although infrequent, endocrine emergencies may present with life-threatening illness as well. This relates to the second point: endocrine emergencies can be easily missed. Many of the disease processes overlap in symptomatology and few have pathognomonic features that can exclude any other diagnosis without confirmatory testing. Third, endocrine and metabolic emergencies are difficult in that even when identified, mismanagement can lead to life-threatening complications. When these emergencies do occur, especially at night, most of our endocrinologist colleagues do not take calls and are unavailable to us.

So, for the practicing emergency physician, we sought to address the topics in a way that highlighted the difficulties in diagnosis and management. We extracted key points from each area and emphasized the approach to diagnosis as well. Treatment options can vary, but we have included evidence-based and guideline-based recommendations (wherever applicable) combining both the best information and our collective years of experience. Finally, we offer a fresh perspective on diabetes in the United States. While more common than the other diseases discussed in this issue, our understanding of how to treat this condition continues to evolve in response to its impact on our patients.

We would like to thank all of the authors and colleagues who contributed to this issue of *Emergency Medicine Clinics of North America*. We would also like to thank Amal

Emerg Med Clin N Am 32 (2014) xvii–xviii
http://dx.doi.org/10.1016/j.emc.2014.03.001
0733-8627/14/$ – see front matter © 2014 Published by Elsevier Inc.

emed.theclinics.com

Mattu, for providing us this wonderful opportunity, and Patrick Manley, for his overwhelming support throughout this endeavor. We hope that all of our readers find the information useful to their practice and that it enhances the care delivered to our patients.

George C. Willis, MD
Department of Emergency Medicine
University of Maryland School of Medicine
Baltimore, MD, USA

1304 Teacher Lane
Severn, MD 21144, USA

M. Tyson Pillow, MD, MEd
Section of Emergency Medicine
Undergraduate Medical Education
Baylor College of Medicine
1504 Taub Loop Road
Houston, TX 77030, USA

San Antonio Military Medical Center
3551 Roger Brooke Drive
Fort Sam
Houston, TX 78234, USA

E-mail addresses:
george.willis.md@gmail.com (G.C. Willis)
tysonpillow@gmail.com (M.T. Pillow)

Hyperthyroidism and Thyrotoxicosis

Danielle Devereaux, MD*, Semhar Z. Tewelde, MD

KEYWORDS

• Hyperthyroidism • Thyrotoxicosis • Thyroid storm • Thyroiditis • Graves disease

KEY POINTS

- Thyroid storm is uniformly fatal if untreated and, even with treatment, mortality ranges from 20% to 50%.
- Consider thyroid storm in any ill patient with signs and symptoms of a hypermetabolic state.
- Be wary in the elderly, children, and pregnant patients who may present with subtle or atypical symptoms of thyroid storm.

Hyperthyroidism is defined as the excess production and release of thyroid hormone by the thyroid gland resulting in inappropriately high serum levels. The disproportionate amount of thyroid hormone leads to an accelerated metabolic state. The most common causes include diffuse toxic goiter (Graves disease), toxic multinodular goiter (Plummer disease), and toxic adenoma.[1] Thyrotoxicosis also refers to a hypermetabolic state that results in excessive amounts of circulating thyroid hormone, but includes extrathyroidal sources of thyroid hormone such as exogenous intake or release of preformed stored hormone. Thyroiditis, inflammation of the thyroid gland resulting in release of stored hormone, is a frequent cause of thyrotoxicosis. The clinical presentation of thyrotoxicosis varies from asymptomatic (subclinical) to life threatening (thyroid storm). Thyroid storm is a true endocrine emergency. The diagnosis is based on history, clinical signs and symptoms, and laboratory analyses including thyroid-stimulating hormone (TSH), free T4 (thyroxine), and T3 (triiodothyroxine).

Thyroid hormone affects virtually every organ system and can result in an amalgam of complaints that can be challenging to identify. However, when undiagnosed, serious complications can occur including delirium, insomnia, anorexia, osteoporosis, muscle weakness, atrial fibrillation, congestive heart failure (CHF), thromboembolism, altered mental status, cardiovascular collapse, and death.[2,3] Populations that are at increased risk for serious sequelae include pregnant women, children, and the elderly.[4] It is

Department of Emergency Medicine, University of Maryland Medical System, University of Maryland, 110 South Paca Street, 6th Floor, Suite 200, Baltimore, MD 21201, USA
* Corresponding author.
E-mail address: danielle.c.devereaux@gmail.com

Emerg Med Clin N Am 32 (2014) 277–292
http://dx.doi.org/10.1016/j.emc.2013.12.001
0733-8627/14/$ – see front matter © 2014 Elsevier Inc. All rights reserved.
emed.theclinics.com

essential that the emergency medicine provider has a high clinical suspicion for hyperthyroidism and thyrotoxicosis in patients with a myriad of seemingly unrelated symptoms, especially when coupled with dysautonomia. Thyroid storm needs to be identified rapidly and treated aggressively to avoid multiorgan dysfunction and death.[5]

EPIDEMIOLOGY

The prevalence of thyrotoxicosis in the United States is estimated at 1.2%, which comprises 0.5% symptomatic and 0.7% subclinical.[6] Occurrences are seen at all ages but presentation peaks between 20 and 50 years of age secondary to the higher prevalence of Graves disease. Toxic multinodular goiter typically occurs after age 50 years, as opposed to toxic adenoma, which presents at a younger age. All forms of thyroid disease are more common in women. Graves disease is the most common cause of thyrotoxicosis in the United States, accounting for 60% to 80% of cases, whereas subacute thyroiditis accounts for 15% to 20%, toxic multinodular goiter accounts for 10% to 15%, and toxic adenoma accounts for 3% to 5%.[7] Of those with thyrotoxicosis only 1% to 2% develop thyroid storm.[8] Although the overall incidence of thyroid storm is low, the morbidity and mortality associated with the diagnosis make it a disease state that all emergency medicine physicians should be adept at identifying and treating.

PATHOPHYSIOLOGY

The production and release of thyroid hormones is regulated by a sensitive negative feedback loop involving the hypothalamus, pituitary gland, and thyroid gland (**Fig. 1**). The hypothalamus releases thyroid-releasing hormone (TRH), which stimulates the pituitary to release TSH, in turn stimulating the thyroid gland to release thyroid hormones, T4 and T3. The increased production of thyroid hormone normally causes inhibition of TRH and TSH release by the hypothalamus and pituitary respectively. Disruption of this delicate system leads to additional production and release of thyroid hormone and subsequent hyperthyroidism.

The production of thyroid hormones in the thyroid gland depends on iodine.[3] Dietary iodide is transported into cells and converted to iodine. The iodine is then bound to thyroglobulin by thyroid peroxidase and subsequently forms monoiodotyrosine (MIT)

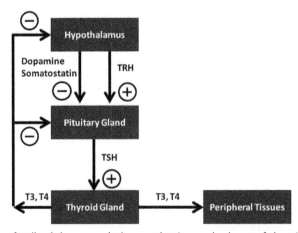

Fig. 1. Negative feedback loop regulating production and release of thyroid hormones.

and diiodotyrosine (DIT).[9] The MIT and DIT are coupled to form T4 and T3 respectively. T3 is more biologically active and is typically formed in the periphery by conversion of T4 to T3. In the serum, thyroid hormone is typically bound to protein and inactive. Any process that increases the amount of unbound (free) thyroid hormone has the potential to cause thyrotoxicosis.

CAUSES

Graves disease is the most common cause of hyperthyroidism in developed countries. It is an autoimmune condition in which antibodies against the TSH receptor cause unopposed stimulation of the thyroid gland. The result is excess production of T4 and T3, an enlarged thyroid gland, and increased iodide uptake. The usual negative feedback loop is not effective because the antibody is directed against the TSH receptor. Individuals with a family history of hyperthyroidism or other autoimmune diseases such as pernicious anemia, myasthenia gravis, type I diabetes mellitus, and celiac disease have an increased propensity of developing Graves.[3]

Toxic multinodular goiter (TMNG) is an important cause of hyperthyroidism. It is caused by unwarranted release of thyroid hormones from multiple autonomously functioning nodules in the thyroid gland. It is more common in areas of dietary iodine deficiency (third-world countries) and in the elderly (poor diet). This condition has an indolent progression and symptoms are typically mild with only slight increase of thyroid hormones above normal. TMNG is more common than Graves disease in the elderly.

Subacute thyroiditis is inflammation of the thyroid gland that typically follows a viral upper respiratory infection and causes additional release of preformed thyroid hormone. Patients typically present with fatigue, sore throat, and upper respiratory symptoms, followed by fever, neck pain, and neck swelling. It is the inflammation of the thyroid gland that causes thyroid hormone to leak into the circulation and subsequent thyrotoxicosis. The disease is usually self-limited but may lead to persistent hypothyroidism.

Toxic nodular goiter (toxic adenoma) is the result of a single nodule in the thyroid gland that is a hyperfunctioning adenoma and produces a surplus of thyroid hormone. Similar to TMNG, this is more common in areas of iodine deficiency. The increased thyroid hormone levels usually decrease TSH, but not to undetectable levels. The normal thyroid gland tissue has no iodine uptake visualized on an iodine uptake study because normal thyroid hormone production is suppressed via the negative feedback loop. However, the adenoma, which functions independently, appears as a single hot nodule with increased iodine uptake.

There are several additional causes of thyrotoxicosis that are rare but deserve consideration. Iodine-induced hyperthyroidism is the result of one or more areas of autonomously functioning thyroid tissue that occur after administration of iodine, classically iodinated contrast material.[10] The excess iodine provides increased substrate for production of thyroid hormones. It is more common in areas with endemic goiter and iodine deficiency. It is possible for iodine to act as an immune stimulator leading to autoimmune thyroid disease and subsequent hyperthyroidism. High iodine intake is associated with increased prevalence of Graves disease.[3] Patients typically present with a painless goiter.

Postpartum thyroiditis is inflammation of the thyroid gland following delivery. It is a transient form of hyperthyroidism that can develop 6 weeks to 6 months postpartum with a significant chance of recurrence in subsequent pregnancies. Patients present with painless goiter and typically have significant family history of autoimmune disease.

Suppurative thyroiditis is an infection of the thyroid gland typically caused by bacteria but can be caused by fungus, mycobacteria, or parasites. It is most common in immunocompromised individuals or those with underlying thyroid disease. It presents with a tender erythematous anterior neck mass, fever, dysphagia, and dysphonia.

Some other rare causes of thyrotoxicosis should be considered in the differential when clinically appropriate.[1] Beta human chorionic gonadotropin (B-hCG) can stimulate the TSH receptor. High levels of B-hCG can be found with molar hydatidiform pregnancies and choriocarcinoma, which can lead to thyrotoxicosis. Follicular thyroid carcinoma, TSH-secreting pituitary tumors, and struma ovarii can all lead to thyrotoxicosis. Thyrotoxicosis factitia is thyrotoxicosis caused by exogenous ingestion of thyroid hormone, either intentionally or accidentally. There have been anecdotal reports of patients inappropriately using thyroid hormone to lose weight.

CLINICAL PRESENTATION

Thyroid hormone increases tissue thermogenesis and basal metabolic rate. Thyrotoxicosis creates a hypermetabolic state in which T3 and free T4 have widespread multiorgan effects. The spectrum of physical manifestations depends on a variety of factors including patient age and duration of illness, and can range from asymptomatic in subclinical disease to life threatening in thyroid storm. The degree of increase of circulating thyroid hormone has not been shown to correlate reliably with symptom severity.[11] Younger patients tend to present with overt symptoms of sympathetic stimulation such as anxiety, restlessness, and tremor, whereas older patients tend to present with less obvious clinical manifestations.[12] Elderly patients may lack adrenergic symptoms and present with depression, fatigue, and weight loss termed apathetic hyperthyroidism. Patients typically have an assortment of complaints varying from specific ailments related to one organ system to nonspecific constitutional symptoms (**Table 1**). There is a wide range of symptoms and differential diagnoses to consider based on clinical presentation.

Hyperthyroidism can have serious effects on the nervous system. Altered mental status and cognitive impairment can present subtly. In one review of elderly patients with hyperthyroidism, dementia and confusion were found in 33% and 18% of patients, respectively. Studies in younger individuals showed that patients with newly diagnosed hyperthyroidism had lower cognitive scores compared with age-matched controls. Seizures, nervousness, anxiety, tremors, and emotional lability are other neurologic consequences.[13] However, patients are frequently misdiagnosed with psychiatric or substance abuse disorders before correct identification of hyperthyroidism. The emergency medicine physician should consider screening patients with new-onset psychiatric symptoms for hyperthyroidism. More than 50% of patients complain of muscle weakness and easy fatigability.[13] The shoulders and pelvic girdle are most severely affected. Patients complain that it is difficult to climb stairs, rise out of the seated position, or comb their hair. These reports can sometimes be mistakenly attributed to neuromuscular disorders. There have even been case reports of hypokalemic periodic paralysis related to thyrotoxicosis that improved with treatment of hyperthyroidism.[14]

Thyroid hormone has significant effects on cardiovascular hemodynamics. Being a lipophilic hormone it easily diffuses across the cytoplasmic membrane of target cells including cardiomyocytes.[15] Hyperthyroidism increases expression of myocardial sarcoplasmic reticulum calcium-dependent adenosine triphosphatase (ATP) increasing myocardial chronotropy (heart rate) and inotropy (contractility), resulting in high left ventricular ejection fraction and cardiac output.[16,17] It remains unclear whether thyroid hormone causes sensitivity to catecholamines, but it alone can alter

Table 1		
Symptoms and signs of thyrotoxicosis		
Symptoms	**Signs**	**Differential Diagnosis**
Constitutional		
Weight loss despite eating	Thin, cachectic	DM, malabsorption, CHF
Heat intolerance, sweating	Diaphoresis, hyperthermia	Hypermetabolic state (pheo, carcinoid), malignancy, infection
Nervousness, restlessness	Anxious appearing	Anxiety, pheo, islet cell tumor
Head, Eyes, Ears, Nose, and Throat		
Neck swelling	Goiter	Thyromegaly, infection
Eyelid swelling, redness, double vision	Proptosis, chemosis, conjunctival injection, lid lag	Ophthalmopathy, conjunctivitis, cellulitis
Cardiac		
Palpitations	Tachycardia, atrial fibrillation	Arrhythmia, pheo, anxiety, drug induced
Respiratory		
Dyspnea	Tachypnea	CHF, angina, deconditioning
Gastrointestinal		
Diarrhea, nausea, vomiting	Abdominal tenderness	Gastroenteritis, malabsorption, IBS
Neuromuscular		
Difficulty rising from chair, difficulty combing hair	Proximal muscle weakness	Myopathy
Extremity shaking	Tremor	Medication side effect, idiopathic
Skin		
Discoloration	Thickening	Pretibial myxedema, Addison disease
Genitourinary/Endocrine		
Amenorrhea, oligomenorrhea	Gynecomastia	Gynecologic disorder
Breast enlargement		Idiopathic, estrogen excess

Abbreviations: DM, diabetes mellitus; IBS, irritable bowel syndrome; pheo, pheochromocytoma.

cardiac metabolism and function independently of beta-adrenergic stimulation.[17] The hypermetabolic state that develops leads to consumption of oxygen, production of metabolic end products such as lactic acid, and arterial smooth muscle relaxation.[15] Systemic vascular resistance consequently decreases, activating the renin-angiotensin system to counteract the decrease and reabsorb sodium, thus expanding the blood volume.[15] The net effect is an increased preload and decreased afterload.[18] Untreated, sustained volume overload and increased cardiac work leads to a compensatory increase in left ventricular mass or hypertrophy.[18] Right heart failure can ensue from the increase in pulmonary artery and right-side filling pressures.[18,19]

Cardiovascular symptoms most commonly include palpitations with an increased resting heart rate and exaggeration during exercise.[19] Sinus tachycardia is most commonly encountered, but atrial fibrillation is the more common dysrhythmia seen with advanced patient age, male sex, valvular disease, and coronary artery disease.[20] Dysrhythmias such as flutter, supraventricular tachycardia, and ventricular tachycardia are uncommon.[15] Long-standing thyroid disease symptoms can include exercise intolerance, dyspnea on exertion, and anginalike chest pain. The cause of this is 2-fold. The surplus of energy needed for exertional activities is limited because of poor cardiac reserve resulting from the resting hypermetabolic demands of the body. Sustained tachycardia inevitably causes decreased cardiac contractility, abnormal diastolic compliance, and pulmonary congestion.[21] Prolonged hemodynamic disarray caused by excessive levels of thyroid hormone can progress to left ventricular dysfunction; however, clinically significant CHF remains a rare event.[20] In severe hyperthyroidism or thyroid storm, CHF occurs predominately in patients with a preexisting heart disease such as ischemic, hypertensive, or alcohol cardiomyopathy, and the increased metabolic demands further impair the already weakened myocardium.[21] Most cases of CHF are reversible and improve with treatment of both the primary hyperthyroid state and the heart failure. First line in controlling the cardiac chronotropic effects of excess thyroid hormone are β-blockers (eg, propranolol). Diuretics (eg, furosemide) are recommended as an adjunctive agent in patients who present with volume overload. In rare circumstances, patients may present with both atrial fibrillation and poor left ventricular function; digoxin may then prove an integral therapy.[21]

Hyperthyroidism can seldom unmask silent conditions. New-onset atrial fibrillation, angina, or heart failure should never be considered solely secondary to thyroid dysfunction until structural disease has been excluded. However, in most patients, symptoms are the result of thyroid disease and not underlying heart disease. Symptoms typically resolve with appropriate thyroid therapy. Cardiovascular ailments have recently been shown to cause an effect on circulating thyroid hormone levels in patients without any thyroid abnormalities.[22] Decreased serum T3 concentrations in patients with heart failure have been found to be proportional to the severity of the New York Heart Association (NYHA) functional classification.[23] Recent studies show that a low T3 level is a powerful predictor of mortality in patients with NYHA class III to IV heart failure.[22,24]

Amiodarone, an antiarrhythmic agent rich in iodine content and structurally similar to levothyroxine, is a well-known culprit of thyroid derangements. Amiodarone-induced hyperthyroidism (AIH) is much more common and challenging to treat than amiodarone-induced hypothyroidism.[25,26] AIH is noteworthy for its 3-fold increased risk for major adverse cardiovascular events.[27] Two forms of AIH exist: type I occurs in patients with preexisting thyroid disease or those living in iodine-deficient areas, and type II is a form of thyroiditis mediated by proinflammatory cytokines.[17] Treatment of AIH with both iodine and antithyroid drugs has marginal effectiveness.[27] Steroid therapy has some proven benefit.[28] Discontinuation of amiodarone and/or total thyroidectomy is often the most effective means of reversal.[29]

The cardiac disorders caused by thyrotoxicosis can subsequently affect the lungs. High-output heart failure can secondarily cause dilatation of the pulmonary artery and precipitate pulmonary arterial hypertension (PAH).[21] Slight increases in pulmonary artery pressure at rest are common in patients with thyrotoxicosis, and the pressure usually increases significantly during exercise. The potential for severe PAH attributable to thyrotoxicosis alone remains unclear. Excess thyroid hormone also alters pulmonary function by weakening respiratory muscles, increasing airway resistance, and decreasing lung compliance.

Thyrotoxicosis can have significant effects on the gastrointestinal tract. Excess sympathetic stimulation can lead to increased motor contractions in the intestine causing increased intestinal transit time and diarrhea. Nausea and vomiting are frequent complaints. Dysphagia can occur as a result of decreased closure of upper esophageal sphincter and decreased propulsion of pharyngeal muscles. Large goiters can physically compress adjacent structures such as the esophagus, leading to dysphagia, and the trachea, leading to respiratory compromise.

Thyrotoxicosis can lead to significant issues with the reproductive system, most notably infertility. Women with excess thyroid hormone can present with anovulation, oligomenorrhea, menometrorrhagia, and amenorrhea. Men have symptoms related to estrogen excess, including gynecomastia, decreased libido, and spider angiomas. Postmenopausal women can have severe osteoporosis, which can predispose to fractures.

CLINICAL EXAMINATION

A detailed and thorough physical examination is important in the evaluation of thyrotoxicosis because it may reveal a specific cause. There are a variety of physical examination findings that, when combined, can lead to diagnosis of thyrotoxicosis (see **Table 1**). Particular attention should be given to the examination of neck and eyes, as well as the neurologic, cardiac, pulmonary, and integumentary systems.[30] The thyroid is a butterfly-shaped gland located in the anterior neck with the isthmus inferior to the cricoid cartilage and the gland wrapping around the trachea. On physical examination it is important to assess size, nodularity, tenderness, and symmetry. The gland is normally soft and nontender. In Graves disease the thyroid is symmetrically enlarged, firm, and a bruit may be auscultated. TMNG reveals an enlarged but soft thyroid. Individual nodules may sometimes be palpated but usually nodules are revealed on ultrasonography. If the examination reveals an enlarged tender gland, then clinicians should consider subacute thyroiditis or suppurative thyroiditis depending on clinical presentation.

Ophthalmologic examination may reveal multiple abnormalities. The classic presentation of Graves disease includes exophthalmos, which is severe proptosis from enlargement of the extraocular muscles. Less significant proptosis can occur with other causes of thyrotoxicosis from sympathetic hyperactivity elevating the levator palpebrae superioris muscle. All patients may appear to stare and have a lid lag, but patients with Graves disease present with unique eye findings. Graves ophthalmopathy or orbitopathy can include proptosis, chemosis, conjunctival injection, periorbital or lid edema, and vasodilation of the conjunctiva. Inability to close the eyelids may lead to corneal ulceration. Diplopia can occur from proptosis and extraocular muscle dysfunction. The presence of increased thyroid hormones and ophthalmopathy strongly suggests the diagnosis of Graves disease.

The neurologic assessment may reveal an agitated, restless, nervous, or anxious patient. In thyroid storm, the alteration of mental status can range from catatonia and depression to frank psychosis. Physical examination may reveal a fine resting tremor that with exertion or an outstretched arm becomes more noticeable and significant. The tremor may also be noted in the feet, tongue, and facial muscles. Muscle group and strength testing may identify decreased bulk and proximal limb weakness, respectively. Hyperreflexia is common. Chronic disease can cause atrophy most notable in the thenar and hypothenar muscles.

Nearly every patient with thyrotoxicosis has a resting tachycardia. Increased blood flow through the aortic outflow tract often leads to a systolic murmur. A systolic scratchy sound, the Means-Lerman scratch, is less common and is thought to result from the hyperdynamic pericardium against the pleura, mimicking pericarditis. In the case of thyroid storm, patients may develop murmurs from significant mitral regurgitation and/or tricuspid regurgitation.[31] Increase in systolic and decrease in dia-stolic blood pressures result in a widened pulse pressure that can extenuate the inten-sity of the normal heart sounds and produce a hyperactive precordium with bounding peripheral pulses. The carotid upstroke is rapid and brisk. In the elderly, an irregularly irregular pulse may be appreciated.

Patient may appear dyspneic from tachypnea secondary to the body's increased oxygen demand and carbon dioxide production. There are case reports of worsening asthma and chronic obstructive pulmonary disease exacerbations in the setting of thyrotoxicosis. Just as patients with pulmonary disease can tire from prolonged res-piratory exacerbations, profound thyrotoxicosis can lead to respiratory muscle weak-ness, diaphragmatic fatigue, and pulmonary decompensation.

Thyrotoxicosis causes deposition of glycosaminoglycans in the dermis of the lower extremities, which causes nonpitting edema, erythema, and thickening of the skin. The skin can resemble an orange peel and is referred to as pretibial myxedema. There is no associated tenderness or pruritus. Pretibial myxedema is a rare finding associated with hyperthyroidism from Graves disease.

UNIQUE POPULATIONS

The diagnosis of hyperthyroidism is difficult in elderly patients because the usual signs and symptoms of a hypermetabolic state may be absent. Elderly patients typically pre-sent with involvement of a single system or have subtle nonspecific symptoms that may be attributed to the natural aging process. Most have small or nonpalpable goiter on physical examination. Apathetic hyperthyroidism, which is uncommon but most frequently seen in the elderly, is characterized by apathetic facies, small goiter, depression, muscle weakness, weight loss, and absence of ophthalmopathy. The diagnosis of thyrotoxicosis in elderly patients is difficult and a high level of suspicion is necessary. Unexplained change in mental status, mood, or behavior; unexplained weight loss; myopathy; new-onset atrial fibrillation or heart failure; and overall incon-gruous symptoms should always prompt further work-up for thyroid dysfunction.

A euthyroid pregnant patient typically experiences resting tachycardia, systolic flow murmur, widened pulse pressure, heat intolerance, increased perspiration, tachyp-nea, dyspnea, and mood changes, all secondary to the normal physiologic changes associated with pregnancy. Therefore, thyrotoxicosis is exceedingly difficult to diag-nose during pregnancy. Hyperthyroidism in pregnancy can be a significant cause of fetal morbidity and mortality. If untreated during pregnancy, it can cause neonatal hy-pothyroidism from TSH antibodies that cross the placenta, destroying the fetal thyroid gland. It can also result in premature labor, low birth weight, and eclampsia. It is impor-tant to consider hyperthyroidism in pregnant patient with goiter, tachycardia greater than 100 beats per minute that does not improve with Valsalva maneuver, weight loss, or onycholysis. Graves disease complicates 1 in 500 pregnancies.

Thyrotoxicosis in the neonate occurs in 1% of pediatric hyperthyroidism cases. It is most commonly secondary to maternal Graves disease and is the result of transpla-cental passage of maternal antibodies. Neonates are typically premature, of low birth weight, and have early skeletal maturation. Affected neonates usually have prominent eyes and small, uniformly enlarged thyroid glands. They may have microcephaly, enlarged ventricles, triangular facies, and frontal bossing. Additional physical findings may include tachycardia, bounding pulses, cardiomegaly, CHF, jaundice, hepatosple-nomegaly, and thrombocytopenia. Clinical manifestations of thyrotoxicosis in children and adolescents include ophthalmopathy (most commonly), failure to thrive, tachy-cardia, increased gastrointestinal motility, muscle weakness, hyperreflexia, sleep disturbance, and distractibility. In addition, children may have acceleration of linear growth and epiphyseal maturation. The most common cause of thyrotoxicosis in children is Graves disease.

THYROID STORM

Thyroid storm is a life-threatening form of thyrotoxicosis that usually occurs following a precipitating event. The most common trigger is infection or sepsis. Patients customarily have a prior history of thyrotoxicosis but thyroid storm can be the initial clinical presentation. Untreated thyroid storm is uniformly fatal. Thyroid storm with treatment has improved outcomes but mortality remains significant at 20% to 50%.[32] The clinical features of thyroid storm are exaggerated signs and symptoms of thyrotoxicosis. Altered mental status is the hallmark. Mental status changes including agitation, emotional lability, delirium, convulsions, and chorealike abnormal movements. Patients can also have autonomic dysfunction depicted by excessive diaphoresis, severe hyperthermia, hypertension, and intractable dysrhythmias. This condition can lead to hypotension and cardiovascular collapse. Other metabolic and electrolyte derangements seen are hyperglycemia from catecholamine-mediated inhibition of insulin, leukocytosis in absence of infection, and hypercalcemia secondary to bone resorption.[33] Specific criteria for identifying thyroid storm were elucidated by Burch and Wartofsky[32] and include hyperpyrexia, tachycardia, atrial fibrillation, CHF, gastrointestinal dysfunction, central nervous system disturbance, and precipitant history (**Fig. 2**). Thyrotoxicosis with concomitant alteration in sensorium or cardiopulmonary decompensation is thyroid storm until proved otherwise.[5]

DIAGNOSTIC ASSESSMENT

Confirming the diagnosis of hyperthyroidism in the emergency department can be achieved by obtaining TSH and free T4 (**Table 2**). Approximately 95% of patients with thyrotoxicosis have an increased T4. A small subset (5%) of patients have normal

Criteria	Points	Criteria	Points
Thermoregulatory dysfunction		**Gastrointestinal-hepatic dysfunction**	
Temperature (°F)		Manifestation	
99.0–99.9	5	Absent	0
100.0–100.9	10	Moderate (diarrhea, abdominal pain, nausea/vomiting)	10
101.0–101.9	15	Severe (jaundice)	20
102.0–102.9	20		
103.0–103.9	25		
≥ 104.0	30		
Cardiovascular		**Central nervous system disturbance**	
Tachycardia (beats per minute)		Manifestation	
100–109	5	Absent	0
110–119	10	Mild (agitation)	10
120–129	15	Moderate (delirium, psychosis, extreme lethargy)	20
130–139	20	Severe (seizure, coma)	30
≥ 140	25		
Atrial fibrillation			
Absent	0		
Present	10		
Congestive heart failure		**Precipitant history**	
Absent	0	Status	
Mild	5	Positive	
Moderate	10	Negative	10
Severe	20		
Scores totaled			
> 45		Thyroid storm	
25–44		Impending storm	
< 25		Storm unlikely	

Fig. 2. Point scale for the diagnosis of thyroid storm. (*From* Burch HB, Wartofsky L. Life-threatening thyrotoxicosis. Thyroid storm. Endocrinol Metab Clin North Am 1993;22(2):263–77; with permission.)

Table 2
Confirmation of the diagnosis of hyperthyroidism in the emergency department using TSH and free T4

Condition	TSH	FT4	FT3	Other Investigation/ Information
Graves disease	Low	High	High	RAIU: increased uptake Thyroid peroxidase antibodies: increased TSH-receptor antibodies: positive
Toxic thyroid adenoma hot nodule	Low	High	High	RAIU: functioning nodule with suppression of other tissue
TMNG	Low	High	High	RAIU: enlarged gland with multiple active nodules
Subacute or granulomatous thyroiditis	Low	High	High	RAIU: low uptake Tg level: markedly raised
Factitious thyroxine-induced thyrotoxicosis	Low	High	High	RAIU: low uptake Tg levels: absent
Iodine-induced hyperthyroidism	Low	High	High	Hx of amiodarone use or exposure to radiocontrast agents RAIU: low uptake
Hyperthyroidism, untreated	Low	High	High	RAIU: high uptake
Hyperthyroidism, T3 toxicosis	Low	Normal	High	RAIU: normal or high uptake
Euthyroid, on exogenous thyroid hormone	Normal	Normal on T4, Low on T3	High on T3, Normal on T4	RAIU: low uptake

Abbreviations: Hx, history; RAIU, radioactive iodine uptake, Tg, thyroglobulin.

T4 and increased T3 only known as T3 toxicosis. Therefore, if the clinical suspicion is high for hyperthyroidism but the T4 is normal, obtain a total T3 because the patient likely has T3 toxicosis. Most cases of hyperthyroidism have suppressed TSH because of the negative feedback loop. However, pituitary-dependent hyperthyroidism has normal TSH with increased T4. Subclinical hyperthyroidism has decreased TSH with normal free T4. It is common for systemic disease to suppress the TSH, so it is important to repeat thyroid studies before starting therapy for subclinical disease. There is no clinical usefulness to obtaining a total T4 in the emergency department. Many drugs interact with thyroid hormone–binding proteins and can confound the diagnosis.

There are additional studies that can be obtained to help confirm the diagnosis in complicated cases. Serum thyroglobulin levels can be obtained to differentiate thyrotoxicosis from factitious thyroid disease. Autoantibodies can be obtained to determine the type of autoimmune disease that is present. Imaging studies can be performed to elucidate the specific cause of hyperthyroidism, but these tests are generally not practical or warranted in the emergency department. Patients who do not fit the clinical picture of Graves disease should have a radioactive iodine uptake study or thyroid scan. Ultrasonography with Doppler flow can be used when radiation exposure is contraindicated, as in pregnancy and breastfeeding. In addition, the use of iodinated contrast studies should be avoided in thyrotoxicosis given that additional iodine substrate can increase serum thyroid levels.[34]

In resource-scarce settings in which imaging may not be available, the ratio of T3 to T4 is useful in assessing cause. When the gland is hyperactive, more T3 than T4 is produced. Therefore, in Graves disease and toxic nodular goiter, the ratio (ng/μg) of T3 to T4 should be greater than 20. Subacute and painless thyroiditis causes release of preformed hormone but does not generate new thyroid hormone, so the ratio of T3 to T4 is less than 20.

MANAGEMENT

Therapy for thyrotoxicosis depends on the underlying cause. Treatment strategies include antithyroid drugs, radioactive iodine, thyroid surgery, and medications for symptom control (**Table 3**).[1] The most commonly used antithyroid drugs are the thionamides, propylthiouracil (PTU) and methimazole (MMI).[35] Thionamides block the synthesis of T4 by inhibiting organification of tyrosine residues. In addition, PTU blocks peripheral conversion of T4 to T3. MMI dosage is 10 to 30 mg per day in once-daily dosing. PTU dosage is 200 to 400 mg per day divided 2 to 3 times per day. Thyroid function tests are repeated every 4 weeks during initial medication management so dosages can be adjusted accordingly. More than one-third of patients go into remission for 10 years or longer after starting antithyroid medication. Common adverse effects of thionamides include abnormal taste, pruritus, urticaria, fever, and arthralgia. Less commonly, patients develop cholestatic jaundice, thrombocytopenia, lupuslike syndrome, hepatitis, and agranulocytosis.

Radioactive iodine therapy can be used in Graves disease, toxic nodules, and TMNGs. It is the most common form of therapy for adults with Graves disease. Therapy is provided by a single oral dose of radioactive iodine that is absorbed by the thyroid gland and causes organ-specific inflammation. Thyroid fibrosis and tissue destruction occur gradually over several months. The major drawback to radioactive iodine is hypothyroidism, which is an expected complication requiring lifelong L-thyroxine replacement therapy. Hypothyroidism occurs within 4 to 12 months of therapy. Radioactive iodine therapy does not require hospitalization and is noninvasive. The thyroid is the only tissue capable of absorbing the iodine so side effects are minimal. Iodine therapy is contraindicated in pregnancy, breastfeeding, and in patients with severe ophthalmopathy.

Thyroid surgery is rapid and effective but invasive and expensive. Patients need to be euthyroid before surgery. It can cause permanent hypothyroidism and transient hypocalcemia requiring calcium supplementation. Surgical complications include recurrent laryngeal nerve damage and permanent hypoparathyroidism. Because of the efficacy of antithyroid medication and radioactive iodine therapy, surgery is performed less frequently. It is generally reserved for pregnant women intolerant of thionamides, children with severe disease, severe ophthalmopathy, amiodarone-induced refractory disease, or unstable cardiac conditions.[1] In the past, stress in the operating room during surgery was the most common cause of thyroid storm, with a mortality of 50%. Thyroid storm during surgery is exceedingly rare now with preoperative therapies including propranolol, antithyroid medication, and iodine.

Symptom control can be achieved with a variety of medications. The American Thyroid Association with the American Association of Clinical Endocrinologists published guidelines for the management of hyperthyroid symptoms.[1] A primary

Table 3
Treatment strategies

Drug	Drug Type	Action	Typical Dosages			
			Neonates	Children	Adults	Thyroid Storm
Antithyroid agents	Propylthiouracil	Prevents production of more T_4 and T_3 in the thyroid, and blocks the conversion of T_4 to T_3 outside the thyroid	5–10 mg/kg/d divided Q8 h PO	Initial: 5–7 mg/kg/d divided Q8 h PO Maintenance: one-third–two-thirds initial dose divided Q8 h	Initial: 100–200 mg PO Q6–8 h Maintenance: 50–100 mg/d	500–1000 mg loading dose, then 250 mg PO/NG/OG or PR Q4–6 h
	Methimazole	Prevents production of more thyroid hormone	NA	Initial: 0.4–0.7 mg/kg/d PO divided Q8 h Maximum: 30 mg/24 h	Initial: 10–20 mg PO Q8-12 h Maintenance: 2.5–10 mg/d	60–80 mg/d PO/NG/OG
Iodides	Lugol solution	Blocks release of stored thyroid hormone from thyroid gland	1 drop PO Q8 h	—	4–8 drops Q6–8 h PO/NG/OG	10 drops Q12 h PO/NG/OG
	Saturated solution of potassium iodide	—	—	1–5 drops Q8 h PO/NG/OG	5–10 drops Q6–8 h PO/NG/OG	5–10 drops Q6–8 h PO/NG/OG
Glucocorticoids	Dexamethasone	Blocks conversion of T_4 to T_3	—	—	2 mg Q6 h PO	2 mg Q6 h IV or PO/NG/OG
	Hydrocortisone	—	—	2 mg/kg PO/IV Q6 h	Prednisone 40–60 mg PO daily × 1 wk then taper	300 mg IV load, then 100 mg IV Q6-8 h
β-Blockers	Propranolol	Reduces symptoms caused by a heightened response to catecholamines; blocks conversion of T_4 to T_3	2 mg/kg/d PO divided Q6-12 h	0.5–1 mg/kg/d divided Q6-12 h	10–40 mg PO Q6-8 h	1 mg/min IV as required, then 60-80 Q4 h PO/NG/OG
	Atenolol	—	—	0.5–1 mg/kg PO daily (maximum dose 100 mg/d)	25–100 mg PO daily (maximum dose 200 mg/d)	NA
	Esmolol	—	100–500 µg/kg IV load then 25–100 µg/kg/min infusion	100–500 µg/kg IV load then 25–100 µg/kg/min infusion	NA	500 µg/kg/min for 1 min, then 50–100 µg/kg/min

Abbreviations: IV, intravenous; NG, nasogastric tube; OG, orogastric tube; PO, by mouth; PR, per rectum; Q, every.

recommendation was to consider β-blockers in all symptomatic patients, especially the elderly and patients with resting heart rates of more than 90 beats per minute. The use of propranolol, atenolol, and metoprolol has been shown to decrease heart rate, systolic blood pressure, muscle weakness, and tremor, and to improve irritability and emotional lability. The calcium channel blockers verapamil and diltiazem have been shown to decrease heart rate in patients for whom β-blockers were contraindicated, but can cause profound hypotension and should be used cautiously.

Treatment of subacute thyroiditis is initially aspirin or other nonsteroidal antiinflammatory medication. Some patients require glucocorticoid therapy given as a once-daily burst for 1 week and then tapered over 4 weeks. β-Blocking medication such as propranolol can be used for symptom control. The thyrotoxicosis typically resolves spontaneously and no further treatment is needed. Subacute thyroiditis should not be treated with antithyroid medication from the emergency department.

Antithyroid medications and β-blockers are the primary treatment of thyrotoxicosis during pregnancy.[1] Radioactive iodine therapy is contraindicated. Surgery is reserved for women who are unable to tolerate antithyroid medication. PTU and MMI can both be used during pregnancy and have similar rates of neonatal hypothyroidism. However, MMI has been associated with scalp defects when used in the first trimester. Therefore, a woman with hyperthyroidism who desires pregnancy should be started on PTU and can be switched to MMI if desired after 12 weeks' gestation.[1] PTU is the drug of choice for breastfeeding mothers given that it is secreted in breast milk to a lesser extent because it is more protein bound. β-Blocking agents can be used for symptom control during pregnancy but risks and benefits must be weighed carefully. β-Blockers cross the placenta and can cause in utero growth restriction, prolonged labor, bradycardia, hypotension, hypoglycemia, and prolonged hyperbilirubinemia in the infant.

Children and adolescents with hyperthyroidism can be treated with antithyroid medication, radioactive iodine, or surgery as clinically indicated. Almost all children requiring antithyroid medication should be treated with MMI. Before initiating therapy, children should have baseline complete blood count and liver function tests. Although MMI has better safety profile than PTU, it is associated with adverse risks including allergic reactions, rashes, myalgias, arthralgias, and rarely agranulocytosis. PTU is associated with hepatoxicity and subsequent liver failure. Its use is contraindicated in children. There have been case reports of fatal fulminant hepatic necrosis.[1] Symptomatic control can be achieved with β-blockers in children (see **Table 3**). Neonatal thyrotoxicosis is almost uniformly a result of maternal Graves disease and the subsequent transplacental passage of maternal thyroid-stimulating antibodies. As a result, hyperthyroidism is usually self-limited because antibodies decline by 3 to 4 months of age. Treatment typically involves symptomatic care (see **Table 3**).

Thyroid storm is a life-threatening hypermetabolic state with significant morbidity and mortality.[6,32] Prompt recognition and initiation of therapy is crucial for good outcomes. Medication management is directed at controlling the overactive thyroid gland and blocking peripheral effects of thyroid hormones (see **Table 3**). These patients are typically critical and should have rapid placement of large-bore intravenous access, supplemental oxygen, and cardiac monitoring. Aggressive volume resuscitation should be started immediately with the exception of patients with concomitant heart failure, in which case use of fluids should be judicious. Because cardiovascular collapse is often the cause of decompensation, β-blockers should be initiated first. β-Blockers control patient symptoms and sympathetic hyperactivity. The initial β-blocker should be propranolol with esmolol infusion as an alternate choice. High-dose steroid should be given early to help augment vascular tone. Both β-blockers and steroids reduce peripheral conversion of T4 to T3. PTU is the preferred medication for thyroid storm because it also decreases peripheral conversion of T4 to T3.[1] It additionally decreases the synthesis of T4 and T3 within the thyroid gland. PTU and MMI are available in oral preparations only. They can be given orally, by nasogastric/orogastric tube, or per rectum as clinically indicated. The initial loading dose for PTU is 600 to 1000 mg, then 250 mg every 4 hours. MMI can be given as 20 mg every 4 hours.

Thionamides are effective at inhibiting synthesis of new thyroid hormone but are ineffective at decreasing preformed stored hormones. Iodine and lithium are effective at blocking release of preformed hormones from the thyroid gland. Iodine should be given 1 hour after PTU or MMI to reduce the risk of increasing thyroid hormone production by providing more substrate.[1] Acetaminophen and cooling devices can be used for hyperthermia. Salicylates should be avoided because they can increase free thyroid hormone levels by decreasing thyroid-binding protein in the serum. If an underlying infectious cause is suspected early broad-spectrum antibiotics must not be forgotten and should be started as early as possible. Patients with refractory life-threatening symptoms can undergo hemodialysis if medical management is ineffective.

DISPOSITION

Patients with thyroid storm require admission to the intensive care unit. Patients with symptomatic thyrotoxicosis may require inpatient admission if initial therapy in the emergency department fails to normalize vital signs, if symptoms are severe, or if the patient does not have adequate follow-up. Patients requiring antithyroid medication who are stable for discharge should be referred to the endocrinology clinic for further evaluation and medication management. Patients with subacute thyroiditis should not be started on antithyroid medication and can followed up with endocrinology for further evaluation and management.

Hyperthyroidism pearls

1. Thyroid storm has a broad differential. Keep the following in mind:
   a. Acute pulmonary edema
   b. Heat stroke
   c. Malignant hyperthermia
   d. Sepsis/septic shock
   e. Sympathomimetic overdose
   f. Serotonin syndrome
   g. Tachyarrhythmias
2. The classic triad of thyroid storm is high fever, exaggerated tachycardia out of proportion to fever, and central nervous system dysfunction or cerebral encephalopathy.
3. Wait at least 1 hour after antithyroid medication before giving iodide or serum thyroid hormone levels may inadvertently be increased, exacerbating the issue.
4. Plasmapheresis, charcoal hemoperfusion, and plasma exchange can be used to rapidly decrease thyroid hormone levels in refractory cases.
5. Do not use aspirin or other salicylates for fever control in thyroid storm because they can increase serum hormone levels.
6. Be careful with β-blockers in patients with concomitant thyroid storm and heart failure.

SUMMARY

Hyperthyroidism and thyrotoxicosis are hypermetabolic conditions that cause significant morbidity and mortality. The diagnosis can be difficult because symptoms can mimic many other disease states leading to inaccurate or untimely diagnoses and management. Thyroid storm is the most severe form of thyrotoxicosis, hallmarked by altered sensorium, and, if untreated, is associated with significant mortality.[32] Thyroid storm should be considered in the differential of any patient presenting with altered mental status.[36] The emergency medicine physician who can rapidly recognize the signs and symptoms of thyrotoxicosis, identify the precipitating event, appropriately and comprehensively begin medical management, and facilitate disposition will undoubtedly save a life.

REFERENCES

1. Bahn R, Burch H, Cooper D, et al. Hyperthyroidism and other causes of thyrotoxicosis: management guidelines of the American Thyroid Association and American Association of Clinical Endocrinologists. Thyroid 2011;21(6):593–645.
2. Larsen PR, Davies TF. Thyrotoxicosis. In: Foster DW, Larsen PR, Kronenberg HM, et al, editors. Williams textbook of endocrinology. 10th edition. Philadelphia: WB Saunders; 2002. p. 374–421.
3. Jameson L, Weetman A. Disorders of the thyroid gland. In: Braunwald E, Fauci A, Kasper D, et al, editors. Harrison's principles of internal medicine. 15th edition. New York: Mc-Graw-Hill; 2001. p. 2060–84.
4. Glauser J, Strange GR. Hypothyroidism and hyperthyroidism in the elderly. Emerg Med Rep 2002;1:1–12.
5. Chong HW, See KC, Phua J. Thyroid storm with multiorgan failure. Thyroid 2010; 20(3):333–6.
6. Hollowell JG, Staehling NW, Flanders WD, et al. Serum TSH, T3 and thyroid antibodies in the United States Population (1988–1994): National Health and Nutrition Examination Survey (NHANES III). J Clin Endocrinol Metab 2002;87:489–99.
7. Lee S. Hyperthyroidism. 2013. Emedicine. Available at: http://emedicine.medscape.com/article/121865-overview. Accessed August 1, 2013.
8. Wogan JM. Selected endocrine disorders. In: Marx JA, Hockberger RS, Walls RM, editors. Rosen's emergency medicine: concepts and clinical practice. 5th edition. St Louis (MO): Mosby; 2002. p. 1770.
9. Bianco AC, Larsen PR. Intracellular pathways of iodothyronine metabolism. In: Braverman LE, Utiger RD, editors. Werner's & Ingbar's the thyroid. 9th edition. Philadelphia: Lippincott Williams & Wilkins; 2005. p. 109–33.
10. Stanbury JB, Ermans AE, Bourdoux P, et al. Iodine-induced hyperthyroidism: occurrence and epidemiology. Thyroid 1998;8(1):83–100.
11. Trzepacz PT, Klein I, Roberts M, et al. Graves' disease: an analysis of thyroid hormone levels and hyperthyroid signs and symptoms. Am J Med 1989;87:558–61.
12. Boelaert K, Torlinska B, Holder RL, et al. Older subjects with hyperthyroidism present with a paucity of symptoms and signs: a large cross sectional study. J Clin Endocrinol Metab 2010;95:2715–26.
13. Kudrjavcev T. Neurologic complications of thyroid dysfunction. Adv Neurol 1978; 19:619–36.
14. Barahona MJ, Vinagre I, Sojo L, et al. Thyrotoxic periodic paralysis: a case report and literature review. Clin Med Res 2009;7(3):96–8.
15. Fadel B, Ellahham S, Ringel M, et al. Hyperthyroid heart disease. Clin Cardiol 2000;23:402–8.

16. Klein I, Danzi S. Thyroid heart disease. Circulation 2007;116:1725.
17. Mintz G, Pizzarello R, Klein I. Enhanced left ventricular diastolic function in hyperthyroidism: noninvasive assessment and response to treatment. J Clin Endocrinol Metab 1991;73:146.
18. Danzi S, Klein I. Thyroid hormone and the cardiovascular system. Med Clin North Am 2012;96:257–68.
19. Napoli R, Biondi B, Guardasole V, et al. Impact of hyperthyroidism and its correction on vascular reactivity on humans. Circulation 2001;104:3076–80.
20. Toft AD, Boon NA. Thyroid disease and the heart. Heart 2000;84:455–60.
21. Dahl P, Danzi S, Klein I. Thyrotoxic cardiac disease. Curr Heart Fail Rep 2008;5: 170–6.
22. Forfar JC, Muir AL, Sawers SA, et al. Abnormal left ventricular function in hyperthyroidism: evidence for a possible reversible cardiomyopathy. N Engl J Med 1982;307:1165–70.
23. Gerdes AM, Iervasi G. Thyroid replacement therapy and heart failure. Circulation 2010;122:385–93.
24. Iervasi G, Pingitore A, Landi P, et al. Low-T3 syndrome: a strong prognostic predictor of death in patient with heart disease. Circulation 2003;107:708–13.
25. Hamilton MA, Stevenson LW, Luu M, et al. Altered thyroid hormone metabolism in advanced heart disease. J Am Coll Cardiol 1990;16:91–5.
26. Martino E, Bartalena L, Bogassi F, et al. The effects of amiodarone on the thyroid. Endocr Rev 2001;22:240.
27. Cohen-Lehman J, Dahl P, Danzi S, et al. Effects of amiodarone on thyroid function. Nat Rev Endocrinol 2010;6:34–41.
28. Bogazzi F, Bartalena L, Cosci C, et al. Treatment of type II amiodarone-induced thyrotoxicosis by either iopanoic acid or glucocorticoids: a prospective, randomized study. J Clin Endocrinol Metab 2003;88:1999–2002.
29. Williams M, Lo Gerto P. Thyroidectomy using local anesthesia in critically ill patients with amiodarone-induced thyrotoxicosis: a review and description of the technique. Thyroid 2002;12:523.
30. Wartofsky L, Ingber SH. Diseases of the thyroid. In: Wilson JD, Brunwald E, Isselbacher KJ, et al, editors. Harrison's principles of internal medicine. McGraw-Hill; 1991. p. 1692–710.
31. Waleed A, Yousef AL, Khamis AH, et al. Thyroid storm with rare cardiac presentations, 10 year intensive care unit experience: case series. Life Sciences Journal 2012;9(4):4555–8.
32. Burch HB, Wartofsky L. Life-threatening hyperthyroidism: thyroid storm. Endocrinol Metab Clin North Am 1993;22:263–77.
33. Mckeown NJ, Tews MC, Gossain VV, et al. Hyperthyroidism. Emerg Med Clin North Am 2005;23:669–85.
34. Rhee C, Bhan I, Alexander E, et al. Association between iodinated contrast media exposure and incident hyperthyroidism and hypothyroidism. Arch Intern Med 2012;172(2):153–9.
35. Cooper DS. Antithyroid drugs. N Engl J Med 2005;352:905–17.
36. American College of Emergency Physicians. Clinical policy for the initial approach to patients presenting with altered mental status. Ann Emerg Med 1999;33:251–81.

Alcoholic Metabolic Emergencies

Michael G. Allison, MD[a,b], Michael T. McCurdy, MD[a,b,*]

KEYWORDS

- Ethanol intoxication • Beer potomania • Alcoholic ketoacidosis
- Alcohol encephalopathy • Wernicke encephalopathy • Korsakoff syndrome

KEY POINTS

- Hypoglycemia in the alcohol intoxicated adult is no more common than the rest of the population; children often have hypoglycemia with alcohol overdose.
- Beer potomania can be treated with simple fluid restriction; isotonic resuscitation should be approached with caution.
- Alcoholic ketoacidosis may not present with ketonemia.
- Alcoholic encephalopathy syndromes, such as Wernicke encephalopathy and Korsakoff syndrome, should be treated with 500 mg intravenous thiamine every 8 hours.

INTRODUCTION

As all emergency providers are aware, habitual users of alcohol frequently find themselves seeking treatment in the Emergency Department (ED). Patients who abuse alcohol, a term that is synonymous with ethanol for the purpose of this article, can present with a myriad of complaints and may exhibit a range of clinical illnesses. Acute alcohol intoxication and withdrawal make up the largest subsets of illnesses stemming from alcohol abuse, and physicians may get lulled into a familiar management pattern for patients with acute alcohol intoxication. However, because of the high risk of significant morbidity if not recognized and treated appropriately, emergency physicians must pay careful attention to the metabolic derangements that plague alcohol abusers. This article discusses how to diagnose efficiently and provide appropriate medical therapy for some key underrecognized alcohol emergencies.

Funding Sources: Nil.
Conflict of Interest: Nil.
[a] Division of Pulmonary and Critical Care Medicine, Department of Medicine, University of Maryland School of Medicine, 110 South Paca Street, 2nd Floor, Baltimore, MD, USA;
[b] Department of Emergency Medicine, University of Maryland School of Medicine, 110 South Paca Street, 6th Floor, Baltimore, MD 21201, USA
* Corresponding author. Department of Medicine, University of Maryland School of Medicine, 110 South Paca Street, 2nd Floor, Baltimore, MD 21201.
E-mail address: drmccurdy@gmail.com

Emerg Med Clin N Am 32 (2014) 293–301
http://dx.doi.org/10.1016/j.emc.2013.12.002
emed.theclinics.com

ALCOHOL INTOXICATION

Acute alcohol intoxication, herein referred to as "intoxication," is defined as the pathologic state produced by the ingestion of alcohol. Blood alcohol levels (BAL) are sometimes used to supplement clinical decision-making in the ED, and a working understanding of the pharmacokinetics of ethanol is helpful in these circumstances. The degree and duration of symptoms of intoxication are governed by the body's absorption, metabolism, and elimination of alcohol over time. Ethanol is absorbed through the gastrointestinal tract and achieves its concentration in the circulation within minutes to a few hours. A standard drink is classified as 14 g of alcohol. Usually this equals about 1.5 ounces of liquor, 5 ounces of wine, or 12 ounces of beer. One serving will increase the BAL by approximately 25 mg/dL. The character of symptoms associated with intoxication varies with every drinker, so reliably predicting blood alcohol level on clinical features alone is difficult.

Ethanol is metabolized via hepatic oxidation by zero-order kinetics, which means that a set amount is metabolized per unit time. Prolonged ethanol exposure induces hepatic enzymatic activity, resulting in increased alcohol degradation in chronic drinkers.[1] Drinkers who do not chronically abuse ethanol eliminate it at a rate of 15 mg/dL/h, whereas chronic abusers eliminate it around 25 mg/dL/h.[1] Observational data from ED patients have found clearance rates of 18 to 20 mg/dL/h with only minor variability among habitual drinkers.[2,3] Although these typically quoted studies provide reasonable estimates of ethanol metabolism, their wide confidence intervals suggest substantial clinical variability among patients. Therefore, acute alcohol intoxication can be diagnosed clinically or by BAL.

To reduce the amount of unnecessary time intoxicated patients spend in the ED for supportive measures, studies have attempted to identify the utility of various therapies to enhance ethanol elimination. Unfortunately, these studies, which have included naloxone, flumazenil, and intravenous fluids, have failed to demonstrate improvement in ethanol clearance with anything other than time.[4–6] Despite a lack of increasing ethanol elimination, intoxicated patients should receive good supportive care until they are lucid and competent and can be safely discharged.

INTOXICATION AND THE ENDOCRINE SYSTEM

Alcohol can cause clinical abnormalities of endocrine function. Its effects on gonadal function, bone and mineral metabolism derangements, and glucocorticoid secretion rarely result in acute illness requiring ED management.[7] However, acute intoxication may result in alterations in glucose metabolism requiring emergency treatment.

Habitual drinkers who consume alcohol in the absence of other nutrition have a theoretical risk of developing hypoglycemia. Fasting states deplete existing glycogen stores, forcing the body to rely on gluconeogenesis to maintain normoglycemia. The metabolism of alcohol by alcohol dehydrogenase creates a molecular milieu that may prevent the normal conversion of amino acids and pyruvate into glucose, allowing the development of hypoglycemia.[7] However, clinical studies of acutely intoxicated patients do not support this theory. Two different cohort studies, using prospective convenience sampling and retrospective laboratory analysis of intoxicated ED patients, found a low incidence of hypoglycemia (4% and 1%, respectively).[8,9] Although intoxicated adults do not seem to have a higher risk of developing hypoglycemia, children who present following acute alcohol ingestion are at risk for hypoglycemia.[10] Finger-stick glucose evaluation should be used in any intoxicated patient, similar to the evaluation in other ED patients with altered mental status.

ELECTROLYTE DERANGEMENTS
Hyponatremia: A Consequence of Beer Potomania

First described in a 1971 case series, beer potomania is alcohol-induced hyponatremia found in alcohol users with concomitant poor nutritional supplementation. A large percentage of the patients in that initial case series consumed greater than or equal to 4 L of beer per day in the days preceding hospitalization.[11] The lone consumption of large quantities of beer causes total body deficiencies in sodium and protein. Because of the kidney's inability to match water excretion with the high volume of hypotonic beer consumption, free water retention occurs, exhibited by a dilutional hyponatremia.

Presentation

Similar to other alcohol-related emergencies, patients with beer potomania often exhibit neurologic abnormalities such as altered mental status, focal neurologic deficits, or seizures. Unfortunately, the diagnosis of beer potomania is elusive due to these similarities in presentation, and patients are often misdiagnosed. For example, alterations in consciousness may also be found with acute intoxication, withdrawal, and delirium tremens. Focal neurologic signs may be seen with alcohol-related head injury. Agitation and disorientation can present as alcohol withdrawal, delirium tremens, or acute psychosis. Seizures may be found with alcohol withdrawal. Only serum electrolyte measurements will reliably differentiate these clinical entities from the hyponatremia associated with beer potomania.

Diagnosis

Hyponatremia in a recent beer drinker, in the absence of a comorbid condition altering sodium levels, is the sine qua non of beer potomania. Because alcoholics are at risk for various causes of hyponatremia, these causes must be ruled out (**Box 1**).[12] In beer potomania, hyponatremia may be particularly dramatic, with some reports citing sodium levels as low as 98 mg/dL.[11] Potassium levels are usually also low, whereas blood urea nitrogen and creatinine levels are typically normal because most patients are euvolemic. Not surprisingly, urine studies reveal low urine osmolality and low urine sodium concentration.[13] Identifying hyponatremia in beer drinkers with these other metabolic abnormalities will lead the clinician on the path to proper therapy.

Management

The safe restoration of intravascular solutes is the cornerstone of managing these patients. Patients with beer potomania are not hypovolemic, and excessively rapid correction of hyponatremia may put a patient at risk for osmotic demyelination syndrome (ODS). Early reports on beer potomania found similar symptom improvement with both 2 to 3 L of isotonic fluid and simple water restriction.[14] The rapid restoration

---

Box 1
Causes of hyponatremia in habitual alcohol drinkers

- Hypovolemia

- Beer potomania

- Pseudohyponatremia—Hypertriglyceridemia or hyperproteinemia

- Syndrome of inappropriate antidiuretic hormone secretion (SIADH)

- Cardiomyopathy

- Cirrhosis

- Cerebral salt-wasting syndrome

of normal sodium concentration with crystalloid, however, may have contributed to the high incidence of ODS in these reports. A form of ODS, central pontine myelinolysis, had been recognized in prior case series of beer potomania before the development of the current understanding of the dangers of rapid sodium correction.[11,15,16] Because ODS/central pontine myelinolysis can occur when the sodium concentration is corrected to greater than 10 mEq/L in the first 24 hours, a more cautious rate of correction may be prudent, such as raising sodium levels by less than or equal to 10 mEq in the first day and less than 18 mEq in the first 48 hours.[13] These authors recommend this careful correction of sodium after finding that 18% of patients with beer potomania developed ODS in a review of the early literature.[13] Life-threatening sequelae of beer potomania (eg, seizures) may warrant the careful administration of small aliquots of hypertonic saline along with close monitoring of serum sodium.[15] However, no benefit exists to treat asymptomatic hyponatremia aggressively because simple water restriction is often sufficient to normalize sodium levels in these patients.

Hypomagnesemia

Hypomagnesemia among alcohol abusers is quite common. Up to 30% of chronic alcoholics and 7% of acutely intoxicated patients will be hypomagnesemic.[17,18] Hypomagnesemia in alcohol abusers can result from a variety of causes, which may include dietary deficiency, gastrointestinal malabsorption, increased urinary excretion, ketosis, and vitamin D deficiency.

Hypomagnesemia clinically manifests as muscle weakness, hyperreflexia, and increased QT intervals, which can predispose patients to dysrhythmias. Acquired long-QT syndrome from electrolyte abnormalities such as hypomagnesemia may predispose patients to the polymorphic ventricular tachycardia known as Torsades de pointes. Magnesium therapy has been shown to be the first-line agent in treating Torsades de pointes in hemodynamically stable patients, even in patients with normal magnesium levels.[19]

Alcoholic Ketoacidosis

The presence of ketoacidosis in nondiabetics was first reported in 1940, and the authors astutely noted that many of the patients recently used alcohol.[20] However, it was not until 1971 that Jenkins and colleagues[21] coined the term "alcoholic ketoacidosis" to describe patients with a similar constellation of symptoms after recent alcoholic binges whose ketosis improved with intravenous hydration. These initial reports helped to lay the foundation for the current understanding of the pathophysiology, diagnosis, and management of alcoholic ketoacidosis.

Pathophysiology

Heavy alcohol use and malnutrition cause ketosis. During an alcohol binge, decreased protein and carbohydrate intake results in the body having to use its glycogen stores. In addition, hepatic alcohol dehydrogenase oxidizes ethanol into acetaldehyde, which favors the reduction of nicotinamide adenine dinucleotide (NAD+) to nicotinamide adenine dinucleotide (reduced form) (NADH).[22] High NADH concentrations impair gluconeogenesis, causing free fatty acid formation. Catecholamine surges and insulin inhibition promote glucagon secretion, which further promotes the conversion of fatty acids into ketones.[23] Acetaldehyde, acetone, and β-hydroxybutyrate (BOHB) are all elevated, but BOHB predominates. High concentrations of ketones cause an anion gap metabolic acidosis. The acidosis is worsened by the concomitant lactic acidosis often present in such patients.[22] In summary, both inadequate stores of energy and high ethanol consumption can cause ketogenesis and acidemia.

Presentation

Patients with alcoholic ketoacidosis generally present with the triad of abdominal pain, nausea, and vomiting.[20,21,24] The general sequence of events is as follows: a recent alcoholic binge causing abdominal pain, which causes cessation of drinking and subsequently leading to the alcoholic acidosis, which causes nausea and vomiting. Clinical signs may include tachypnea, tachycardia, and hypotension from volume depletion. Similar to diabetic ketoacidosis, the abdominal examination can elicit tenderness without guarding or rebound. The nonspecific symptoms and signs associated with alcoholic ketoacidosis often warrant ruling out concomitant anatomic causes as well (**Box 2**).

Diagnosis

The diagnosis of alcoholic ketoacidosis requires appropriate clinical signs and symptoms in the presence of classic metabolic derangements on laboratory investigation. Patients typically have an elevated anion gap acidosis, ketonuria, and occasionally ketoacidemia. BOHB, the predominant ketone in the disease, is present in much higher concentrations than in diabetic ketoacidosis.[25] BOHB is not routinely tested in most commercial serum or urine ketone assays, resulting in its underidentification. Because alcohol consumption has typically ceased days before presentation, BAL is often negative.[22] Serum pH may also be normal due to the presence of a mixed metabolic derangement, namely a ketoacidosis and a contraction alkalosis.[22]

Management

Early and proper recognition of alcoholic ketoacidosis is important because the treatment is highly efficacious. Before this clinical entity was better understood, practitioners used insulin and bicarbonate in select patients; however, these therapies are no longer recommended because of their lack of benefit.[20,21] A seminal paper on the treatment of alcoholic ketoacidosis compared saline infusions to 5% dextrose containing solutions for volume loading.[26] All patients in the study did well and resolved their ketoacidosis, but patients receiving dextrose-containing solutions cleared their ketoacidosis in half the time. Current therapy for alcoholic ketoacidosis should use isotonic volume expansion with dextrose-containing fluids, such as 5% dextrose in normal saline.

Alcoholic Encephalopathy

As a consequence of carbohydrate-heavy alcohol consumption at the expense of vitamin-rich food consumption, chronic alcohol abusers are at particular risk for encephalopathy resulting from thiamine (Vitamin B1) deficiency. In 1880s, Wernicke[27] described a syndrome characterized by confusion, ataxia, and ophthalmoplegia,

---

Box 2
Differential diagnosis of abdominal pain in patients consuming alcohol

- Pancreatitis
- Alcoholic hepatitis
- Gastritis/esophagitis
- Intra-abdominal sepsis
- Pneumonia
- Spontaneous bacterial peritonitis

and Korsakoff[28] separately identified a syndrome of mental disturbance in patients with either acute illness or alcohol abuse. The mental disturbance in Korsakoff's patients took many forms, but often included confabulation. The syndromes became linked in the mid-1900s when characteristic cerebral lesions were found in both disorders. Wernicke encephalopathy (WE), a reversible form of the encephalopathy and the Korsakoff syndrome (KS), a persistent state of encephalopathy characterized by confabulation, are still present today and are underdiagnosed in the emergency setting.

Cause and pathophysiology

Thiamine depletion occurs in 2 to 3 weeks in the absence of vitamin-rich foods or supplementation. Because of an increased appreciation of thiamine deficiency as the cause for both WE and KS, many countries now supplement their food with the vitamin, which has decreased the number of cases by 40% in some instances.[29] Resulting from policies enacted to supplement grains, alcohol abusers are now the most notable risk group for alcoholic encephalopathy due to poor intake, decreased absorption, and impaired storage of thiamine.[30]

For unknown reasons, thiamine deficiency selectively damages certain parts of the brain that anatomically correlate with the clinical symptoms associated with WE and KS. Classically, the mammillary bodies are the most affected, but other areas are also prone to develop lesions, including the dorsomedial thalamus, ocular motor nuclei, vestibular nuclei, locus ceruleus, and peri-aqueductal gray matter.[30]

Diagnosis

The diagnosis of WE and KS remains difficult. Some case series have found WE is first diagnosed during autopsy 80% of the time.[31] Often patients with the mental status manifestations of WE and KS can be misdiagnosed as primarily psychiatric, resulting in improper therapy and delayed diagnosis.[32] A high level of suspicion must be maintained when evaluating alcohol abusers with altered mental status.

Because the classic triad of mental status changes, ophthalmoplegia, and ataxia is not universally present, an operational definition has been established. The diagnostic criteria for WE include the presence of any 2 of the following 4 conditions in a known alcohol abuser: (1) nutritional deficiency, (2) ocular findings, (3) ataxia, and (4) mental status changes.[33] These 4 criteria for WE increase the diagnostic sensitivity of WE at the expense of decreased specificity, resulting in potential overdiagnosis.

Thiamine levels have no role in the diagnosis of WE or KS in the ED. The tests take days to perform and are rarely available when making diagnostic and treatment decisions. Likewise, imaging studies should not be routinely used for making the diagnosis of WE. A noncontrast brain magnetic resonance image will be able to determine if pathologic lesions exist in the mammillary bodies or other areas characteristic for the disease; however, this risks underdiagnosis because magnetic resonance image has a low sensitivity of 53%. Computed tomographic scan performs even worse with a sensitivity of 13%.[34] Basing treatment decisions on imaging alone would miss a large number of WE cases. WE remains a clinical diagnosis and, given the benign nature of its treatment with thiamine replacement, emergency physicians should not worry about the potential for overdiagnosis because the consequences of underdiagnosis can be severe.

Treatment

Standard therapy for WE and KS is thiamine supplementation, although optimal dosing remains elusive despite decades of experience treating these conditions. Because of the risk of decreased intestinal absorption in alcoholics, most experts recommend parenterally administering thiamine; however, a *Cochrane Review* found inadequate evidence to recommend a particular dose or duration of thiamine supplementation.[35] In the only prospective study on the subject, patients responded most favorably to a dose of 200 mg intramuscular injection, which happened to be the highest dose given in the study.[36] Despite the lack of evidence, some national guidelines suggest dosing thiamine at 500 mg 3 times a day.[37] Higher doses of thiamine pose no known risk, so emergency providers may wish to treat with the larger recommended doses.

A commonly held belief by physicians is that glucose administration before thiamine repletion in patients with suspected thiamine deficiency and hypoglycemia may precipitate WE or KS. On a cellular level, thiamine acts as a cofactor for glycolysis and the ultimate production of ATP. Concerns about timing of glucose and thiamine therapy stem from the fact that giving a glucose load to a thiamine-deplete person potentially risks the utilization of all remaining thiamine stores, thus precipitating WE. The origins of these concerns are a variety of case reports and case series, in which patients were given dextrose-containing solutions over many days without any thiamine repletion.[38–40] There is no clear human evidence that glucose loading before thiamine supplementation results in acute deterioration of mental status, although animal studies have shown documented cerebral changes after an acute glucose load in thiamine-deficient rats.[41,42] The authors of a literature review on the subject note there is not good evidence evaluating this clinical question in humans in an acute setting. Given the dangers of acute hypoglycemia, the authors suggest providing emergent glucose supplementation followed by prompt thiamine supplementation.[43]

SUMMARY

The spectrum of metabolic derangements due to the habitual and recreational use of alcohol is vast. Emergency physicians must be vigilant when treating the intoxicated and altered patient. Many of the disease states previously discussed are curable if managed in a timely fashion. Furthermore, many of the conditions discussed within this article are preventable with abstinence from alcohol; as physicians, we should always attempt to engage our patients in discussions regarding health maintenance and the need to seek help with addictions.

REFERENCES

1. Jones AQ. Disappearance rate of ethanol from the blood of human subjects: implications in forensic toxicology. J Forensic Sci 1993;28:104.
2. Gershman H, Steeper J. Rate of clearance of ethanol from the blood of intoxicated patients in the emergency department. J Emerg Med 1991;9:307–11.
3. Brennan DF, Betzelos S, Reed R. Ethanol elimination rates in an ED population. Am J Emerg Med 1995;13:276–80.
4. Nuotto E, Palva ES, Seppala T. Naloxone-ethanol interaction in experimental and clinical situations. Acta Pharmacol Toxicol 1984;54:278–84.
5. Lheureux P, Askenasi R. Efficacy of flumazenil in acute alcohol intoxication; double blind placebo-controlled evaluation. Hum Exp Toxicol 1991;10:235–9.
6. Li J, Mills T, Erato R. Intravenous saline has no effect on blood ethanol clearance. J Emerg Med 1999;17:1–5.
7. Adler RA. Clinically important effects of alcohol on endocrine function. J Clin Endocrinol Metab 1992;74:957–60.
8. Sporer KA, Ernst AA, Conte R, et al. The incidence of ethanol-induced hypoglycemia. Am J Emerg Med 1992;10:403–5.

9. Sucov A, Woolard RH. Ethanol associated hypoglycemia is uncommon. Acad Emerg Med 1995;2:185–9.
10. Lamminpaa A. Acute alcohol intoxication among children and adolescents. Eur J Pediatr 1994;153:868–72.
11. Demanet JC, Bonnyns M, Bleiberg H, et al. Coma due to water intoxication in beer drinkers. Lancet 1971;2(7734):1115–7.
12. Liamis GL, Milionis HJ, Rizos EC, et al. Mechanisms of hyponatremia in alcohol patients. Alcohol Alcohol 2000;35:612–6.
13. Sanghvi SR, Kellerman PS, Nanovic L. Beer potomania: an unusual cause of hyponatremia at high risk of complications from rapid correction. Am J Kidney Dis 2007;50:673–80.
14. Hilden T, Svendsen TL. Electrolyte disturbances in beer drinkers: a specific hypoosmolality syndrome. Lancet 1975;2(7928):245–6.
15. Joyce SM, Potter R. Beer potomania: an unusual cause of symptomatic hyponatremia. Ann Emerg Med 1986;15:745–7.
16. Ayus JC, Krothapalli RK, Ariess AI. Changing concepts in treatment of severe symptomatic hyponatremia. Rapid correction and possible relation to central pontine myelinolysis. Am J Med 1985;78:897–902.
17. Heaton FW, Pyrah LN, Beresfor CC, et al. Hypomagnesemia in chronic alcoholism. Lancet 1962;2:802–5.
18. Wu C, Kenny MA. Circulating total and ionized magnesium after ethanol ingestion. Clin Chem 1996;42:625–9.
19. Tzivoni D, Banai S, Schuger C, et al. Treatment of torsade de pointes with magnesium sulfate. Circulation 1988;77:392.
20. Dillon ED, Dyer WW, Smelo LS. Ketone acidosis of non-diabetic adults. Med Clin North Am 1940;24:1813–22.
21. Jenkins DW, Eckle RE, Craig JW. Alcoholic ketoacidosis. JAMA 1971;217:177–83.
22. Halperin ML, Hammeke M, Josse RG, et al. Metabolic acidosis in the alcoholic: a pathophysiologic approach. Metabolism 1983;12:381–9.
23. McGuire LC, Cruickshank AM, Munro PT. Alcoholic ketoacidosis. Emerg Med J 2006;23:417–20.
24. Adams SL, Mathews JJ, Flaherty JJ. Alcoholic ketoacidosis. Ann Emerg Med 1987;16:90–7.
25. Umpierrez GE, Digirolamo M, Turlin JA, et al. Differences in metabolic and hormonal milieu in diabetic and alcoholic induced ketoacidosis. J Crit Care 2000;15:52–9.
26. Miller PD, Heinig RE, Waterhouse C. Treatment of alcoholic acidosis: the role of dextrose and phosphorus. Arch Intern Med 1978;138:67–72.
27. Wernicke C. Die akute hämorrhagische polioencephalitis superior. Fischer Verlag, Kassel. Lehrbuch der Gehirnkrankheiten für Ärzte und Studierende 1881;II: 229–42.
28. Korsakoff SS. Psychic disorder in conjunction with peripheral neuritis. Translated by Victor M, Yakovlev PI. Neurology 1955;5:394–406.
29. Rolland S, Truswell AS. Wernicke-Korsakoff syndrome in Sydney hospitals after 6 years of thiamin enrichment of bread. Public Health Nutr 1998;1:117–22.
30. Donnino MW, Vega J, Miller J, et al. Myths and misconceptions of Wernicke's encephalopathy: what every emergency physician should know. Ann Emerg Med 2007;50:715–21.
31. Harper C. The incidence of Wernicke's encephalopathy in australia – a neuropathological study of 131 cases. J Neurol Neurosurg Psychiatry 1983;46:593–8.

32. Isenberg-Grezeda E, Kutner HE, Nicolson SE. Wernicke-Korsakoff syndrome. Under-recognized and under-treated. Psychosomatics 2012;53:507–16.
33. Caine D, Halliday GM, Kril JJ, et al. Operational criteria for the classification of chronic alcoholics: identification of Wernicke's encephalopathy. J Neurol Neurosurg Psychiatry 1997;62:51–60.
34. Antunez E, Estruch R, Cardenal C, et al. Usefulness of CT and MR imaging in the diagnosis of acute Wernicke's encephalopathy. AJR Am J Roentgenol 1998;171: 1131–7.
35. Day E, Bentham PW, Callaghan R, et al. Thiamine for prevention and treatment of Wernicke-Korsakoff syndrome in people who abuse alcohol. Cochrane Database Syst Rev 2013;(7):CD004033.
36. Ambrose ML, Bowden SC, Whelan G. Thiamine treatment and working memory function of alcohol-dependent people: preliminary findings. Alcohol Clin Exp Res 2001;25:112–6.
37. Thompson AD, Cook CC, Touquet R, et al. The Royal College of Physicians report on alcohol: guidelines for managing Wernicke's encephalopathy in the accident and emergency department. Alcohol Alcohol 2002;37:513–21.
38. Phillips GB, Victor M, Adams RD, et al. A study of the nutritional defect in Wernicke's syndrome; the effect of a purified diet, thiamine, and other vitamins on the clinical manifestations. J Clin Invest 1952;31:859–71.
39. Drenick EJ, Joven CB, Swendseid ME. Occurrence of acute Wernicke's encephalopathy during prolonged starvation for the treatment of obesity. N Engl J Med 1966;274:937–9.
40. Watson AJ, Walker JF, Tomkin GH, et al. Acute Wernickes encephalopathy precipitated by glucose loading. Ir J Med Sci 1981;150:301–3.
41. Jordan LR, Zelaya FO, Rose SE, et al. Changes in the hippocampus induced by glucose in thiamin deficient rats detected by MRI. Brain Res 1998;791:347–51.
42. Zimitat C, Nixon PF. Glucose loading precipitates acute encephalopathy in thiamin-deficient rats. Metab Brain Dis 1999;14:1–20.
43. Schabelman E, Kuo D. Glucose before thiamine for Wernicke encephalopathy: a literature review. J Emerg Med 2012;42:488–94.

Hypothyroidism
Causes, Killers, and Life-Saving Treatments

Sarah B. Dubbs, MD[a],*, Ryan Spangler, MD[b]

KEYWORDS

- Thyroid • Hypothyroidism • Myxedema • Levothyroxine
- Thyroid-stimulating hormone • Coma

KEY POINTS

- Iodine deficiency is the most common cause of hypothyroidism worldwide.
- Hashimoto thryoiditis is the most common cause in the United States.
- Hypothyroidism is more common in elderly, white women.

INTRODUCTION

Hypothyroidism is one of the most frequently encountered endocrinology disorders. Although most of the time this disease does not require immediate emergency evaluation and treatment, the emergency department is often the first point of care for many patients. This truth makes it essential that emergency physicians have an understanding of basic thyroid function, pathophysiology of thyroid-related disorders, and treatment methodology.

The overarching disease of hypothyroidism can have multiple causes and several presentations (thus its reputation as a mimicker), but treatment is rather straightforward. The mainstay of treatment is thyroid hormone supplementation. Outpatient follow-up and treatment are necessary for complete and accurate treatment of these patients, but early intervention and referral from the emergency department can be easy to initiate, and in some severe cases lifesaving.

Myxedema coma, otherwise known simply as myxedema, is the rare but deadly manifestation of severe hypothyroidism. The extremely high mortality rate (historically as high as 80%, but still up to 60%) associated with myxedema makes it necessary for early recognition and treatment by emergency physicians.[1] Although it is not commonly encountered, a healthy degree of suspicion of the "worst first" mentality must be maintained to prevent poor outcomes in these patients.

---

[a] Department of Emergency Medicine, University of Maryland School of Medicine, 110 South Paca Street, 6th Floor Suite 200, Baltimore, MD 21201, USA; [b] Emergency Medicine Residency Program, University of Maryland Medical Center, 110 South Paca Street, 6th Floor Suite 200, Baltimore, MD 21201, USA
* Corresponding author.
E-mail address: sdubbs@umem.org

Emerg Med Clin N Am 32 (2014) 303–317
http://dx.doi.org/10.1016/j.emc.2013.12.003
0733-8627/14/$ – see front matter © 2014 Elsevier Inc. All rights reserved.

In a study by Chen and colleagues[2] it was noted that in a series of patients admitted to the hospital with overt hypothyroidism only 21% was diagnosed on admission. Perhaps more concerning was that 50% of patients in the study ultimately diagnosed with myxedema went undiagnosed. This study indicates that hypothyroid crisis is not well recognized by emergency physicians. In fact, it can be argued that the main job of the emergency physician is to identify thyroid disorders whenever possible. Higher-risk populations include elderly patients and those with cardiovascular and neuropsychiatric illness because thyroid function can be closely tied to these entities.

EPIDEMIOLOGY

In the developed world, thyroid disease is often found to be associated with autoimmune disease and is approximately 5 to 10 times more common in women than in men.[3,4] In Europe, studies have shown that the incidence of hypothyroidism may also be increasing, although it is unclear if this is from increased awareness or an overall increase in autoimmune disorders.[3] The National Health and Nutrition Examination Survey III found subclinical hypothyroidism to be present in 4.3% and overt hypothyroidism in 0.3% of the US population. Other studies indicate that up to 15% of older women may have subclinical hypothyroidism. Higher thyroid-stimulating hormone (TSH) and antithyroid antibodies are found in women, the elderly, whites, and Mexicans (compared with African Americans).[5] A trend has also been found in increased prevalence of autoimmune disorders and subsequently hypothyroidism.[3] Much of these studies focused on chart review and treatment of hypothyroidism, suggesting that an even higher number of subclinical and unidentified patients may be present.

Hypothyroidism can be classified into three categories: (1) primary (thyroid gland), (2) secondary (pituitary gland), or (3) tertiary (hypothalamus). Causes of primary hypothyroidism vary by location, but it is the most common type of hypothyroidism.[4] Worldwide, iodine deficiency is the most common cause. However, in the United States and other iodine-replete areas, chronic thyroiditis, also known as Hashimoto thyroiditis, is the most common cause.[6] Central hypothyroidism has even lower rates, and is thought to be approximately 1 in every 1000 cases of hypothyroidism, most frequently caused by pituitary adenoma.[7] It is a common side effect of treatment of several other conditions and can be seen in 20% to 50% of patients irradiated for nasopharyngeal and paranasal sinus tumors. However, the affects tend to show up several years later rather than immediately.[4,7] Sheehan syndrome and traumatic brain injury can also cause central hypothyroidism through direct or indirect mechanisms. **Table 1** summarizes the types and etiologies of hypothyroidism.

PATHOPHYSIOLOGY

Overall, the production and regulation of thyroid hormones is a relatively simple feedback system. The biochemical synthesis at a cellular and molecular level is somewhat more complex and not as immediately relevant to an emergency physician's goals. The process begins in the hypothalamus with the production of thyrotropin-releasing hormone (TRH). TRH then stimulates the anterior pituitary to secrete TSH.[8] After TSH is released, this stimulates the thyroid to release synthesize, and secrete trioiodothryonine (T3) and thyroxine (T4) from the thyroid itself. T3 and T4 both feed back to the hypothalamus and the pituitary to inhibit TRH and TSH. This feedback mechanism allows for very tight control of TSH levels in the serum.[9,10] **Fig. 1** shows the relationships between the hormones.

Centrally, TRH and TSH are secreted according to a circadian rhythm, with a nocturnal surge in the early nighttime hours. This can be affected by derangements

Table 1 Causes of hypothyroidism	
Primary (thyroid gland dysfunction)	Iodine deficiency Autoimmune thyroiditis • Hashimoto thyroiditis • Atrophic autoimmune thyroiditis Medication-induced (see **Table 2**) Congenital hypothyroidism • Thyroid aplasia or hypoplasia • Defective synthesis of thyroid hormones Iatrogenic • Thyroidectomy • Cancer treatments
Central Secondary (pituitary dysfunction)/tertiary (hypothalamic dysfunction)	Pituitary adenoma Craniopharyngioma Traumatic brain injury Sheehan syndrome Iron overload Sarcoidosis Syphilis Tuberculosis

Data from Vaidya B, Pearce S. Management of hypothyroidism in adults. BMJ 2008;337:a801; and Persani L. Central hypothyroidism: pathogenic, diagnostic and therapeutic challenges. J Clin Endocrinol Metab 2012;97(9):3068–78; with permission.

in gonadal hormones, leptin, and other feeding- and sleep-related hormones, which can affect hypothalamic-pituitary feedback. This results in the condition of central hypothyroidism, which can be difficult to detect, because TSH can be normal, or even slightly elevated in some patients. This is because it is not always a matter of decreased quantity, but also secretion of dysfunctional TSH.[4]

Most T4 produced is stored in the bloodstream and body attached to thyroxine-binding globulin (TBG), albumin, transthyretin (prealbumin), and other lipoproteins. While attached to these molecules, the T4 is not biochemically active but provides

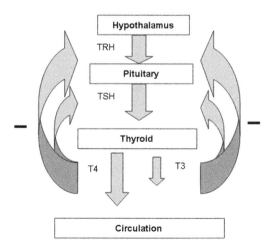

Fig. 1. Thyroid feedback loop.

a reservoir of stored T4, capable of maintaining function for days even if thyroid function were to cease. The protein binding further provides buffer against overactivity of thyroid hormones.[11]

Although T3 is also produced in the thyroid, only a small percentage of T3 is actually made in the thyroid itself. About 80% is produced in extrathyroidal tissues by deiodination of T4. The primary sites of conversion occur in the liver and the kidneys, but most tissues are capable of performing this. T3 is also bound by TBG, albumin, and transthyretnin, ready for immediate use and storage as needed.[11]

When T4 is released and peripherally converted into the bioactive T3, the overall effect is to increase metabolism. There is a direct action of increased peripheral oxygen consumption and thermogenesis. Also, T3 has direct cardiovascular effects to increase ionotropy and chronotropy. Increased cardiac output is somewhat of an indirect result. In hypothyroidism, the end result is the opposite. The exaggerated responses of hypothermia, bradycardia, and hypotension seen in myxedema are an example of this.[1]

Primary hypothyroidism, as seen in Hashimoto thyroiditis, is the result of cell and antibody-mediated destruction of thyroid tissue. Antibodies to thyroperoxidase, thyroglobulin, TSH receptors, and TSH blocking antibodies can all contribute. Because the thyroid needs iodine to build T4 and T3, iodine deficiency causes thyroid deficiency. A transient hypothyroidism can be seen with iodine excess, and is known as Wolff-Chaikoff effect. Frequently, medications can cause hypothyroidism. Frequently cited medications are amiodarone and lithium, with incidence of hypothyroidism of 14% to 18% and 10%, respectively. Overuse of antihyperthyroid medications propothiouracil and methimazole can lead to hypothyroidism. Other common causes are thyroidectomy or radioactive iodine treatment (see **Table 1**; **Table 2**).[7]

EMERGENCY DEPARTMENT PRESENTATION

The hypothyroid patient most frequently presents to the emergency department with multiple, vague complaints of insidious onset, and has a nonspecific physical examination. These circumstances can make the diagnosis elusive even to the attentive physician. The presenting symptoms and signs often vary with age and gender, and the severity of these clinical features varies greatly. Despite the difficulty of diagnosis, routine screening is not recommended in the emergency department because of the effects of nonthryoidal illnesses on thyroid function tests, and national guidelines vary on how best to approach screening in the United States.[4,12]

CLINICAL FEATURES

The hypothyroid state's multitude of manifestations is a result of every organ system relying on thyroid hormone for normal function. The insufficient level of the hormone causes a spectrum of depression in the function of these systems. See **Table 3** for

Table 2	
Medication effects on native thyroid function	
Decreased TSH secretion	Dopamine, glucocorticoids, octreotide, metformin, opiates
Decreased thyroid hormone secretion	Lithium, iodine/iodinated contrast, amiodarone
Increased thyroid hormone metabolism	Phenobarbital, rifampin, phenytoin, carbamazepine

Table 3 Clinical features of hypothyroidism	
Symptoms	**Signs**
Fatigue	Goiter
Weight gain	Nonpitting edema
Cold intolerance	Coarse, dry skin and hair
Hoarse voice	Brittle nails
Dry skin and hair	Macroglossia
Constipation	Slowed relaxation phase of reflexes
Irregular menses and/or menorrhagia	Psychosis
Sexual dysfunction	Bruising/bleeding
Impaired fertility	Pericardial or pleural effusion
Difficulty with concentration	Ascites
Myalgias and arthralgias	**Hypothermia**
Paresthesias	**Hypotension**
Memory deficits	**Hypoglycemia**
Depression	**Altered mental status/coma**

Signs of myxedema coma are shown in boldface.

a summary of the signs and symptoms of hypothyroidism. **Box 1** lists some examples of common presentations of hypothyroidism. The most extreme end of this spectrum is myxedema coma. Although it is rare, myxedema coma is life-threatening and must be recognized and treated emergently.

Symptoms

Symptoms of progressive fatigue and malaise are almost always present with hypothyroidism. Weight gain is another frequent and typical symptom, caused by decreased metabolic rate and oxygen consumption.[4] Other common symptoms include cold intolerance, voice changes, dry skin, hair loss, constipation, irregular menses, difficulty concentrating, memory problems, and depression. Patients also report myalgias, arthralgias, and paresthesias. Some may even present with sexual dysfunction or impaired fertility. A child may manifest hypothyroidism with impaired growth or delayed puberty.

Box 1 Common patient presentations associated with hypothyroidism
Elderly patients
• With new psychiatric complaints
• With cramping, constipation
Patient with combination of weakness, weight gain, and/or hyponatremia
History of depression, weight gain, hoarseness
Young "anemic" woman with frequent episodes of heavy vaginal bleeding
Patient with history of hypertension who develop sudden hypotensive episodes, even after reduction of medication
Refractory hypotension not responsive to routine treatments
Adapted from Tews MC, Shah SM, Gossain VV. Hypothyroidism: mimicker of common complaints. Emerg Med Clin North Am 2005;23:654; with permission.

Physical Examination Findings and Signs

Head and neck

The hypothyroid patient presents with coarse facial features, dry skin, and pallor. His or her hair may be coarse as well, with visible thinning. Facial edema, especially periorbital, can be caused by hypothyroidism. Some patients have macroglossia, which can affect their speech, in addition to a hoarse, deep voice. Finally, goiter, if present, is a fairly obvious and sensitive sign of thyroid dysfunction.

Cardiovascular

Vital signs reveal bradycardia, diastolic hypertension, and in severe cases hypotension as a result of depressed cardiac output. Diastolic hypertension is attributable to increased systemic vascular resistance. Overall cardiac output is decreased, secondary to the slower heart rate and decreased contractility.[13,14]

Signs of pericardial effusion, such as muffled heart sounds, rubs, and jugular venous distention, pulsusparadoxis may be present on physical examination. Bedside ultrasound examination quickly confirms the presence or absence of effusion and tamponade physiology.

Respiratory

Breath sounds may be decreased or abnormal because of hypoventilation and/or pleural effusions.

Abdominal

As with the cardiovascular and respiratory examinations, the abdominal examination may reveal effusion in the form of ascites. Abdominal ascites is relatively rare, occurring in approximately 4% of patients with thyroid disease.[15] Hypothyroidism may also cause constipation and ileus. Thus, bowel sounds may be hypoactive on auscultation and the patient may have mild, diffuse tenderness on palpation.

Dermatologic

Hypothyroid patients have fluffy, nonpitting edema, also known as myxedema. Myxedema derives from the Greek word for mucous, describing the glycosaminoglycans deposition that causes this distinctive edema.[16]

The skin may also take on a pallor appearance caused by hypothyroid-induced anemia. The skin is dry and coarse, nails brittle as well, and hair is coarse with areas of alopecia. There have been some reports of psoriasiform lesions related to severe hypothyroidism.[17]

Neurologic

Many of the neurologic findings associated with hypothyroidism center around cognitive functions, such as orientation, memory, and higher-order thinking.

Patients may also display muscle hypertrophy, proximal muscle weakness, and easy fatigability of strength.[18] Nerve entrapment syndromes, such as carpel tunnel syndrome, can occur as a result of edema. This finding is revealed on examination when pain and paresthesias are reproduced with maneuvers, such as with the Tinel test and Phalen sign.[19] A delayed relaxation phase in deep tendon reflexes (also known as the myxedema reflex or Woltman sign) has also been reported frequently in the literature.[20,21]

Psychiatric

Hypothyroid patients may suffer from depression, reflecting in the physical examination as a slow, flat affect. Some may even display signs of psychosis by responding to internal stimuli or expressing delusional thoughts, a state often referred to as "myxedema madness." In general, laboratory evaluation in psychiatric patients is guided by the history and physical examination. However, with the possibility of subclinical hypothyroidism and the subtlety of symptoms, a screening TSH should be considered in this patient population. See **Box 1** for several examples of clinical scenarios that should trigger a hypothyroidism work-up.

LABORATORY FINDINGS
Diagnosis of Hypothyroidism

This difficulty in diagnosing hypothyroidism does not lie in the laboratory studies themselves; it lies in the shrewdness of the physician to include it on the list of differential diagnoses despite the vague and nebulous symptoms and signs with which patients present.

The first-line diagnostic tool to diagnose hypothyroidism in the emergency department is serum thyrotropin testing. Most facilities are able to perform an ultrasensitive monoclonal antibody test for TSH. These have been shown to be quick, reliable, and reproducible.[22] An abnormal TSH should lead to further testing of the active thyroid hormones T4 and T3. Free thyroxine levels can be measure in two ways. Total thyroxine refers to the combined amount of protein-bound and nonbound hormone. The free T4 level (FT4) refers only to the unbound form, and as the metabolically active moiety[23] is preferred over the total thyroxine level.[12]

High TSH

An elevated TSH indicates some level of hypothyroidism, determined by the level of circulating T4 and T3. When the FT4 level is low, the disease process is classified as *primary hypothyroidism*.

When the FT4 and T3 levels are normal in the setting of low TSH, the disease is classified as *subclinical hypothyroidism*. Subclinical hypothyroidism has multiple etiologies. It can stem from an incomplete autoimmune process that will eventually lead to total thyroid failure. Inadequate dosing or absorption in patients who are on thyroxine replacement medications may also be the cause of these abnormal laboratory values; however, it must be noted that the TSH can be persistently elevated for up to 6 weeks after initiating thyroxine therapy.[24,25] Other times, it can be part of the normal recovery phase in nonthyroidal illness as the body tries to compensate for low thyroid hormone synthesis during the illness. Finally, the TSH can be elevated with normal T4 and T3 levels during acute psychiatric illness and with abuse of amphetamines.[26]

Elevated TSH with elevated FT4 and T3 points to a primary TSH problem, usually a TSH-secreting adenoma in the pituitary gland causing hyperthyroidism.

Normal TSH

A normal TSH level is a fairly reliable indicator of normal thyroid function. Therefore, other nonthyroidal etiologies must be investigated for the patient's symptoms when TSH levels are normal. In the rare case of *central hypothyroidism*, TSH levels can be inappropriately normal, accompanied by low levels of T4.[26]

Low TSH

Low TSH is almost always associated with hyperthyroidism. In the setting of hypothyroid symptoms, an abnormally low level of TSH can result from overall reduced TSH production, called *secondary hypothyroidism*. In patients who are on thyroxine therapy for hypothyroidism, it can be caused by a dose that is too high. Finally, certain medications, such as dopamine and corticosteroids, have been shown to depress TSH levels.[27]

Associated Laboratory Findings

The global effects of thyroid dysfunction cause a wide variety of other laboratory abnormalities in hypothyroid patients. Anemia is frequently encountered in association with hypothyroidism. Depressed red blood cell production causes a normochromic, normocytic anemia. If significant menorrhagia is playing a role, the patient may display an iron-deficiency anemia with a hypochromic, microcytic picture. Many hypothyroid patients also have an autoimmune-related pernicious anemia, resulting in a macrocytic anemia.

Severely hypothyroid patients may also develop coagulopathy, with abnormal clotting times and international normalized ratio. Platelet counts may be normal despite abnormal function.

Renal free water secretion is reduced in hypothyroidism, causing hyponatremia.[28,29] Renal insufficiency is also present in severe hypothyroidism, reflected in elevated brain urea natriuretic peptide and creatinine levels.

Decreased gluconeogenesis and reduced insulin clearance leads to hypoglycemia. This process may be solely caused by the hypothyroid state; however, it may be attributed to a more serious process, adrenal insufficiency. Hypoglycemia (and the concurrent hypotension and other symptoms and signs) related to adrenal insufficiency must be identified as such to be treated appropriately.

Increased muscle membrane permeability allows muscle enzymes to leak into the serum. Creatine kinase levels are elevated to reflect this process.

Decreased respiratory drive is reflected on an arterial blood gas analysis as hypercapnia and hypoxemia with respiratory acidosis.

Other abnormal laboratory values associated with hypothyroidism are elevated transaminases, lactate, and cholesterol. When lumbar puncture is performed as part of the diagnostic process, elevated opening pressure and cerebrospinal fluid protein levels can be present with profound hypothyroidism.[30]

TREATMENT
Hypothyroidism

Although there are many causes of hypothyroidism, the main goal of treatment is to replace the thyroid hormones that are lacking, T3 and T4. Generally, this involves a synthetic compound levothyroxine. Levothyroxine is identical to T4, and is converted to T3 in extrathyroidal tissue the same way endogenously produced T4 is converted. Levothyroxine has a half-life of 7 days so it reaches a steady state rapidly when started on 1.6 µg/kg/day dosing as recommended. Special note should be taken for patients older than age 60 and those with ischemic cardiovascular disease, and should start at a lower dose. There is some discussion of combination therapy with T4 and T3, but there has been no demonstrated benefit over simple levothyroxine therapy.[6]

This one medication approach seems very simple and straightforward; however, different brand preparations of this medication tend to vary slightly in available drug concentrations and switching manufacturers can result in inadequate or overtreatment based on prior regimens. In addition, in one study 40% to 48% of patients on levothyroxine were either overtreated or undertreated.[6] For patients with a known history of hypothyroidism presenting with worsening symptoms, a thorough medication history should be obtained for possible recent pharmacy changes.[23,31]

The American Association of Clinical Endocrinologists suggests a mean dose of 1.6 µg/kg of ideal body weight.[23] However, each individual may be different depending on the degree of thyroid dysfunction, concurrent medications, and general responsiveness. Titration of medication is based on normalization of TSH levels, and should be first analyzed at approximately 6 weeks, with slow titration of 12.5 to 25 µg adjustments and repeat TSH every 1 to 2 weeks.[23] Obviously 6-week follow-up in the emergency department is not a feasible plan for continued care, but it may be important to take into account for patients recently started on levothyroxine with possible overtreatment or undertreatment.

Patients starting levothyroxine or being prescribed new medications need to be aware of possible drug interactions and their effect on levothyroxine dosing. Many drugs can affect levothyroxine at various aspects of its therapeutic course. Common drugs, such as aluminum hydroxide, ferrous sulfate, and calcium, can potentially affect absorption of levothyroxine in the gastrointestinal tract. Other drugs, such as rifampin and sertraline, can affect metabolism and require a higher dosing. Anticonvulsants, birth control pills, and other protein-bound medications can affect the binding of levothyroxine to TBG, albumin, and other proteins that can alter the amount of active drug in the bloodstream.[23] **Table 4** summarizes the effects that some common medications have on levothyroxine.

Subclinical Hypothyroidism

Although in the emergency department it is rare to order screening tests, the chance of identifying subclinical hypothyroidism may still occur (elevated TSH, normal T3/T4). Treatment of subclinical hypothyroidism is controversial, because with normal T4 levels there are generally no symptoms as this is the bioactive compound. The American Association of Clinical Endocrinologists recommends treatment of TSH levels greater than 10, with presence of goiter, or antithyroid peroxidase antibodies because these patients have been shown to be the most likely to progress to true hypothyroidism. It is recommended that a lower dose be used to treat subclinical levels, starting at 35 to 50 µg daily, with standard follow-up.[23]

Pregnancy

Treatment of hypothyroidism in pregnant patients is of particular importance, and TSH screening is recommended as a routine prepregnancy and prenatal work-up. In pregnancy some women may develop thyroid antibodies that can increase the chance for spontaneous abortion regardless of treatment. Untreated hypothyroidism, even mild, in pregnant women increases the risk of several complications including preeclampsia, anemia, postpartum hemorrhage, fetal death, low birth weight, and others. Studies do suggest that cognitive dysfunction of offspring can be prevented with treatment. Levothyroxine is pregnancy class A (also safe in lactation) and it is recommended to initiate, or continue appropriate treatment in pregnant patients. It is also important to note that in general the course of a patients hypothyroidism during pregnancy is unpredictable. In those with chronic hypothyroidism, some improve their symptoms and some get worse.[32]

DISPOSITION

In general, the disposition status of the hypothyroid patient presenting to the emergency department is straightforward. Many of these patients can be discharged home, with the caveat that follow-up is required, particularly if long-term levothyroxine therapy has been started. The recommended follow-up window is 6 weeks after

Table 4
Drug effects on levothyroxine treatment

Mechanism of Effect	Agents
Interference with absorption	Bile acid sequestrants
	Sucralafate
	Cationexchance resins (Kayexelate)
	Oral bisphosphonates
	Proton pump inhibitors
	Raloxifene
	Ferrous sulfate
	Phosphate binders
	Calcium
	Chromium picolinate
	Charcoal
	Orlistat
	Ciprofloxacin
	H$_2$ receptor antagonists
	Grapefruit juice, espresso coffee, high fiber, soy products
Increased clearance	Phenobarbitol
	Primidone
	Phenytoin
	Carbamazepine
	Oxacarbazepine
	Rifampin
	Growth hormone
	Sertraline
	Tyrosine kinase inhibitors
	Quetiapine
	Stavudine
	Nevirapine
Peripheral metabolism	**Glucocorticoids**
	Amiodarone
	Propylthiouracil
	β-Blockers
	Iodinated contrast
	Interleukin-6
	Clomipramine

Agents that are frequently used in the emergency department are shown in boldface.
Data from Garber J, Cobin R, Gharib H, et al. Clinical practice guidelines for hypothyroidism in adults: cosponsored by the American Association of Clinical Endocrinologists and the American Thyroid Association. Endocr Pract 2012;18(6):1004.

initiation to reevaluate TSH levels. Some patients exhibiting severe hypothyroidism may require admission to the hospital if it is believed by the physician that the patient is unsafe to be discharged home to reliably follow-up and take medication. If the patient's disease is thought to be medication-induced, the risks and benefits of continuing or discontinuing the offending medication must be carefully considered. As always, the patient's mental status and psychological status is an important factor in the disposition decision.

MYXEDEMA COMA

Myxedema coma, or simply myxedema, is the most severe manifestation of hypothyroidism with a mortality rate of 30% to 60%, a decrease from almost 80% in the past.[33] Its incidence is rare, and exact numbers are not known based on difficulty of specific definition and possible underrecognition. A frequently cited contributory clue is change in weather, with up to 90% of cases occurring during winter months. It is theorized that this is caused by altered temperature regulation in the severely hypothyroid patient. Myxedema coma is more common among older women and almost never occurs in individuals younger than age 60. Also, there are little data on incidence of myxedema in the equatorial regions, which may be the result of underreporting, but it is hypothesized that the lack of seasonality may play a role.[34,35]

The cardinal signs of myxedema coma are depressed mental status and hypothermia. If a history is available, the patient or family may report the signs and symptoms of undiagnosed hypothyroidism, as described previously; or, the patient may even already carry the diagnosis. The cardiovascular, respiratory, gastrointestinal, renal, and hematologic manifestations of hypothyroidism are at the severe end of the spectrum. Severe hypotension and shock may be the result of depressed cardiac contractility, tamponade, or bradydysrhythmias. Myxedema has even been reported to cause prolongation of the Q-T interval, predisposing patients to torsades de pointes.[36] Hypoventilation can be so profound that acid-base status is disturbed. Patients may have associated gastrointestinal bleeding caused by myxedema-associated coagulopathy.[37] The physical findings associated with myxedema coma are, again, on the extreme end of the hypothyroid symptoms described previously: dough-like nonpitting edema, dry and brittle skin and hair, delayed reflexes, and of course altered sensorium. Some of the most common precipitating events of myxedema coma are listed in **Box 2**.

Laboratory testing should not only focus on diagnosing the hypothyroidism with TSH and thyroxine levels; it should include investigation into the wide differential of altered mental status. Furthermore, a wide net should be cast to identify possible precipitating and aggravating factors in the myxedema state. Common precipitators of myxedema coma are infections, strokes, congestive heart failure, exposure to low ambient temperature, trauma, gastrointestinal bleeding, and metabolic disturbances. Medications, such as anesthetics, sedatives, narcotics, amiodarone, lithium, and changes to levothyroxine-replacement therapy, are also known to precipitate myxedema coma.[38]

Treatment of patients with myxedema coma can vary among practitioners and there is not a consistent or proved method of treatment. Largely because of the rarity of the

---

Box 2
Precipitating events causing myxedema coma

Infection or sepsis

Gastrointestinal hemorrhage

Hypoglycemia

Hypothermia

CO_2 retention

Burns or trauma

Medications

Stroke

Data from Klubo-Gwiezdzinska J, Wartofsky L. Thyroid emergencies. Med Clin North Am 2012;96(2):385–403; and Wall CR. Myxedema coma: diagnosis and treatment. Am Fam Physician 2000;62(11):2485–90.

illness, there are no large studies, and certainly no randomized controlled trials investigating this treatment. Controversy exists in treatment with T4 versus T3, intravenous (IV) versus oral based on bioavailability of each drug.[39] However, there is some literature present noting that using T3 can result in increased mortality, although the cause is not clear and most studies are small case reports. Most sources, because of this, recommend treatment of IV or oral levothyroxine, because evidence does not seem to indicate significant difference between the two.[1]

General recommendations suggest the use of 100 to 500 μg of IV levothyroxine. Dosing tends to vary based on different studies, some recommending lower dosing for older, frailer patients, especially those with cardiovascular disease. Other sources recommend a size-base dosing calculating total body distribution of levothyroxine and administering a distribution size dose of 6 μg/dL (70-kg man, 7-L distribution area, 420-μg dose of levothyroxine). This initial loading dose should be followed by 50 to 100 μg of IV levothyroxine daily until the patient is able to be converted to an oral formulation.[40]

Those in favor of using T3 suggest a loading dose of 10 to 20 μg followed by 10 μg every 4 hours for 24 hours, then 10 μg every 6 hours for 1 to 2 days until the patient can continue with oral medication. An eight-patient case series by Yamamoto and co-workers[41] suggests that although dosing ranges are large, overdosing should be avoided because doses of levothyroxine greater than 500 μg and T3 greater than 75 μg were both associated with increased mortality. Combination therapy of levothyroxine and T3 may be useful, with a loading dose of 4 μg/kg ideal body weight of levothyroxine, followed by 100 μg in 24 hours, then 50 μg daily, IV or orally. T3 would be started simultaneously with doses of 10 μg every 8 to 12 hours until the patient can take oral maintenance doses of levothyroxine.[41]

Although the initial loading dose and exact medication to be used for thyroid replacement is not well established, the use of IV hydrocortisone is consistently recommended throughout the literature. Because of the potential of secondary hypothyroidism and concurrent hypopituitarism, there is strong potential for associated adrenal insufficiency. A dose of 100 mg every 8 hours IV hydrocortisone is suggested to be continued until adrenal insufficiency is ruled out. Some sources suggest a random cortisol level be drawn before treatment to assess adrenal function, and if necessary a corticotropin stimulation test can be performed later. Most recommend discontinuing the hydrocortisone without taper needed once adrenal insufficiency is ruled out.[33]

Further treatment of myxedema coma is necessary to treat the precipitating cause. This can be environmental, infectious, medication induced, or otherwise. Many recommendations suggest immediate septic work-up up including broad-spectrum antibiotics after cultures have been sent. Lumbar puncture is also likely to be necessary in these patients to rule out meningitis as a cause of altered mental status and hypothermia. Special thought needs to be given to finding the precipitating event because this in and of itself can potentially be life threatening.

Critical care treatment of patients with myxedema coma is often necessary because of the severity of illness. Intubation in these patients may be necessary, and has the potential of being a difficult procedure. Patients with hypothyroidism can often be overweight, coupled with the potential for airway myxedema, making airway management difficult. The patients may also have already developed hypercapnia caused by hypoventilatory effects of their illness, have reduced lung volumes, and in severe cases, pleural and pericardial effusions, which can lead to cardiovascular and respiratory collapse if not managed appropriately.[42] Furthermore, external airway anatomy, such as a large goiter, may cause tracheal deviation, and certainly obstruct normal

---

Box 3
Summary of recommendations for patients with suspected myxedema coma

Interventions

   Airway control

   Fluid resuscitation

Diagnostics

   Complete blood count

   Basic metabolic panel

   TSH and free T4 levels

   Blood/urine/sputum cultures

   Lumbar puncture

   Electrocardiogram

   Chest radiograph

   Head computed tomography

   Echocardiogram

Medications

   Levothyroxine, 100–500 µg IV loading; then 50–100 µg IV daily (until patient can take oral medication)

   or

   Triiodiodothyronine, 10–20 µg loading; then 10 µg q 4 hours for 24 hours, then 10 µg q 6 hours for 1–2 days until the patient can take oral medication

   and

   Hydrocortisone, 100 mg IV q 8 hours

   Broad-spectrum antibiotics

   Vasopressors as needed

---

cervical anatomy needed to easily perform an emergent cricothyrotomy if necessary. These recommendations are summarized in **Box 3**.

Patients with suspected myxedema coma by definition have altered mental status and should always be admitted to the hospital with strong consideration for an intensive care unit level admission. These patients can present very sick because their inherent compensatory mechanisms are dysfunctional due to the severe hypothyroid state. In addition, the precipitating factor for their myxedema can be severe, such as sepsis, myocardial infarction, or stroke. Mortality for myxedema tends to increase in hypothermic patients based on the severity of their hypothermia.[43] A study by Dutta and colleagues[44] also noted that patients that were noncompliant with previously prescribed thyroid-replacement medication tended to have higher mortality than those with first-time diagnoses. This study also found that an elevated sequential organ failure assessment (SOFA) score was shown to predict higher mortality.[44]

SUMMARY

Hypothyroidism, one of the most common endocrine disorders encountered, is likely to be directly or indirectly related to frequent patient visits to primary care physicians and emergency physicians. The clinical signs and symptoms can be broad, nonspecific, and subtle at times. Myxedema coma can be equally ambiguous but much more deadly. Early suspicion, recognition, and treatment can improve patient outcomes for any range of the hypothyroid disorders.

REFERENCES

1. Mills L, Lim S. Identifying and treating thyroid storm and myxedema coma in the emergency department. Emerg Med Pract 2009;11(8):1–26.
2. Chen T, Hou S, How C, et al. Diagnosis of unrecognized primary overt hypothyroidism in the ED. Am J Emerg Med 2010;28:866–70.
3. Flynn RW, MacDonald TM, Morris AD, et al. The thyroid epidemiology, audit, and research study: thyroid dysfunction in the general population. J Clin Endocrinol Metab 2004;89(8):3879–84.
4. Devdhar M, Ousman Y, Burman K. Hypothyroidism. Endocrinol Metab Clin North Am 2007;36:595–615.
5. Hollowell J, Staehling N, Flanders W, et al. Serum TSH, T4, and thyroid antibodies in the United States Population (1988 to 1994): National Health and Nutrition Examination Survey (NHANES III). J Clin Endocrinol Metab 2002;87(2):489–99.
6. Vaidya B, Pearce S. Management of hypothyroidism in adults. BMJ 2008;337: a801.
7. Persani L. Central hypothyroidism: pathogenic, diagnostic and therapeutic challenges. J Clin Endocrinol Metab 2012;97(9):3068–78.
8. Magner JA. Thyroid-stimulating hormone: biosynthesis, cell biology, and bioactivity. Endocr Rev 1990;11:354.
9. Shupnik MA, Ridgway EC, Chin WW. Molecular biology of thyrotropin. Endocr Rev 1989;10:459.
10. Dyess EM, Segerson TP, Liposits Z, et al. Triiodothyronine exerts direct cell-specific regulation of thyrotropin-releasing hormone gene expression in the hypothalamic paraventricular nucleus. Endocrinology 1988;123:2291.
11. Mendel CM, Weisiger RA, Jones AL, et al. Thyroid hormone-binding proteins in plasma facilitate uniform distribution of thyroxine within tissues: a perfused rat liver study. Endocrinology 1987;120:1742.
12. Garber J, Cobin R, Woeber K, et al. Clinical practice guidelines for hypothyroidism in adults: cosponsored by the American Association of Clinical Endocrinologists and the American Thyroid Association. Endocr Pract 2012;18(6):989–1028.
13. Klein I, Ojamaa K. Thyroid hormone and the cardiovascular system. N Engl J Med 2001;344(7):501–9.
14. Coceani M. Heart disease in patients with thyroid dysfunction: hyperthyroidism, hypothyroidism and beyond [English]. Anadolu Kardiyol Derg 2013;12(1):62–6.
15. Krishnan S, Philipose Z, Rayman G. Lesson of the week: hypothyroidism mimicking intra-abdominal malignancy. BMJ 2002;325(7370):946.
16. Smith TJ, Bahn RS, Gorman C. Connective tissue, glycosaminoglycans, and diseases of the thyroid. Endocr Rev 1989;10:366–92.
17. Kwinter J, Weinstein M, Bargman H. Psoriasiform lesions and abscesses as initial manifestations of severe hypothyroidism in a previously healthy 15-year old girl. Pediatr Dermatol 2007;24(3):321–3.
18. Cruz MW, Tendrich M, Vaisman M, et al. Electroneuromyography and neuromuscular findings in 16 primary hypothyroidism patients. Arq Neuropsiquiatr 1996;54:12–8.
19. Sabeen A, Allan G. Musculoskeletal manifestations of thyroid disease. Rheum Dis Clin North Am 2010;36:637–46.

20. Houston C. The diagnostic importance of the myxœdema reflex (Woltman's sign). Can Med Assoc J 1958;78(2):108.
21. Burkholder D, Klaas J, Kumar N, et al. The origin of Woltman's sign of myxoedema. J Clin Neurosci 2013;20(9):1204–6.
22. Mirapurkar S, Samuel G, Sivaprasad N. Development of an immunoenzymometric assay (IEMA) for the estimation of human thyroid stimulating hormone (hTSH) in serum. J Immunoassay Immunochem 2010;31(4):290–300.
23. Mendel CM. The free hormone hypothesis: a physiologically based mathematical model. Endocr Rev 1989;10:232–74.
24. Smith SA. Commonly asked questions about thyroid function. Mayo Clin Proc 1995;70:573–7.
25. Khandelwal D, Tandon N. Overt and subclinical hypothyroidism. Drugs 2012; 72(1):17–33.
26. Dayan CM. Interpretation of thyroid function tests. Lancet 2001;357:619–24.
27. Surks MI, Sievert R. Drugs and thyroid function. N Engl J Med 1995;333(25): 1688–94.
28. DeRubertis FR Jr, Michelis MF, Bloom ME, et al. Impaired water excretion in myxedema. Am J Med 1971;51:41–53.
29. Hanna FW, Scanlon MF. Hyponatraemia, hypothyroidism, and role of arginine-vasopressin. Lancet 1997;350:755–6.
30. Swanson JW, Kelly JJ Jr, McConahey WM. Neurological aspects of thyroid dysfunction. Mayo Clin Proc 1981;56:504–12.
31. Garber J, Cobin R, Gharib H, et al. Clinical practice guidelines for hypothyroidism in adults: cosponsored by the American Association of Clinical Endocrinologists and the American Thyroid Association. Thyroid 2012;22(12):1200–35.
32. Gharib H, Cobin R, Dickey R. Subclinical hypothyroidism during pregnancy: position statement from the American Association of Clinical Endocrinologists. Endocr Pract 1999;5(6):367–8.
33. Wall CR. Myxedema coma: diagnosis and treatment. Am Fam Physician 2000; 62(11):2485–90.
34. Davis PJ, Davis FB. Hypothyroidism in the elderly. Compr Ther 1984;10:17–23.
35. Bailes BK. Hypothyroidism in elderly patients. AORN J 1999;69:1026–30.
36. Schenck JB, Rizvi AA, Lin T. Severe primary hypothyroidism manifesting with torsades de pointes. Am J Med Sci 2006;331:154–6.
37. Fukunaga K. Refractory gastrointestinal bleeding treated with thyroid hormone replacement. J Clin Gastroenterol 2001;33:145–7.
38. Klubo-Gwiezdzinska J, Wartofsky L. Thyroid emergencies. Med Clin North Am 2012;96(2):385–403.
39. Arlot S, Debussche X, Lalau JD, et al. Myxoedema coma: response of thyroid hormones with oral and intravenous high-dose L-thyroxine treatment. Intensive Care Med 1991;17:16–8.
40. Mandel S, Brent G, Larsen PR. Levothyroxine therapy in patients with thyroid disease. Ann Intern Med 1993;119:492–502.
41. Yamamoto T, Fukuyama J, Fujiyoshi A. Factors associated with mortality of myxedema coma: report of eight cases and literature survey. Thyroid 1999;9(12):1167–74.
42. Mathew V, Misgar RA, Ghosh S, et al. Myxedema coma: a new look into an old crisis. J Thyroid Res 2011;2011:493462.
43. Kearney T, Dang C. Diabetic and endocrine emergencies. Postgrad Med J 2007; 83:79–86.
44. Dutta P, Bhansali A, Masoodi SR, et al. Predictors of outcome in myxedema coma: a study from a tertiary care centre. Crit Care 2008;12:R1.

The Changing Face of Diabetes in America

Omoyemi Adebayo, MD[a], George C. Willis, MD[b],*

KEYWORDS

- Childhood • Diabetes • Obesity • Epidemic • LADA • Autoimmune

KEY POINTS

- Due to the increasing prevalence of childhood obesity and other environmental factors, juvenile-onset type 2 diabetes mellitus (T2DM) is a quickly spreading disease.
- Similar to treatment in adult patients with T2DM, treatment of juvenile-onset T2DM involves oral medications and lifestyle modifications.
- Latent autoimmune diabetes of adults (LADA) manifests clinically like T2DM but has an element of autoimmunity, leaving patients at risk of developing diabetic ketoacidosis (DKA).
- Oral medications for the treatment of LADA work initially, but treatment often requires initiation of insulin therapy early as the disease progresses.

INTRODUCTION

Over the past few decades, consumers have been constantly bombarded with enticements to get bigger food portions, especially via the marketing industry. As a result, the temptation for caloric overload is greater than ever and, unfortunately, so is the growing prevalence of one of America's deadliest diseases, diabetes mellitus. Growing in more ways than one, diabetes is now claiming new classifications, shifts in affected populations, and changes in treatment algorithms.

Diabetes mellitus is an endocrine disorder characterized by dysregulation of insulin production, insulin sensitivity, and glucose control. Centers for Disease Control and Prevention (CDC) data from 2010 indicate that this disorder accounts for more than 37 million ambulatory care visits each year and was listed as the 7th leading cause of death.[1] Diabetes is traditionally classified in 2 subsets: type 1 diabetes mellitus (T1DM), which consists of an autoimmune etiology, and T2DM, which consists of an

Disclosures: No financial disclosures or conflicts of interest to disclose.
[a] Department of Emergency Medicine, University of Maryland Medical Center, 110 South Paca Street, 6th Floor, Suite 200, Baltimore, MD 21201, USA; [b] Department of Emergency Medicine, University of Maryland School of Medicine, 110 South Paca Street, 6th Floor, Suite 200, Baltimore, MD 21201, USA
* Corresponding author.
E-mail address: george.willis.md@gmail.com

Emerg Med Clin N Am 32 (2014) 319–327
http://dx.doi.org/10.1016/j.emc.2013.12.004
0733-8627/14/$ – see front matter © 2014 Published by Elsevier Inc.

emed.theclinics.com

insulin sensitivity problem. Typically, T1DM patients are diagnosed in childhood. They tend to have a lower body mass index (BMI) and are dependent on insulin due to destruction of pancreatic beta cells and subsequent absolute insulin deficiency. T2DM patients are typically diagnosed in adulthood and usually after the age of 40. They tend to have a high BMI and can be managed with oral medications and lifestyle modifications until resistance becomes so high they require insulin for management.

There have been recent discoveries, however, that exhibit changes in diabetic presentations that require further innovative investigation. Latent autoimmune diabetes of adults (LADA) and juvenile-onset T2DM represent some of these changes in the field. Unfortunately, these 2 entities are increasing in prevalence. Due to their atypical presentations, mismanagement can result, especially if an emergency provider is not aware of them.

Because diabetes is associated with both microvascular and macrovascular complications, appropriate diagnosis, referral, and treatment are paramount in assuring that diabetic patients receive the appropriate treatment and referral in emergency departments (EDs) around the country. Despite that diabetes has been researched for many years, downfalls in American diet, physiologic evolution in today's children, and advances in genetic mapping have meant that providers have needed to find new methods of keeping up with the ever-changing faces of diabetes.

JUVENILE-ONSET TYPE 2 DIABETES MELLITUS

T2DM is commonly regarded as a disease of obese adults who have led sedentary lifestyles or have genetic predisposition to developing diabetes. Patients with this disease require a combination of diet, exercise, and medications, either an oral hypoglycemic or parenteral insulin injections, for treatment.

It is unlikely that in the majority of medical school textbooks and medical reference material there is any discussion of T2DM being a rapidly devastating disease of children. There has been, however, a shift in the pathogenesis of T2DM, a disease once relegated to middle-aged and elderly patients, to where it is becoming more commonplace in America's children than anyone ever anticipated. The SEARCH for Diabetes in Youth Study reports that the incidence rate of T2DM in patients between the ages of 10 and 19 is approximately 10 cases per 100,000 person-years.[2] Although this overall prevalence sounds unimpressive, emergency providers must take note because this marks a greater than 20% increase since the 2001 statistics, making childhood T2DM one of the nation's most aggressively expanding health crises. Although it is still currently behind T1DM in terms of shear numbers of children affected, T2DM is likely to catch and surpass its autoimmune counterpart in the United States.[3] In Japan, the patterns childhood diabetes are beginning to mirror those of adult diabetes in the United States, with T2DM accounting for more than 80% of all of their childhood cases.[4]

Risk Factors

T2DM in childhood has been linked to a host of risk factors associated with maternal health patterns that are present, even preconception. Similarly, as in adult-onset T2DM, the causes of the disease are multifactorial, including a host of environmental factors. The American Diabetes Association asserts that the prevalence of T2DM in a parent of a T2DM child is as high as 90% in some regions of the country.[5] Other major risks for developing T2DM in children include female gender, lack of exercise, gestational diabetes exposure, and obesity—obesity both in children and in the mother.[5]

Adamo and colleagues[6] analyzed several studies that positively correlate maternal gestational/preconception health and the risk for development of childhood insulin resistance and ultimately juvenile-onset T2DM. One study, in the *American Journal of Clinical Nutrition*, found that prematernal obesity was the single greatest predictor of childhood insulin and other metabolic dysregulation.[6,7] Prevention of this disease does not begin with early childhood interventions in kindergarten or preschool, as some studies have urged. On the contrary, intervention should take place in future pregnant patients who are not even aware they will become pregnant; as a result of their preconception weight and dietary and lifestyle choices, their children may suffer from dramatically increased odds of developing T2DM.

Childhood obesity is another risk factor that deserves mention because it, along with lower levels of activity in the youth population, also contributes to an increased incidence of juvenile-onset T2DM. The prevalence of severe childhood obesity has increased by greater than 300% since the 1970s, with rates as low as 0.8% in 1976.[8,9] Prior to 2000, the CDC defined all children with a BMI over the 95th percentile as "overweight." There was no classification of "obesity" prior to this. Now, the CDC defines a child as overweight when the BMI is over the 85th percentile but less than the 95th percentile, adjusted for age and gender.[10,11] Obesity is defined as a BMI over the 95th percentile.[10,11] The advent of this new definition has provided the opportunity for earlier intervention and has shone a spotlight on this rapidly growing problem. Approximately 1 of every 3 children in the United States today meets the definition of overweight or obese. These numbers are proposed to double, to equate to 60 million children, by 2020.[11]

Childhood obesity has several problems aside from the development of diabetes. In 2008, all obesity in the United States was linked to $148 billion in health care costs.[12] Compared with just 10 years prior, in 1998, these costs were almost half, yet still staggering at $78 billion a year.[12] From 1979 to 1999, childhood obesity–related hospital costs were greater than $90 million in 20 years.[13] As in adults, childhood obesity has also been correlated with an increased risk of development of diabetes, heart disease, vascular disease, and other health problems.

It is now known that all ethnic groups are at risk for the development of obesity. Mexican American and non-Hispanic blacks, however, still carry the highest numbers of obese children per capita compared with all other ethnic groups in the United States.[14] Park and colleagues[15] examined the cross-sectional data of the National Health and Nutrition Examination Survey group from 1999 to 2008 and found that not only are there race-specific risk factors but also age- and gender-specific risks. These factors supersede race as a risk factor for the development of obesity and its complications in the case of this age group of children.[14,15]

Maternal and perinatal health problems are also thought to play an integral role in the development of obesity in childhood. In a study performed to identify risk factors for obesity development in kindergarteners, researchers found that severe maternal obesity and maternal gestational diabetes were both associated with a 3-times risk increase for kindergarten obesity.[8] This same study found that advanced maternal age at first live birth and previous birth weight of greater than 4000 g had a negative association with childhood obesity development.[8]

Pathophysiology

Pediatric endocrine research has revealed over the past 10 to 15 years that although there is much overlap between child-onset and adult-onset T2DM patients, there are several key differences between these 2 populations.

Essentially all cases of T2DM, in adults or children, begin as a problem with impaired glucose tolerance before progressing toward overt disease. On average, time of onset from impaired glucose tolerance to outright diabetes is approximately 10 years in adults,[16] which occurs because of an approximately 7% decline in pancreatic beta cell function per year.[16] Comparing these figures with those of obese children who go on to develop childhood diabetes, the mean time from prediabetes to disease is 2.5 years or 7.5 faster than it takes adults to develop the disease.[16] Beta cell destruction in this population occurs at a rate of approximately 15% each year.[16] Research is still unclear as to why there is such a stark contrast between the 2 groups.

Another manner in which diabetes in the young varies from the traditional adult disease is that the presence of acanthosis nigricans, a thickening and hyperpigmentation of the nape of the neck, is far more common in children than adults and often can serve as a precursory marker for impending diabetes and an opportunity for early intervention.[5,16,17] As many as 90% of children with acanthosis nigricans have some degree of insulin resistance.[17] The disease process in both adults and children imposes similar risks of accelerated disease to the various organ systems. Cardiovascular disease and pulmonary disease, especially in this population heavily afflicted with reactive airway disease, are real concerns in children with T2DM. This population represents patients for whom providers must have moderate to high suspicion for more adult diagnoses when they present to an ED. Cardiovascular complications, such as acute coronary syndrome, are certainly plausible in this population and should not be eliminated from the differential diagnosis simply based on age.

Treatment

Although the defining objective parameters and definitions of T2DM are the same in children as they are in adults, the recommendations for treatment of children have different focuses than those for adults. A treatment guideline exists by way of the American Academy of Pediatrics, which, in conjunction with the American Diabetes Association, the Pediatric Endocrine Society, the American Academy of Family Physicians, and the Academy of Nutrition and Dietetics, produced 6 key points that practitioners who are involved in the management and monitoring of children with T2DM should use to guide their clinical decision making.[18]

To summarize the proposals, first, they recommend that anyone with evidence of severe disease (ie, DKA, hemogloblin [Hb]A_{1C} >9%, or random blood glucose $\geq$250 mg/dL) should have insulin therapy initiated immediately. Second, in children diagnosed with mild or moderate diabetes, lifestyle modifications and metformin therapy should be initiated together at the time of diagnosis.[18] This treatment strategy is confirmed by the results of the Treatment Options for Type 2 Diabetes in Adolescents and Youth (TODAY) trial, which found that pharmacologic therapy was more effective than lifestyle changes when each was tested in isolation and had even better effectiveness when the 2 were combined in treatment of children with T2DM.[19] Metformin is the only oral medication approved by the Food and Drug Administration for the treatment of childhood diabetes. Results found, however, that even with dual oral hypoglycemic therapy there was an almost 40% failure rate to achieve adequate glycemic control.[16,19] This underwhelming result likely means a shorter time until insulin is required for adequate treatment of the disease. The remainder of the recommendations includes a focus on the frequency of monitoring of blood sugar and HbA$_{1C}$ by primary physicians and references to other society guidelines for optimal lifestyle changes needed for proper glycemic control.[18] The treatment guidelines are outlined in **Table 1**.

The TODAY study also revealed that several children and adolescents who were diagnosed with T2DM were found to have comorbidities, such as microalbuminemia, dyslipidemia, and hypertension.[20] This population is at a higher risk for early development of long-term vascular complications, such as atherosclerosis and

Table 1
Key action statements for treatment and management of T2DM in children

Key Action Proposed	Level of Evidence Supporting Key Action
(1) Immediate insulin therapy in (a) ketosis, (b) DKA, (c) random blood glucose $\geq$250 mg/dL, or (d) HbA$_{1c}$ >9%.	C
(2) In all other cases, initial therapy includes lifestyle modification AND immediate initiation of metformin.	B
(3) Recommend pediatricians trend HbA$_{1c}$ every 3 mo and intensify therapy for patients not meeting treatment goals.	D
(4) Patients should monitor their blood glucose if they are (a) taking insulin or other hypoglycemic drugs, (b) initiating or changing therapy for their diabetes, (c) are not meeting their treatment goals, or (d) have intercurrent illness.	D
(5) Suggest primary doctors incorporate the *Academy of Nutrition and Dietetics Pediatric Weight Management Evidence-Based Nutrition Practice Guideline* in counseling patients with T2DM at point of initial diagnosis.	D
(6) Recommend at least 60 min of vigorous physical activity daily and limiting nonacademic electronic screen viewing time to <2 h daily.	D

cardiovascular disease. Diabetic pediatric patients who present to an ED with hypertension benefit from close follow-up with their pediatrician for management of these comorbidities.

Primary prevention should also be considered in at-risk populations. Patients who present to an ED with unrelated complaints and have evidence of acanthosis nigricans benefit from a referral to their pediatrician for evaluation of impaired glucose control. Lifestyle modifications should be encouraged early in this patient population.

LATENT AUTOIMMUNE DIABETES OF ADULTS

LADA is another diabetic conundrum that has developed and grown in the past few years. The disease goes by one of several eponyms, including diabetes 1.5, slow-onset T1DM, and slow-onset insulin-dependent diabetes mellitus.[21] Although the existence of this form of diabetes has been described as early as 1986, widespread knowledge of this peculiar entity is nonexistent.[22]

LADA is a form of diabetes that is a hybrid of T1DM and T2DM.[23–25] The Immunology of Diabetes Society (IDS) has laid the foundation for diagnostic criteria, which include (1) onset of diabetes after 30 years of age (some groups have proposed that the cutoff age be as low as 25 or as high as 35), (2) identification of active islet cell autoantibodies (typically glutamic acid decarboxylase autoantibody [GADA]), and (3) insulin-independent treatment for at least 6 months after diagnosis of diabetes.[26,27]

Despite that the IDS diagnostic criteria stands as the most accepted, there are studies that suggest a new definition should be developed to mirror the ever-changing population affected by the disease.[28] Points are made against each of the diagnostic criteria for why they should be modified. With regard to the age criteria, some studies have argued that GADA antibodies are present in patients less than 30 years old who present phenotypically as T2DM.[25] Lack of consistently sensitive and widespread availability of autoantibody assays causes ripples of confusion and disagreement surrounding the second diagnostic criterion. As for the insulin-free treatment period requirement, some investigators bring up the fact that the report to start a patient on insulin is dependent on a patient's primary physician's practice beliefs and patterns. Another practitioner may start a patient, who may not be started on insulin after a year by one doctor, on insulin after only a month after failed oral therapy simply because of different practice styles.[27] It soon becomes clear why so much confusion exists over the precise diagnostic criteria.

Prevalence and Proposed Mechanisms

Most studies to establish incidence or prevalence have been done abroad, in locations such as China, Korea, India, and Europe. Some studies have shown that the incidence of LADA ranges from 5% to 10% of the general population.[23,25] Even so, these figures may be underestimated because many patients with LADA are misdiagnosed as either T2DM or T1DM because the process of LADA is not universally known among general practitioners. Further studies have shown that 10% to 30% of patients diagnosed with T2DM also test positive for autoantibodies and should be diagnosed with LADA.[29]

The reason LADA is so difficult to diagnose is because it possesses so many properties of both T1DM and T2DM. A point of major debate is just how closely LADA resembles the metabolic syndrome patterns of T2DM. Most patients with LADA fit the phenotypic profile of a T2DM patient: they have a higher BMI, have a later onset of diabetes, and are not dependent on insulin.[30] Clinically, patients who fit this profile are most likely diagnosed with T2DM at the onset of hyperglycemia and treated with oral hypoglycemic and lifestyle modifications. There are differences, however, between patients with LADA and patients with T2DM. Mollo and colleagues[24] found in their cross-sectional study that there was a statistically higher rate of metabolic syndrome in LADA patients (37%) than in patients with T1DM but the rate was lower than in patients with T2DM (67%). In another larger prospective observational study, similar differences were found between groups; however, percentages of metabolic syndrome were greater overall across all groups.[31] Research has not determined if the genetics of LADA is most similar to T1DM or T2DM because there are studies that have shown evidence of genetic homogeneity to both.[23,24,27,31–33] Similar to the rate of acceleration of islet cell dysfunction in children with T2DM, patients with LADA experience an extremely rapid progression to insulin dependence for glycemic control.[23,24]

Clinical Presentation

Because of the significant overlap between patients with LADA and T2DM, making the diagnosis in an ED is often difficult. As discussed previously, patients with LADA share many characteristics with patients that have adult-onset T2DM. They have a higher BMI and are not initially dependent on insulin.[30] Common symptoms of hyperglycemia, such as polyuria and polydipsia, can be present. Several of these patients may already have been diagnosed with T2DM and started on oral medications by their primary practitioner. They may be compliant with diet and lifestyle modifications and still have refractory hyperglycemia. Consequently, this patient population is likely to be diagnosed with LADA.

Contrary to T2DM patients, because of the element of insulin deficiency due to the rapid decline in pancreatic beta cells, LADA patients often require insulin at an earlier stage in their disease progression. As a result, they often experience treatment failures with the oral regimens alone, even when coupled with lifestyle modifications. Subsequently, because of the insulin deficiency, patients with LADA are also prone to developing DKA. Therefore, a young adult patient with DKA who was recently on oral diabetic medications is more likely to be suffering from LADA, which is contrary to the standard teaching of DKA being primarily a T1DM complication.

Treatment

In general, the traditional model for LADA is similar to that of T1DM and T2DM, depending on whether a patient is in the insulin resistance phase or islet cell failure stage of disease. As with the broader subsets of diabetes, initial focus should be on weight reduction and caloric restriction and the use of oral hypoglycemics during the insulin-independent phase (first 6 months after diagnosis).[21]

Differences arise in the question of how soon insulin therapy should be initiated. Studies in T2DM patients using early insulin therapy in place of sulfonylureas have shown that this intervention can drastically slow down the destruction of islet cell function.[34,35] This theory was further tested in a small study by Kobayashi and colleagues,[36] which found that early administration of insulin in these patients caused an immunomodulatory response where levels of C-peptide were actually sustained compared with the sulfonylurea group, which again progressed quickly to insulin dependence. This has been shown to occur only with the sulfonylureas. The insulin sensitizers, such as metformin and the thiazolidinediones, have been shown to be safe and have a role in preserving beta cell function initially.[35] If oral medications are initiated in an ED, patients suspicious of having LADA need much closer follow-up to observe for early signs of treatment failure and early initiation of insulin therapy.

Insulin therapy should be considered in patients who exhibit refractory hyperglycemia despite compliance with oral medications. As their pancreatic beta cells continue to decline, their basal insulin levels start to decrease and they become more predisposed to developing complications, such as DKA. Long-acting insulin therapies have been shown effective in the management of LADA.[37]

Patients with LADA who present in DKA should be treated as any other DKA patient. Intravenous fluids and insulin are mainstays of therapy. Unlike the majority of T1DM diabetic patients, however, patients with LADA have more circulating insulin than T1DM diabetic patients and less insulin resistance than T2DM diabetic patients.[38] Therefore, they respond extremely well to insulin infusions and often have shorter ICU stays and subsequent hospitalizations.

SUMMARY

A lot has changed recently regarding standard management of diabetes. Diabetes is becoming an ever-changing disease with global impacts on the field of medicine. With diabetes foundations projecting 333 million people globally to be affected by 2025, it is imperative that emergency providers continue to stay ahead. Early interventions have proved key in decreasing the amount of childhood obesity, which has indisputably been identified as one of the greatest risk factors for child-onset T2DM. Studies have shown that even earlier efforts focused on preconception maternal health have benefits in the role of preventing juvenile-onset T2DM. When these efforts have failed, however, and T2DM is present in a child, recognition that initiation of therapy includes both lifestyle and immediate pharmacologic therapy institution is key if glycemic control is to be achieved at all. Recognition and adequate treatment of T2DM are paramount in diminishing the inevitable cardiovascular risks involved with this endocrine disorder.

LADA is a commonly misdiagnosed entity in diabetes that may present in EDs as noncompliant T2DM patients, when in actuality they are suffering from this autoimmune variant. Prompt institution of insulin therapy may provide some of the best protection against islet cell destruction, as some early studies have indicated. At this juncture, a couple of facts are clear: diabetes mellitus is not going anywhere and is getting worse. Modifying the societal impact of this burden must be done from all levels of life, including political, social, medical, and, most impactful, individual.

REFERENCES

1. Xu J, Kochanek K, Murphy S, et al. Deaths: final data for 2007. Natl Vital Stat Rep 2010;58(19):1–136.
2. Writing Group for the SEARCH for Diabetes in Youth Study Group, Dabelea D, Bell RA, et al. Incidence of diabetes in youth in the United States. JAMA 2007; 297(24):2716–24.
3. Alberti G, Zimmet P, Shaw J, et al. Type 2 diabetes in the young: the evolving epidemic: the international diabetes federation consensus workshop. Diabetes Care 2004;27(7):1798–811.
4. Cockram C. The epidemiology of diabetes mellitus in the Asia-Pacific region. Hong Kong Med J 2000;6(1):43–52.
5. Kaufman F. Type 2 diabetes in children and young adults: a "New Epidemic". Clin Diabetes 2002;20:217–8.
6. Adamo KB, Ferraro ZM, Brett KE. Pregnancy is a critical period for prevention of obesity and cardiometabolic risk. Can J Diabetes 2012;36(3):133–41.
7. Catalano PM, Farrell K, Thomas A. Perinatal risk factors for childhood obesity and metabolic dysregulation. Am J Clin Nutr 2009;90(5):1303–13.
8. Flores G, Lin H. Factors predicting severe childhood obesity in kindergarteners. Int J Obes 2013;37(1):31–9.
9. Skelton JA, Cook SR, Auinger P, et al. Prevalence and trends of severe obesity among US children and adolescents. Acad Pediatr 2009;9:322–32.
10. Barlow SE, Expert Committee. Expert committee recommendations regarding the prevention, assessment, and treatment of child and adolescent overweight and obesity: summary report. Pediatrics 2007;120(Suppl 4):S164–92.
11. de Onis M, Blössner M, Borghi E. Global prevalence and trends of overweight and obesity among preschool children. Am J Clin Nutr 2010;92:1257–64.
12. Finkelstein EA, Trogdon JG, Cohen JW, et al. Annual medical spending attributable to obesity: payer-and service-specific estimates. Health Aff (Millwood) 2009;28(5):w822–31.
13. Lytle L. Dealing with the childhood obesity epidemic: a public health approach. Abdom Imaging 2010;37(5):719–24.
14. Long J, Mareno N, Shabo R, et al. Overweight and obesity among white, black, and Mexican American children: implications for when to intervene. J Spec Pediatr Nurs 2012;17(1):41–50.
15. Park M, Falconer C, Viner R, et al. The impact of childhood obesity on morbidity and mortality in adulthood: a systematic review. Obes Rev 2012;13(11):985–1000.
16. Santoro N. Childhood obesity and type 2 diabetes: the frightening epidemic. World J Pediatr 2013;9(2):101–2.
17. Wilson V. Type 2 diabetes: an epidemic in children. Nurs Child Young People 2013;25(2):14–7.
18. Copeland K, Silverstein J, Flinn S, et al. Management of newly diagnosed type 2 diabetes mellitus (T2DM) in children and adolescents. Pediatrics 2013; 131(2):364–82.
19. TODAY Study Group, Zeitler P, Hirst K, et al. A clinical trial to maintain glycemic control in youth with type 2 diabetes. N Engl J Med 2012;366(24):2247–56.

20. Copeland K, Zeitler P, Geffner M, et al. Characteristics of adolescents and youth with recent-onset type 2 diabetes: the TODAY cohort at baseline. J Clin Endocrinol Metab 2011;96(1):159–67.
21. Stenström G, Gottsäter A, Bakhtadze E, et al. Latent autoimmune diabetes in adults: definition, prevalence, beta-cell function, and treatment. Diabetes Care 2005;54(Suppl 2):S68–72.
22. Groop LC, Bottazzo GF, Doniac D. Islet cell antibodies identify latent type1 diabetes in patients aged 35–75 years at diagnosis. Diabetes 1986;35:237–41.
23. Zhou Z, Xiang Y, Leslie R, et al. Frequency, immunogenetics, and clinical characteristics of Latent Autoimmune Diabetes in China (LADA China Study): a nationwide, multicenter, clinic-based cross-sectional study. Diabetes 2013;62(2): 543–50.
24. Mollo A, Hernandez M, Mauricio D, et al. Latent autoimmune diabetes (LADA) is perched between type 1 and type 2: evidence from adults in one region of Spain. Diabetes Metab Res Rev 2013;29(6):446–51.
25. Brahmkshatriya P, Mehta A, Saboo B, et al. Characteristics and prevalence of Latent Autoimmune Diabetes in Adults (LADA). ISRN Pharmacol 2012;2012:1–8.
26. Fourlanos S, Dotta F, Greenbaum CJ, et al. Latent autoimmune diabetes in adults (LADA) should be less latent. Diabetologia 2005;48(11):2206–12.
27. Liao Y, Xiang Y, Zhou Z. Diagnostic criteria of latent autoimmune diabetes in adults (LADA): a review and reflection. Front Med 2012;6(3):243–7.
28. Redondo M. LADA: time for a new definition. Diabetes 2013;62(2):339–40.
29. Turner R, Stratton I, Horton V, et al. UKPDS 25: auto-antibodies to islet-cell cytoplasm and glutamic acid decarboxylase for prediction of insulin requirement in type 2 diabetes. UK Prospective Diabetes Study Group. Lancet 1997; 350(9087):1288–93.
30. Torn C, Landin-Olsson M, Ostman J, et al. Glutamic acid decarboxylase antibodies (GADA) is the most important factor for prediction of insulin therapy within 3 years in young adult diabetic patients not classified as Type 1 diabetes on clinical grounds. Diabetes Metab Res Rev 2000;16(6):442–7.
31. Hawa MI, Thivolet C, Mauricio D, et al. Metabolic syndrome and autoimmune diabetes: action LADA 3. Diabetes Care 2009;32(1):160–4.
32. Roh M, Jung C, Kim B, et al. The prevalence and characteristics of latent autoimmune diabetes in adults (LADA) and its relation with chronic complications in a clinical department of a university hospital in Korea. Acta Diabetol 2013;50(2):129–34.
33. Djekic K, Mouzeyan A, Ipp E. Latent autoimmune diabetes of adults is Phenotypically similar to type 1 diabetes in a minority population. J Clin Endocrinol Metab 2012;97(3):E409–13.
34. Alvarsson M, Sundkvist G, Lager I, et al. Beneficial effects of insulin versus sulphonylurea on insulin secretion and metabolic control in recently diagnosed type 2 diabetic patients. Diabetes Care 2003;26(8):2231–7.
35. Cernea S, Buzzetti R, Pozzilli P. Beta-cell protection and therapy for latent autoimmune diabetes in adults. Diabetes Care 2009;32(Suppl 2):S246–52.
36. Kobayashi T, Nakanishi K, Murase T, et al. Small dose of subcutaneous insulin as a strategy for preventing slowly progressive cell failure in islet cell antibody-positive patients with clinical features of NIDDM. Diabetes 1996;45(5):622–6.
37. Maruyama T, Tanaka S, Shimada A, et al. Insulin intervention in slowly progressive insulin-dependent (type 1) diabetes mellitus. J Clin Endocrinol Metab 2008;93(6): 2115–21.
38. Leslie RD, Kolb H, Schloot NC, et al. Diabetes classification: grey zones, sound and smoke: action LADA 1. Diabetes Metab Res Rev 2008;24(7):511–9.

Derangements of Potassium

Laura Medford-Davis, MD[a,b,*], Zubaid Rafique, MD[a,b]

KEYWORDS

- Potassium • Hypokalemia • Hyperkalemia • Peaked T waves

KEY POINTS

- Potassium balance regulates the excitability of cardiac cells, and both hypokalemia and hyperkalemia can cause cardiac arrest when severe.
- Treatment of hyperkalemia includes cardiac membrane stabilization, transcellular shifting, and total body potassium elimination. Sodium bicarbonate and Kayexalate are not recommended for management.
- Treatment of symptomatic hypokalemia consists of repletion with potassium chloride, which is available in liquid, pill, and intravenously (IV) administrable forms. Magnesium should be repleted simultaneously to potentiate potassium absorption and avoid further potassium losses.
- Determine and treat the underlying cause of potassium derangement to prevent recurrence.
  o Avoid potentiating medications.
  o Consider the dietary potassium contribution.
  o Consider problems with potassium excretion from the gastrointestinal (GI) tract or kidneys.
  o Consider transcellular potassium shifts across cell membranes.

INTRODUCTION AND PATHOPHYSIOLOGY

About 98% of total body potassium (K+) is intracellular,[1,2] and 75% of the intracellular potassium is contained in skeletal muscle cells.[3,4] The body maintains the remaining 2% extracellular component within a tight range of 3.5 to 5.0 mEq/L (1 mmol equals 1 mEq K+).[3] The main mechanism for maintaining this transcellular ratio is the sodium-potassium (Na-K) adenosine triphosphatase (ATPase) pump, which uses energy in the form of adenosine triphosphate to drive K+ into cells in exchange for sodium (Na). The resulting K+ gradient creates a resting membrane potential that determines cardiac and neuromuscular cell excitability and signal conduction.

[a] Division of Emergency Medicine, Baylor College of Medicine, 1 Baylor Plaza, Houston, TX 77030, USA; [b] Department of Emergency Medicine, Ben Taub General Hospital, Ben Taub General Hospital Emergency Center, 1504 Taub Loop, Houston, TX 77030, USA
* Corresponding author. Department of Emergency Medicine, Ben Taub General Hospital Emergency Center, 1504 Taub Loop, Houston, TX 77030.
E-mail address: medford.davis@gmail.com

Emerg Med Clin N Am 32 (2014) 329–347
http://dx.doi.org/10.1016/j.emc.2013.12.005
0733-8627/14/$ – see front matter © 2014 Elsevier Inc. All rights reserved.

Because the extracellular K+ level is proportionally so much less than the intracellular level, even a small change in the extracellular level significantly alters the resting membrane potential. Hyperkalemia is less tolerated by the body and causes more significant extracellular shifts than hypokalemia. A 100 mEq excess of total body K+ increases extracellular levels by 0.5 mEq, whereas a 100 mEq deficit decreases extracellular levels by just 0.3 mEq.[3] Three different mechanisms alter the extracellular K+ concentration: K+ intake, K+ excretion, and transcellular shift of K+ into or out of cells.[3] Many common medications affect one of these 3 mechanisms and can provoke a potassium imbalance (**Boxes 1** and **2**).

Usually the body's regulatory mechanisms can resist large fluctuations in daily potassium intake. However, over time or in those persons predisposed to K+ disorders, diet can affect the extracellular K+ level. Patients with altered total-body potassium stores, who chronically take medications that alter K+ balance, or who have a disease predisposing them to K+ imbalance may need to either increase or avoid intake of potassium-rich foods (**Box 3**).

Excretion of K+ from the body is primarily managed by the kidneys, which are responsible for 90% of excretion in normal physiology.[2,4] The other 10% is excreted mostly by the intestine into stool, with a small contribution from sweat. In cases of severe burns or extreme exercise, sweat and skin losses increase. Similarly, in end-stage renal disease when the kidneys no longer function, the gut upregulates to perform 25% of excretion.[2]

Box 1
Medications causing hyperkalemia

Inhibit excretion

  Decrease aldosterone

    Angiotensin converting enzyme inhibitors

    Angiotensin receptor blockers

    Potassium-sparing diuretics (spironolactone)

    Nonsteroidal antiinflammatory drugs (NSAIDs)

    Heparin

    Nonselective β-blockers

  Block sodium channels

    Potassium-sparing diuretics (amiloride, triamterene)

    Antibiotics (trimethoprim, pentamidine)

Transcellular shift

  Inhibit Na-K ATPase pump

    Digoxin (dose dependent)

    NSAIDs

    Nonselective β-blockers

    Anesthetics (succinylcholine, suxamethonium)

Data from Alfonzo AV, Isles C, Geddes C, et al. Potassium disorders—clinical spectrum and emergency management. Resuscitation 2006;70:10–25; and Pepin J, Shields S. Advances in diagnosis and management of hypokalemic and hyperkalemic emergencies. Emerg Med Pract 2012;14(2):1–17.

| **Box 2** |
| **Medications causing hypokalemia** |

Transcellular Shift

Insulin

β-Agonists

  Bronchodilators

  Tocolytics

Synthroid

Phosphodiesterase inhibitors

  Caffeine

  Theophylline

Overdose

  Verapamil

  Barium

Decongestants

Increased K+ Excretion

Thiazide diuretics

Loop diuretics (furosemide and bumetanide)

Mineralocorticoids (fludrocortisone)

High-dose glucocorticoids (prednisone)

High-dose penicillins

Aminoglycosides

Cisplatin

Amphotericin

Data from Refs.[2–4,13]

Na-K ATPase exchangers are present both in the intestine and in the distal renal nephron to excrete K+. In the kidney, high amounts of urine and sodium arriving to the distal nephron stimulate the Na-K ATPase to excrete more K+,[4] as does aldosterone. Low renal perfusion, hypovolemia, low sodium levels, or high potassium levels trigger renal renin release, which leads to aldosterone release by the adrenal glands,[3] increasing renal excretion of K+.

Finally, certain physiologic states and medications affect the transport of K+ across the cell membrane, leading to transcellular shifts that can alter extracellular K+ levels. These shifts can be caused by alterations in the Na-K ATPase pump, pH and acid-base status in the body, and tonicity of the serum.[4] Hyperglycemia and hypernatremia are 2 examples of hypertonic states that drive potassium out of cells.[3]

The symptoms of potassium alterations are typically vague, so a careful history is important to raise clinical suspicion of the diagnosis. Symptoms of both hypokalemia and hyperkalemia affect the cardiac, muscular, and GI systems. The rate of change in extracellular K+ levels is more important than the absolute K+ level in determining severity of symptoms and risk for deterioration, so symptoms are unreliable predictors of absolute K+ values. Workup of any patient whose history suggests potassium

Box 3
Foods rich in potassium

Legumes and grains
  Whole-grain bread
  Wheat bran
  Granola
  Beans (kidney, pinto, black, navy, and lima)
  Nuts, nut butter
Vegetables
  Potato
  Yam, sweet potato
  Tomato
  Spinach
  Beets
  Broccoli
  Brussel sprouts
  Bamboo shoots
  Winter squash (acorn, butternut, pumpkin)
  Cabbage
  Carrots (raw)
  Spinach
  Canned mushrooms
  Pickles
Fruits
  Banana, plantain
  Fig
  Prune
  Raisin
  Date
  Apricot (especially dried)
  Avocado
  Melon (cantaloupe and honey dew)
  Kiwi
  Mango
  Citrus (nectarine and orange)
  Pear
Dairy
  Milk (soy and regular)
  Yogurt

Meats

  Beef

  Clams

  Sardines

  Scallops

  Lobster

  Salmon

  White fish

Other

  Sports beverages and supplements

  Imitation salt (low-sodium products)

  Molasses

  Chocolate

Data from Bakris GL, Olendzki B. Patient information: low potassium diet (beyond the basics). Available at: www.uptodate.com/contents/low-potassium-diet-beyond-the-basics. Accessed September 26, 2012.

imbalance should include electrocardiography (ECG), basic metabolic panel (with electrolyte and creatinine levels), complete blood count, and urinalysis. If symptoms are severe, blood gas analysis to determine pH and urine electrolyte levels to differentiate the causes are also suggested (**Box 4**).[4] Magnesium levels need to be checked in cases of hypokalemia. The ECG may show specific abnormalities that can help make the diagnosis and suggest risk of cardiac deterioration, but it is not sensitive and absence of ECG changes does not rule out a significant potassium abnormality.

HYPERKALEMIA
Etiology

Hyperkalemia, extracellular K+ levels greater than 5.0 mEq/L or 5.5 mEq/L depending on the laboratory assay,[1–4] can be caused by failure to excrete enough K+, leading to total body excess, transcellular shifts, or measurement error (**Box 5**). Many common medications inhibit K+ excretion or shift it out of cells and into the extracellular space (see **Box 1**). Patients with underlying disorders predisposing them to hyperkalemia

| Box 4 |
Diagnostic workup
ECG
BMP/Chem7
Magnesium[a]
CBC
UA
Blood gas, Urine electrolytes[b]
[a] In hypokalemia
[b] In severe cases

Box 5
Disorders causing hyperkalemia

Failure of excretion

Decreased glomerular filtration rate

   Renal insufficiency

   Renal failure

Heart failure

Obstructive uropathy

Low aldosterone level

   Adrenal insufficiency (Addison disease)

   Low renin level

Type 4 renal tubular acidosis

Medications that inhibit Na-K ATPase in the distal nephron (see **Box 1**)

Transcellular shifts (Na-K ATPase pump)

Hemolysis

   Rhabdomyolysis

   Tumor lysis syndrome

   Hematoma reabsorption

Medications that inhibit Na-K ATPase pump (see **Box 1**)

Insulin deficiency

   Diabetes mellitus

   Prolonged fasting

Hypertonicity

   Hyperglycemia

   Hypernatremia

Acidosis

Hyperkalemic periodic paralysis (mutation of skeletal muscle Na-K pump)

   Fasting

   Intense exercise

   High-K+ meal

Measurement error (pseudohyperkalemia)

Hemolysis during blood draw

   Prolonged tourniquet use

   Small needle caliber

   Excessive fist clenching

   Excessive plunger force to pull blood into a syringe

Hemolysis before laboratory analysis

   Delay between blood draw and analysis

   Aggressive sample shaking

Hyperviscosity

    Extreme leukocytosis

    Extreme thrombocytosis

    Polycythemia vera

Patient hyperventilation during blood draw (respiratory alkalosis causing transient K+ shift)

Large, rapid potassium load

Massive blood transfusion protocol

High-dose potassium penicillin

Poisoning/ingestion

Data from Refs.[1–4]

---

are much more sensitive to initiation of these medications. Ingesting too much K+ rarely causes hyperkalemia except in patients with preexisting K+ homeostasis abnormalities.

Renal disorders are the most common cause of hyperkalemia, followed by cell lysis, which releases large intracellular K+ stores.[2] High K+ levels stimulate aldosterone secretion, which acts on the renal tubules to increase K+ excretion into the urine, but in primary mineralocorticoid deficiency this homeostasis mechanism fails to activate, whereas in renal failure the kidney is unable to respond to aldosterone.[4] High plasma K+ levels also stimulate insulin secretion from the pancreas, which drives K+ intracellularly,[4] although patients with diabetes mellitus may not have sufficient insulin production capacity to counteract high K+ levels.

Clinical Presentation

Patients with hyperkalemia may be completely asymptomatic or may have cardiac, muscular, or GI complaints. Hyperkalemia depolarizes the cardiac membrane, slowing conduction.[5] Patients may experience palpitations or generalized fatigue and malaise. Muscle cramps,[4] paresthesias, and weakness are common.[2] Weakness can progress to a flaccid paralysis.[2] Nausea, vomiting, and diarrhea can also occur.[4]

Physical examination findings include bradycardia and/or irregular cardiac rhythm with frequent premature ventricular contractions.[2] Neurologic examination may reveal decreased deep tendon reflexes and decreased strength with intact sensation.[2,3,5]

Diagnostic Testing

An ECG is the first step in the workup of a patient with hyperkalemia. Hyperkalemia increases myocyte sensitivity in different areas of the heart progressively as K+ levels rise:[2]

1. Atria
2. Ventricles
3. Bundle of His
4. Sinoatrial node
5. Interatrial tracts

Therefore, the ECG progresses through several phases that are loosely correlated with absolute serum K+ levels and with the rate of increase in serum K+ levels.[2,6] The first and most common sign is tall, "peaked" T waves with a narrow base (**Fig. 1**). These occur most frequently in the precordial leads V2-V4. A sensitive sign

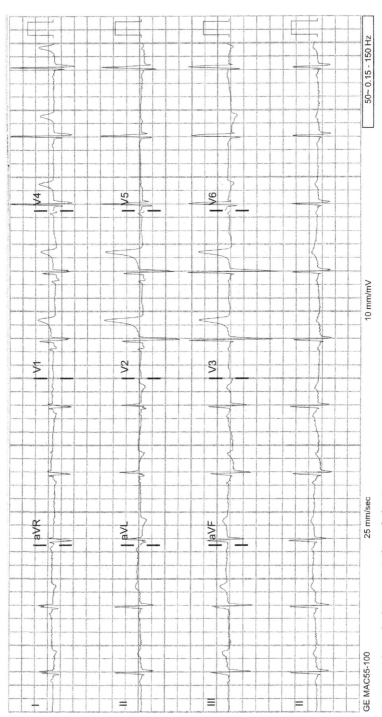

Fig. 1. ECG with peaked T waves in hyperkalemia.

is if the amplitude of the T exceeds the amplitude of the R.[7] As the atria are affected the PR interval lengthens, and as the ventricles are affected the QRS widens. When hyperkalemia affects the conduction system, the P waves decrease in amplitude until the ECG develops a "nodal" rhythm with absent P waves (**Fig. 2**). The QRS continues to widen until the S and T waves merge into a "sine wave" pattern (**Fig. 3**). The sine wave pattern usually shortly precedes ventricular fibrillation (VFib) and cardiac arrest.

However, research has shown poor sensitivity for these changes, with only 32% of ECGs in known hyperkalemia having peaked T waves and only 52% exhibiting any ECG change. If strict measurement criteria were used, just 18% of ECGs displayed a change despite hyperkalemia.[8] When limited to hyperkalemia greater than 6.0 mEq/L rather than 5 mEq/L, 46% to 64% had changes, suggesting a nonsignificant trend with degree of hyperkalemia.[1]

Treatment

Most experts agree that ECG changes and/or symptoms should be treated expeditiously, but because these can occur at varying absolute K+ levels and some patients can have K+ levels greater than 7.5 mEq/L without ECG changes or symptoms, it is still undecided whether an absolute K+ threshold exists whereby risk of arrhythmia necessitates treatment in the asymptomatic patient.

In the setting of ECG changes, cardiac membrane stabilization is the first priority to prevent arrhythmias and cardiac arrest. Calcium is the mainstay of cardiac stabilization to restore resting membrane potential, either as gluconate or chloride compounds.[4] Calcium chloride has approximately 3 times more elemental calcium than calcium gluconate (6.8 mEq/10 mL vs 2.2 mEq/10 mL),[2] and it has greater bioavailability because calcium gluconate has to be metabolized into an active form.[4] However, calcium gluconate has less risk of tissue necrosis, which allows faster transfusion.[4] There is no randomized evidence supporting one or the other,[9] and decision on which agent to use remains provider and facility dependent.

Next, potassium levels can be lowered either temporarily by medications that cause an intracellular shift of K+ or by therapies that eliminate K+ from the body to decrease total body stores (**Table 1**). Insulin and β-agonists stimulate the Na-K ATPase pump to pull more K+ into cells[4] and are the mainstays of evidence-based therapy for transcellular shift. The 2 medications are synergistic, so using both in combination results in a larger reduction of extracellular K+ than using either alone.[5,9,10] There is no difference in inhaled or IV forms of β-agonists, although IV forms are not currently available in the United States, nor is there a difference between albuterol and levalbuterol.[9] Both metered-dose inhalers and nebulizers are also equally effective, although it may be easier to deliver consistent dosing with the nebulized form.[4]

Sodium bicarbonate has been used to promote intracellular shift of K+, but no good evidence supports its routine use in hyperkalemia. It is significantly less effective than insulin or β-agonists, with a maximum effect of 0.4 mEq/L,[10] and it has only been helpful in patients with a nongap metabolic acidosis.[2,4] Furthermore, several studies have found no effect compared with placebo[9] and no additional effect compared with insulin or β-agonists alone.[1]

Reduction of total body K+ can be accomplished by enhancing the body's renal or GI elimination. Loop diuretics are useful in patients who still produce urine.[3,5] Sodium polystyrene, or Kayexalate, has been commonly used in practice since studies suggesting its efficacy were published in 1961, with the presumed mechanism of increased Na-K exchange across the bowel wall.[2,11] Onset of action is delayed by 2 to 6 hours, decreasing its utility in the management of acute hyperkalemia in the

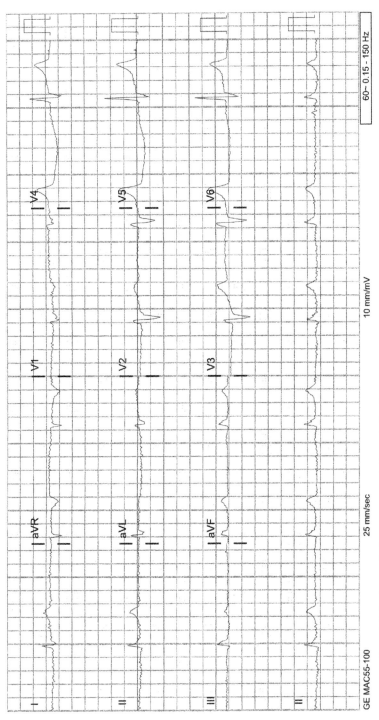

Fig. 2. ECG with nodal rhythm and absent T waves in hyperkalemia.

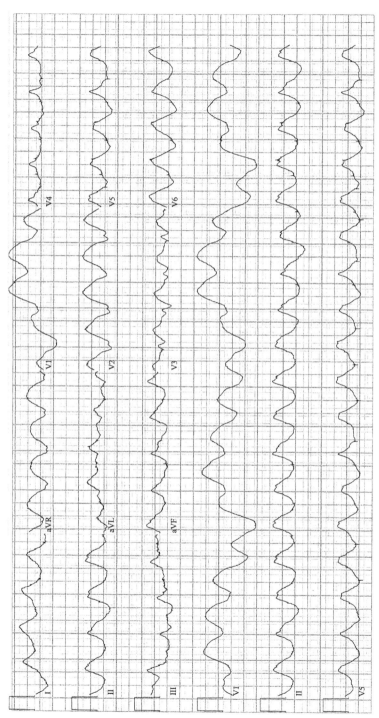

Fig. 3. ECG with sine wave pattern in hyperkalemia. (*Courtesy of Elizabeth Arrington, MD, Houston, TX.*)

Table 1
Treatment of hyperkalemia

Medication	Dose	Time to Onset (min)	Magnitude of K+ Reduction (mEq/L)	Duration of Effect (h)	Caveats
Calcium	1–2 g (10 mL)	Immediate	No effect on K+	0.5–1[2,4,5]	• May potentiate arrhythmias in digoxin toxicity • Extravasation can cause tissue damage and phlebitis
β-Agonists (albuterol)	20 mg	Within 30[2–5,9,10]	0.5–1.5[1,2,4,5,9]	2–6[1–5]	• Patients taking nonselective β-blockers may be resistant to this effect[2,5] • Tremors, anxiety
Insulin	10 units	15–30[2,4,5,9,10]	0.6–1.2[2–5,10]	2–6[2,5,10]	• Give with Dextrose 50%; monitor glucose closely for hypoglycemia • Patients with ESRD are more susceptible to hypoglycemia because of decreased excretion of insulin
Loop diuretics (Lasix, Bumex)		15[5]		1–3[3,5]	Not effective in patients with ESRD who no longer make urine
Dialysis	N/A	Immediate	1–2[2,5]	2–6[2,5]	

Abbreviations: ESRD, end-stage renal disease; N/A, not applicable.

emergency department.[4,5] It also causes significant constipation and so is usually administered in combination with a stool softener. However, subsequent research has not replicated the 1961 results, instead showing that Kayexalate makes no difference in serum K+ levels[9,10,12] and that stool softeners alone are equally effective.[5] A dangerous side effect of Kayexalate is intestinal necrosis, and the US Food and Drug Administration has issued a warning against administering it in combination with the stool softener sorbitol, which is thought to increase the incidence of intestinal necrosis.[4,5] In light of its delayed onset of action, uncertain efficacy, and high-risk side-effect profile, Kayexalate is not recommended in the treatment of hyperkalemia.[9]

Finally, dialysis is the definitive treatment for removing potassium from the body. Most of the K+ elimination occurs during the first 2 hours of dialysis.[1] However, dialysis only filters the extracellular compartment, minimizing its effect on total body K+ stores, and in cases of elevated total body K+ stores, the body quickly reequilibrates to a hyperkalemic state. Within 6 hours, extracellular K+ returns to 70% of its predialysis levels.[2] In situations of resuscitation from cardiac arrest, case reports have demonstrated successful return of spontaneous circulation and good neurologic outcomes despite prolonged arrest when dialysis is initiated during cardiopulmonary resuscitation (CPR) to correct hyperkalemia.[2]

Key Points

- Treatment of hyperkalemia includes
  - Cardiac membrane stabilization
  - Transcellular shifts
  - Total body potassium elimination
- Changes in practice
  - Sodium bicarbonate is not an indicated therapy; can consider its use in acidotic patients with hyperkalemia
  - Do not give Kayexalate
  - In cases of cardiac arrest due to hyperkalemia, perform prolonged CPR until K+ level is corrected; the patient should not be pronounced dead until their K+ level is normalized.
- Next steps
  - Repeat serial K+ measurements to monitor for rebound hyperkalemia
  - Prevent recurrence
    - Avoid potentiating medications (see **Box 1**)
    - Determine and treat underlying cause (see **Box 5**)
      - Failure to excrete enough K+ to maintain a balance
      - Transcellular shifts
      - Suspect measurement error in otherwise normal patients and repeat laboratory analysis before initiating treatment

HYPOKALEMIA
Etiology

Hypokalemia, extracellular K+ concentration less than 3.5 mEq/L, can be caused by increased K+ loss from the body, transcellular shifts, decreased K+ intake, and sometimes by magnesium depletion (**Box 6**).[2] K+ is excreted into the stool via Na-K ATPase exchange pumps in the GI tract, and any disease state (eg, diarrhea) or medication (eg, laxatives) that increases stool output increases GI K+ losses.

The kidneys are primarily responsible for maintaining K+ balance via the Na-K ATPase exchange pumps in the distal nephron. Anything that activates these pumps or increases the flow of Na or urine through the distal nephron increases renal K+ losses.[4] Low magnesium (Mg) levels stimulate Na-K ATPase activity. Some drugs such as amphotericin, aminoglycosides, and cisplatin lower Mg, which secondarily lowers K+ (see **Box 2**).[13] If Mg remains low, any K+ intake is quickly excreted by the kidneys despite a total body K+ deficit.

Aldosterone via the renin-angiotensin-aldosterone system is a primary activator of the Na-K ATPase pump in the distal nephron.[3] High aldosterone levels occur during dehydration in reaction to hypovolemia and in cases of high cortisol and adrenocorticotropic hormone or aldosterone-secreting tumors (Cushing syndrome; Conn syndrome).[4]

High-urine-flow states increase renal excretion of K+. Diuresis, whether drug induced or driven by the body's elimination of other substances such as excess glucose or water, therefore increases K+ losses. A high-sodium diet and drugs

Box 6
Disorders causing hypokalemia

Excessive loss

GI tract

  Diarrhea

  Laxative abuse

  Fistula

  Ileostomy

Renal

  Increased Na+ delivery to the distal nephron

    High-sodium diet

    Drugs (eg, penicillins)

  Increased urinary flow

    Hyperglycemia

    Mannitol

    High-volume IV normal saline

  Activation of Na-K ATPase

    Hypomagnesemia

    Renal tubular acidosis types 1 and 2

    Liddle syndrome

    High aldosterone levels

      Primary

        Conn syndrome

        Cushing syndrome

      Secondary

        Hypovolemia (eg, vomiting)

        Bartter syndrome

        Gitelman syndrome

        Excessive licorice intake (with glycyrrhizic acid, not sold in the United States)

Cutaneous

  Excessive sweating

  Extensive burns

Transcellular shift

Alkalosis

Hypernatremic hypokalemic paralysis

Thyrotoxic periodic paralysis

Other

Low dietary intake (when chronic)

Data from Refs.[2–4,13]

such as penicillins also increase renal K+ excretion by delivering more Na to the distal nephron where the Na gradient drives the Na-K ATPase exchange.[3] Cutaneous losses are usually negligible except in cases of excessive sweating as happens during extreme exercise or heat exhaustion or when large-surface-area burns break down the skin barrier.[4]

Several common medications can shift K+ intracellularly, causing an apparent hypo-kalemia despite normal total body K+ stores (see **Box 2**). Alkalosis, respiratory or meta-bolic, also drives K+ intracellularly. In addition to stimulating renal losses, a high aldosterone level leads to a metabolic alkalosis, which can perpetuate hypokalemia by simultaneously shifting K+ intracellularly, further reducing extracellular levels.[4] Renal tubular acidosis types 1 and 2 are the only cases in which hypokalemia occurs in the setting of an acidosis rather than an alkalosis.[4] The body can compensate for a low-K+ diet by severely limiting renal excretion of potassium, but if a low-potassium diet continues chronically, it can eventually lead to clinically significant hypokalemia.

Clinical Presentation

Like in hyperkalemia, most hypokalemic patients are asymptomatic, particularly at K+ levels greater than 3.0 mEq/L. Patients with heart failure are more likely to be symp-tomatic, and it is recommended that their levels should remain 4.0 mEq/L or more to prevent arrhythmias.[2] Muscular symptoms include generalized malaise, fatigue, lethargy, and weakness.[2] Fasciculations and tetany also occur.[4] Severe cases may present as an ascending paralysis that can include respiratory muscles.[2] GI com-plaints include ileus due to impaired smooth muscle activity, which can cause nausea, vomiting, and constipation.[2,4] Inability to concentrate the urine can also create a neph-rogenic diabetes insipidus presentation with polyuria and polydipsia.[3]

On examination, weakness may be evident, with decreased strength typically more pronounced in proximal muscles and lower extremities.[3] Mental status and orientation remain intact. Abdominal examination may reveal distention in cases of ileus.[4]

Diagnostic Testing

An ECG is an initial diagnostic test with immediate results that can be used to guide further treatment. Hypokalemia predisposes to several arrhythmias, including first-degree heart block with a prolonged PR interval, second-degree heart block, and atrial fibrillation.[4] These rhythms can deteriorate into ventricular tachycardia (VTach), VFib, torsades de pointes, and cardiac arrest. Patients taking digitalis are more susceptible to arrhythmias in the setting of hypokalemia.[2,4]

In addition to arrhythmias such as first-degree atrioventricular block with an increased P wave amplitude,[3] there are several more specific signs of hypokalemia that can appear on ECG. The first sign of hypokalemia is usually decreased T wave amplitude, followed by ST depressions or T wave inversions.[3] U waves are the clas-sically taught abnormality and are best seen in V2 and V3 (**Fig. 4**). As they enlarge, they can merge with and mimic T waves (which are simultaneously decreasing in amplitude), giving the false impression of a prolonged QT. Sometimes U waves grow so tall that they appear similar to the peaked T waves of hyperkalemia, but U waves usually have a broader base.

Additional testing should include a blood gas and pH analysis. In hypokalemia, the kidney cannot excrete bicarbonate and instead excretes protons and chloride, causing a metabolic alkalosis (or perpetuating an existing alkalosis, which may have caused the hypokalemia via transcellular shift initially).[3] All patients with hypokalemia should have a magnesium level checked because of the strong correlation between hypomagnesemia and hypokalemia.[3] It is helpful to determine total body K+ stores

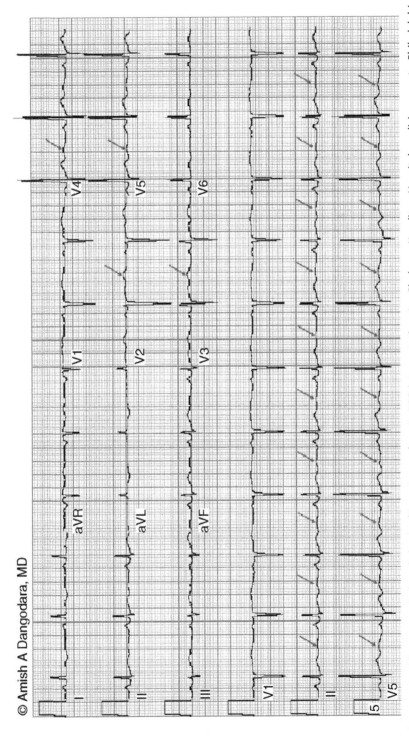

Fig. 4. ECG with U waves in hypokalemia. (*From* Dangodara A. ECG interpretation. In: Glasheen JJ, editor. Hospital medicine secrets. Philadelphia: Mosby/Elsevier, 2007; with permission.)

to differentiate between transcellular shifts and total K+ loss, but measuring total body K+ requires a 24-hour urine collection.[13]

Treatment

Treatment of hypokalemia includes both potassium and magnesium repletion. Hypomagnesemia is frequently found in patients with hypokalemia because hypomagnesemia causes hypokalemia via renal wasting, and other common causes of hypokalemia such as diarrhea and diuretic use also cause a simultaneous hypomagnesemia.[3,4,7] However, in severe cases of symptomatic hypokalemia, concurrent Mg repletion is recommended even with normal Mg levels because Mg activates the Na-K ATPase pump to promote cellular uptake of dosed K+.[4]

Although asymptomatic hypokalemia greater than 3.0 mEq/L can be safely discharged with a high-K+ diet (see **Box 3**) and close follow-up after addressing the cause, any symptomatic hypokalemia should be repleted in the emergency department. Patients with recent myocardial infarction or with heart failure should be repleted to levels of at least 4.0 mEq/L.[3,4] As a guide, a 0.3-mEq/L drop in extracellular K+ levels represents a 100-mEq/L total body deficit.[4] When K+ is rechecked after repletion but before transcellular equilibration, 10 mEq of K+ is expected to increase extracellular levels by 0.1 mEq/L.

The maximum recommended dose of potassium chloride in low-risk hypokalemia with minimal symptoms and without arrhythmia is 20 to 80 mEq/d.[4] It is important to consider the likely cause of the hypokalemia, as aggressive repletion in cases of transcellular shift can lead to overcorrection of total body K+ and rebound hyperkalemia once the cause of the shift is resolved. K+ levels should be rechecked periodically during and after repletion to prevent overcorrection.[4]

Patients with minimal symptoms who are tolerating intake by mouth can receive pill or liquid potassium chloride, which has the advantage of a single large dose. If patients present with nausea or vomiting and are unable to tolerate intake by mouth, IV correction is recommended at a rate of 10 to 20 mEq/h. Patients should be monitored on a telemetry monitor during IV infusion for the development of dysrhythmias. In patients with significant dysrhythmias (VTach) as a presenting symptom, 20 mEq can be pushed over 3 to 10 minutes to prevent deterioration into cardiac arrest.[2,4] IV potassium chloride causes burning and discomfort at the IV site and can cause phlebitis.[4] A central line is recommended for rates greater than 10 mEq/h.

Key Points

Hypokalemia is a common disorder, but is well tolerated by the body relative to hyperkalemia. However, severe cases of hypokalemia can cause dysrhythmias and cardiac arrest.

- Treatment of symptomatic hypokalemia consists of repletion with potassium chloride
  - Intake by mouth in pill or liquid forms
  - IV
    - Max rate 10 to 20 mEq/h
    - Push rapidly over 5 to 10 minutes in cases of cardiac arrest or impending arrest (VFib, VTach)
- Next steps
  - Repeat serial K+ measurements to monitor for recurrence and prevent overcorrection
  - Remember to replete Mg along with K+

- ○ Prevent recurrence
  - ■ Avoid potentiating medications (see **Box 2**)
  - ■ Determine and treat underlying cause (see **Box 6**)
    - • Increased K+ losses from the body
      - ○ GI
      - ○ Renal
      - ○ Cutaneous
    - • Transcellular shifts
    - • Decreased K+ intake

SUMMARY

Changes in potassium elimination, primarily due to the renal and GI systems; shifting potassium between the intracellular and extracellular spaces; and dietary potassium intake are the 3 major causes of potassium derangements. Several common medications can contribute to either hyperkalemia or hypokalemia. False laboratory results regarding elevations in potassium value are also a common cause for hyperkalemia, and the test should be repeated if suspicion for pseudohyperkalemia exists. Symptoms of potassium derangement are vague but can be cardiac, musculoskeletal, or GI. There are no absolute guidelines for when to initiate treatment of potassium derangement, but it is generally recommended when the patient is symptomatic and/or has changes on the ECG attributable to potassium derangement. Treatment of hyperkalemia includes cardiac membrane stabilization with IV calcium, pushing potassium intracellularly using insulin (which should be given in combination with glucose to avoid hypoglycemia) and β-antagonists, and removing potassium from the body entirely with dialysis. Neither sodium bicarbonate nor Kayexalate are recommended as evidence-based therapies. Treatment of symptomatic hypokalemia consists of repletion with potassium chloride either by mouth or IV. Magnesium should be repleted when repleting potassium. Repeat potassium levels should be checked after treatment of potassium derangement to monitor effect and guide further therapy. Medications and diet should be adjusted to prevent recurrence, especially in patients predisposed by renal insufficiency.

REFERENCES

1. Putcha N, Allon M. Management of hyperkalemia in dialysis patients. Semin Dial 2007;20(5):431–9.
2. Alfonzo AV, Isles C, Geddes C, et al. Potassium disorders—clinical spectrum and emergency management. Resuscitation 2006;70:10–25.
3. Schaefer TJ, Wolford RW. Disorders of potassium. Emerg Med Clin North Am 2005;23:723–47.
4. Pepin J, Shields S. Advances in diagnosis and management of hypokalemic and hyperkalemic emergencies. Emerg Med Pract 2012;14(2):1–17.
5. Weisberg LS. Management of severe hyperkalemia. Crit Care Med 2008;36(12): 3246–51.
6. Webster A, Brady W, Morris F. Recognising signs of danger: ECG changes resulting from an abnormal serum potassium concentration. Emerg Med J 2002;19: 74–7.
7. Slovis C, Jenkns R. ABC of clinical electrocardiography: conditions not primarily affecting the heart. BMJ 2002;324:1320–3.
8. Montague B, Ouellette JR, Buller GK. Retrospective review of the frequency of ECG changes in hyperkalemia. Clin J Am Soc Nephrol 2008;3:324–30.

9. Mahoney BA, Smith WA, Lo D, et al. Emergency interventions for hyperkalemia [review]. Cochrane Database Syst Rev 2005;(2):CD003235.

10. Elliott MJ, Ronksley PE, Clase CM, et al. Management of patients with acute hyperkalemia. CMAJ 2010;182(15):1631–5.

11. Scherr L, Ogden DA, Mead AW, et al. Management of hyperkalemia with a cation-exchange resin. N Engl J Med 1961;264:115–9.

12. Gruy-Kapral C, Emmett M, Santa Ana CA, et al. Effect of single dose resin-cathartic therapy on serum potassium concentration in patients with end-stage renal disease. J Am Soc Nephrol 1998;9:1924–30.

13. Cohn JN, Kowey PR, Whelton PJ, et al. New guidelines for potassium replacement in clinical practice. Arch Intern Med 2000;160:2429–36.

Calcium, Magnesium, and Phosphate Abnormalities in the Emergency Department

Wan-Tsu W. Chang, MD[a], Bethany Radin, DO[b],
Michael T. McCurdy, MD[a,b],*

KEYWORDS

- Hypercalcemia • Hypocalcemia • Hypermagnesemia • Hypomagnesemia
- Hyperphosphatemia • Hypophosphatemia

KEY POINTS

- Disorders of calcium, magnesium, and phosphate are relatively common clinical problems, especially among critically ill patients.
- Because of their crucial role in cellular physiology, particularly for neuromuscular function and cardiac conduction, severe derangements of these minerals can be fatal.
- Understanding the complex physiologic role of these minerals in the human body is essential to promptly identify the problem, initiate appropriate therapy, and provide an adequate disposition.

INTRODUCTION

Disorders of calcium, magnesium, and phosphate are relatively common clinical problems encountered by emergency medicine providers. Because of their crucial role in cellular physiology, particularly for neuromuscular function and cardiac conduction, severe derangements of these minerals can be fatal. Understanding the complex physiologic role of these minerals in the human body is essential to promptly identify the problem, initiate appropriate therapy, and provide an adequate disposition. This article focuses on the physiology and pathophysiology of these mineral disorders.

The authors have nothing to disclose.
[a] Department of Emergency Medicine, University of Maryland School of Medicine, 110 South Paca Street, 6th Floor, Suite 200, Baltimore, MD 21201, USA; [b] Division of Pulmonary and Critical Care Medicine, Department of Medicine, University of Maryland School of Medicine, 110 South Paca Street, 2nd Floor, Baltimore, MD 21201, USA
* Corresponding author. Division of Pulmonary and Critical Care Medicine, Department of Medicine, University of Maryland School of Medicine, 110 South Paca Street, 2nd Floor, Baltimore, MD 21201.
E-mail address: drmccurdy@gmail.com

Emerg Med Clin N Am 32 (2014) 349–366
http://dx.doi.org/10.1016/j.emc.2013.12.006
0733-8627/14/$ – see front matter © 2014 Elsevier Inc. All rights reserved.

emed.theclinics.com

EPIDEMIOLOGY

Abnormalities of calcium, magnesium, and phosphate are common in hospitalized patients and are associated with increased morbidity and mortality rates.[1,2] Both acute, severe electrolyte disorders in hospitalized patients as well as chronic, mild electrolyte abnormalities in the general population are associated with adverse outcomes.[3] Risk factors for electrolyte disturbances include older age, diabetes mellitus, renal disease, diuretic use, and malnutrition.[3]

Calcium abnormalities are associated with many pathologic states, most notably malignancy. Twenty percent to 30% of patients with cancer experience hypercalcemia during the course of their disease, and malignancy accounts for more than 30% of emergency department visits for hypercalcemia.[4,5] Conversely, hypocalcemia is found in 88% of patients in intensive care units.[6]

Although approximately 75% of Americans have magnesium-deficient diets, less than 2% of the general population is actually hypomagnesemic.[7] Certain groups, such as people with coronary disease, have a relatively high incidence of this deficiency.[8] Hypomagnesemia, also common in hospitalized and critically ill patients,[9,10] is associated with longer hospitalizations and a higher mortality rate than in those with normal magnesium levels.[11]

Hypophosphatemia is found in up to 5% of hospitalized patients and is particularly prevalent among those with diabetic ketoacidosis, chronic obstructive pulmonary disease, malignancy, malnutrition, and sepsis.[12] Severe deficiency contributes to the mortality rate among these groups.[12,13] Hyperphosphatemia is a risk factor for death among patients with chronic kidney disease as well as among kidney transplant recipients.[1,14,15] The serum phosphate level is associated with cardiovascular risk even in individuals without kidney disease.[16]

NORMAL PHYSIOLOGY

Bone contains almost all of the calcium and phosphate and more than half of the magnesium in the human body. Small amounts of these ions are present in extracellular fluid and intracellular space, and they play important roles in normal physiology. Extracellular calcium is the principal substrate for bone mineralization and a cofactor for many extracellular enzymes. Calcium ions function as signaling molecules for many intracellular processes, including the contraction of cardiac, skeletal, and smooth muscles; neurotransmitter release; and various endocrine and exocrine secretions. Intracellular magnesium is an essential cofactor of enzymatic reactions and stabilizer of DNA, RNA, and ribosomes. Extracellular magnesium is crucial for normal neuromuscular excitability and nerve conduction. Organic phosphate is an integral constituent of nucleic acids; phospholipids; structural, signaling, and enzymatic phosphoproteins; and nucleotide cofactors for enzymes and proteins. Cytosolic phosphate directly regulates intracellular reactions such as those involved in glucose transport, lactate production, and ATP synthesis.

Calcium is the most abundant mineral in the human body. Ninety-nine percent of total body calcium resides in bone, of which 99% is in the mineral phase and 1% is rapidly exchangeable. Approximately half of total serum calcium is bound to proteins, mainly albumin and globulins. The normal ionized calcium concentration in serum is 1.1 to 1.4 mmol/L (4.5–5.6 mg/dL). Intracellularly, 99% of calcium exists in complexes within the mitochondrial compartment, with the cytosolic free calcium concentration being approximately 100 nmol/L. This large extracellular-to-intracellular gradient of calcium is maintained by Ca^{2+}- and H^{+}-ATPases as well as Na^{+}/Ca^{2+} exchangers.[17] Clinically, measuring the total serum calcium concentration usually suffices because it generally parallels the ionized concentration, except in patients with alterations in serum protein concentration or binding properties.

Magnesium, which is found in bone, muscle, and soft tissues, is the fourth most common mineral and second most abundant intracellular cation in the human body. Approximately half of the magnesium in bone is not sequestered in the mineral phase but is freely exchangeable. The normal concentration of magnesium in serum is 0.7 to 1.0 mmol/L (1.7–2.0 mg/dL). Approximately one-third of serum magnesium is protein bound, 15% is loosely complexed with phosphate or other anions, and 55% is present as the free ion. Intracellularly, more than 95% of magnesium is bound to other molecules, most notably ATP. The cytosolic free magnesium concentration is approximately 0.5 mmol/L, maintained by a sodium-magnesium antiporter.[17]

Eighty-five percent of phosphate in the body is in the mineral phase of bone. In serum, inorganic phosphorus is present at a concentration of 0.81 to 1.45 mmol/L (2.5–4.5 mg/dL) and exists almost entirely in the ionized phosphate form as either $H_2PO_4^-$ or HPO_4^{2-}. Only 12% of serum phosphate is protein bound. Intracellular free phosphate concentrations are comparable with extracellular concentrations, although the negative electrical potential inside cells creates a significant energy requirement for translocation of phosphate into cells, which is accomplished through sodium-phosphate cotransport driven by the transmembrane sodium gradient.[17]

Abnormalities of calcium, magnesium, and phosphate are collectively called disorders of mineral metabolism. Two major hormones, parathyroid hormone (PTH) and vitamin D, regulate the serum levels, intracellular levels, and optimal bone mineral content of these electrolytes. Disease processes involving the intestine, kidney, bone, and parathyroid gland affect this homeostasis.

MAINTAINING HOMEOSTASIS

Calcium, magnesium, and phosphate homeostasis is tightly controlled to maintain normal cellular physiology. In serum, protein-bound and free fractions of these minerals exist in equilibrium with the biologically active ionized form. PTH, calcitonin, and vitamin D hormonally regulate absorption, excretion, and resorption of these minerals in the intestine, kidneys, and bone.

PTH controls the concentration of ionized calcium in the blood and extracellular fluid. Low calcium levels trigger PTH release, which promotes bone mineral dissolution and increases renal reabsorption of calcium. PTH also increases renal hydroxylation of inactive vitamin D to calcitriol (1,25[OH]₂), the hormonally active form of vitamin D, which then enhances gastrointestinal absorption of dietary calcium. Increased serum calcium and calcitriol levels inhibit PTH secretion from the parathyroid glands. Parathyroid cells respond to both the absolute concentration and the rate of change of the serum calcium concentration. This negative feedback loop responds more dramatically both to hypocalcemia than hypercalcemia and to acute drops in serum calcium.[17] Because of their responsiveness to PTH and ability to decrease calcitriol synthesis, normal-functioning kidneys prevent calcium overload.

Calcitonin is a thyroid hormone released in response to high calcium concentrations. As opposed to PTH, calcitonin inhibits bone resorption of calcium and renal reabsorption of calcium and phosphate.

The homeostasis of phosphate is closely linked to that of calcium, with both minerals being deposited in and resorbed from bone together. In response to low serum phosphate concentration, calcitriol increases gastrointestinal phosphate absorption and the kidneys decrease phosphate excretion. In contrast, when serum levels are elevated and exceed the renal threshold phosphate concentration (ie, creating a serum concentration that surpasses the absorptive capabilities of the kidney), PTH and phosphatonins promote rapid renal phosphate excretion. In response to alkalosis, phosphate shifts intracellularly, acting as a buffer for maintenance of the body's pH.[12]

Normal homeostasis for magnesium, like calcium, is regulated by the intestine, bone, and kidneys. Dietary magnesium is mainly absorbed in the small intestine via a passive mechanism, with the quantity absorbed largely dependent on its electrochemical gradient (ie, the lower the serum magnesium level is, the more dietary magnesium is absorbed).[18] The kidney controls the serum magnesium level by determining the degree of its reabsorption in the thick ascending limb of the loop of Henle and, to a lesser extent, in the distal tubules. Similar to its intestinal absorption, the degree of magnesium reabsorption is passively regulated by its serum concentration and only minimally by hormonal triggers.[18,19]

Most of the total body stores of calcium and phosphate are located in bone in the form of hydroxyapatite, $Ca_{10}(PO_4)_5(OH)_2$. At any given time, approximately 15% of the bone surface undergoes remodeling, controlled by many cytokines and hormones, including PTH and calcitriol.[20] Thus, alterations in bone remodeling greatly affect calcium and phosphate homeostasis.

PATHOPHYSIOLOGY OF CALCIUM, MAGNESIUM, AND PHOSPHATE DISORDERS

Disorders of calcium, magnesium, and phosphate homeostasis occur with disruptions in the hormonal regulation by PTH, calcitonin, and vitamin D as well as diseases of the intestine, kidney, and bone. Catecholamines, magnesium, and other stimuli can affect PTH secretion, though the major regulator of PTH secretion is the ionized calcium concentration.[21] Glucocorticoids stimulate PTH synthesis and release, which might be significant during prolonged stress or with pharmacologic glucocorticoid administration. PTH release stimulated by glucocorticoids cannot be reversed by either calcitriol or elevated serum calcium, which could explain, at least in part, the role of glucocorticoids in the cause of osteoporosis.[22] A variety of malignancies produce PTH-related peptide (PTHrP), which mimics the biologic effects of PTH in an unregulated fashion to cause severe bone degradation and hypercalcemia.

In excess, magnesium competitively inhibits presynaptic acetylcholine release and calcium influx into the presynaptic nerve channels via voltage-dependent calcium channels. This process inhibits neuromuscular transmission, thereby causing hypoexcitability of the nervous system.

Phosphatonins are a group of proteins identified in genetic and cancer-related disorders of renal phosphate wasting. They induce non–PTH-mediated urinary excretion of phosphate.[19] In hyperphosphatemia, phosphate complexes with calcium, which reduces the amount of available ionized calcium and, thus, triggers PTH release, inducing secondary hyperparathyroidism and increased bone turnover.

CALCIUM ABNORMALITIES
Hypercalcemia

Definition and classification
Normal serum calcium concentration is 8.5 to 10.5 mg/dL. Hypercalcemia is defined as a total serum calcium (Ca^{2+}_{total}) concentration greater than 10.5 mg/dL or an ionized calcium ($Ca^{2+}_{ionized}$) greater than 1.4 mmol/L (5.6 mg/dL). Hypercalcemia can be classified by severity. Mild hypercalcemia is Ca^{2+}_{total} 10.5 to 11.9 mg/dL or $Ca^{2+}_{ionized}$ 1.4 to 2.0 mmol/L (5.6–8.0 mg/dL). Moderate hypercalcemia is Ca^{2+}_{total}

12.0 to 13.9 mg/dL or $Ca^{2+}_{ionized}$ 2.0 to 2.5 mmol/L (8–10 mg/dL). Severe hypercalcemia is Ca^{2+}_{total} 14 mg/dL or more or $Ca^{2+}_{ionized}$ more than 2.5 mmol/L (>10 mg/dL).

Cause

Malignancy and hyperparathyroidism account for more than 80% of cases of hypercalcemia.[4,23] In malignancy, hypercalcemia can result from (1) direct osteolysis by metastatic disease[20] (eg, breast cancer, multiple myeloma); (2) production of circulating factors, such as PTHrP, which stimulate osteoclastic resorption of bone; or (3) increased production of calcitriol, which stimulates gastrointestinal absorption of calcium (eg, Hodgkin lymphoma[24]).

Hyperparathyroidism is most commonly caused by a benign adenoma that autonomously secretes PTH. Less commonly, it may be a component of the constellation of symptoms of multiple endocrine neoplasia. Secondary hyperparathyroidism is caused by diffuse hyperplasia of the parathyroid gland in response to hypocalcemia or hyperphosphatemia. Tertiary hyperparathyroidism often results from secondary hyperparathyroidism resulting from years of chronic kidney disease, causing hyperplastic glands to become unresponsive to calcium levels over time.[25]

Other causes of hypercalcemia include thyrotoxicosis, granulomatous disease, medications, total parenteral nutrition, immobilization, and a wide variety of medications (**Boxes 1–4**, **Table 1**).[26]

Signs and symptoms

Vague, nonspecific symptoms usually develop when the Ca^{2+}_{total} concentration is greater than 12 mg/dL. Severity of symptoms is related to not only the absolute calcium level but also the rate of increase in serum calcium.[26]

Hypercalcemia affects nearly every organ system in the body but particularly the central nervous system and kidneys. Neurologic symptoms begin with fatigue, depression, weakness, and confusion and can progress to hallucination, disorientation, hypotonicity, seizures, and coma. Renal effects include nephrolithiasis; calcium deposition can lead to nephrogenic diabetes insipidus as well as acute kidney injury. Patients might also experience gastrointestinal manifestations, such as anorexia, nausea, vomiting, and constipation, as well as nonspecific musculoskeletal tenderness.[26]

Cardiovascular signs and symptoms of hypercalcemia vary. Calcium has a positive inotropic effect until levels reach more than 15 mg/dL, at which time myocardial depression ensues. The QT interval typically shortens, and the PR and QRS intervals are prolonged when the serum calcium concentration is more than 13 mg/dL (**Fig. 1**).[26] Many patients with hypercalcemia develop hypokalemia, further contributing to dysrhythmia risk. Atrioventricular block may develop and progress to complete heart block and even cardiac arrest when Ca^{2+}_{total} is 15 to 20 mg/dL.

Management

The treatment of hypercalcemia depends on the severity of symptoms and the underlying cause. In general, volume repletion with isotonic sodium chloride is an effective short-term treatment. Once patients are euvolemic, loop diuretics can be administered to block sodium and calcium reabsorption, thereby facilitating renal excretion of calcium.[26] Replacing diuresis-induced potassium and magnesium losses should also be considered.

Bisphosphonates (eg, zoledronic acid, pamidronate), which bind to hydroxyapatite to impede osteoclastic bone resorption, are the first-line therapy for malignancy-related hypercalcemia. Calcitonin also decreases bone resorption and

---

Box 1
Causes of hypercalcemia

Solid tumors

- Breast
- Head and neck
- Lung
- Urologic system

Hematologic malignancies

- Acute myeloid leukemia
- Adult T-cell leukemia/lymphoma
- Myeloma
- Hodgkin lymphoma
- Non-Hodgkin lymphoma

Sarcoid disease

Paget disease

Rhabdomyolysis

Mycobacterium infection

Endocrine disorders

- Adrenal insufficiency
- Hyperparathyroidism
- Pheochromocytoma
- Thyrotoxicosis

Medications

- Antacids
- Lithium
- Theophylline
- Thiazide diuretics
- Vitamin A
- Vitamin D

Congenital causes

Childhood cancers

Immobility

Data from National Cancer Institute. Hypercalcemia (PDQ). 2010. p. 1–25. Available at: http://cancer.gov/cancertopics/pdq/supportivecare/hypercalcemia/HealthProfessional. Accessed October 28, 2013.

---

increases renal calcium excretion; however, tachyphylaxis might develop after several days of use. Less used treatments for severe malignancy-related hypercalcemia are gallium nitrate and plicamycin, which inhibit osteoclastic bone resorption; these drugs are not used often because of their toxicity and the availability of better alternatives.[26,27]

| **Box 2** |
| **Causes of hypomagnesemia** |

Medications

- Aminoglycosides
- Amphotericin B
- Cisplatin
- Cyclosporin
- Digoxin
- Diuretics
- Insulin
- Tacrolimus
- Proton pump inhibitors

Inflammation

- Infection/sepsis
- Postoperative period
- Trauma

Gastrointestinal

Diarrhea

- Gastric suctioning
- Intestinal fistula
- Malnutrition
- Pancreatitis

Renal

- Diuretic phase of ATN
- Postobstructive diuresis

Endocrine

- Diabetes
- Hyperparathyroidism
- Hyperthyroidism
- Hyperaldosteronism

Alcoholism

PRBC transfusion

Hungry bone syndrome

Data from Refs.[10,11,31,32]

Practical first-line considerations for hypercalcemia include the elimination of inciting medications (see **Box 1**) as well as a decrease in dietary calcium intake. More aggressive therapies include peritoneal dialysis and hemodialysis, which are both highly effective in lowering serum calcium levels.[26] A discussion of definitive treatment of the underlying cause (dietary changes, surgical resection of the parathyroid gland, or chemotherapy) is beyond the scope of this article.

> **Box 3**
> **Causes of hyperphosphatemia**
>
> - Acromegaly
> - Acute renal failure
> - Antacids
> - Bisphosphonates
> - Bowel ischemia
> - Bowel prep solutions
> - Chronic kidney disease
> - Hemolysis
> - Hypoparathyroidism
> - Malignant hyperthermia
> - Phosphate enemas
> - Rhabdomyolysis
> - Supplements
> - Tumor lysis syndrome
> - Total parenteral nutrition
> - Vitamin D excess

Hypocalcemia

Definition and classification

Hypocalcemia is defined as a Ca^{2+}_{total} concentration of less than 8.5 mg/dL or a $Ca^{2+}_{ionized}$ concentration of less than 1.1 mmol/L (4.5 mg/dL). Because half of serum calcium is bound to albumin, a low Ca^{2+}_{total} level could simply reflect hypoalbuminemia but not the serum level of the metabolically active ionized calcium. Therefore, using a formula (eg, $Ca^{2+}_{corrected} = Ca^{2+}_{measured} + 0.8 \times [4 - albumin_{measured}]$) to correct for hypoalbuminemia helps to distinguish factitious hypocalcemia from true hypocalcemia. However, simply checking an ionized calcium level is the most accurate method of identifying true hypocalcemia.

Cause

True hypocalcemia warrants a more thorough search into the underlying cause. PTH deficiency from hypoparathyroidism can be hereditary or acquired. Acquired hypoparathyroidism may result from neck irradiation, parathyroidectomy, infiltrative disease, or autoimmune disease. PTH receptor or downstream signaling abnormalities cause PTH resistance or pseudohypoparathyroidism.[26,28,29]

Severe hypomagnesemia and vitamin D deficiency also cause hypocalcemia by their effects on PTH. Because phosphate avidly binds calcium, hyperphosphatemia (eg, from rhabdomyolysis) can cause acute hypocalcemia. Acute pancreatitis can be associated with hypocalcemia primarily by precipitation of calcium soaps in the abdomen. Medications associated with hypocalcemia include chemotherapeutic drugs, anticonvulsants, foscarnet, sodium phosphate preparations, proton pump inhibitors, and histamine-2 receptor blockers.[26,28,29]

More transient decreases in $Ca^{2+}_{ionized}$ can be seen with the administration of calcium binders, such as the citrate in transfused blood products and intravenous bicarbonate. Additionally, acute respiratory alkalosis can decrease the hydrogen ion concentration, thereby freeing up binding sites on albumin to increase protein binding of $Ca^{2+}_{ionized}$, causing hypocalcemia.[26,28,29]

Signs and symptoms

Most patients with mild hypocalcemia are asymptomatic. Symptom severity is related to the rapid rate of change. The most specific symptoms of hypocalcemia are perioral numbness and carpopedal spasms of the hands and feet. In some patients, these spasms can progress to tetany. Chvostek and Trousseau signs highlight the neuromuscular hyperexcitability of these patients. The Chvostek sign is the facial muscle spasm elicited by tapping the facial nerve. The Trousseau sign is described as a carpopedal spasm seen with inflation of a sphygmomanometer cuff. In addition, patients can present with irritability, confusion, hallucinations, movement disorders, and seizures.[26,28,29]

Acute hypocalcemia can lead to syncope, congestive heart failure, and angina because of diminished myocardial contractility.[30] QT prolongation leading to ventricular arrhythmias can also be seen (**Fig. 2**).[31] Smooth muscle contraction can lead to laryngeal stridor, dysphagia, and bronchospasm. Dermatologic manifestations of chronic hypocalcemia include coarse hair, brittle nails, dry skin, and poor dentition.

Management

Treatment of hypocalcemia depends on the cause, severity, and presence of symptoms. Intravenous calcium is indicated only in the setting of symptomatic hypocalcemia and should not be given to patients with hyperphosphatemia because of the risk of precipitation. Intravenous calcium comes in the form of calcium gluconate (a 10-mL vial = 94 mg of elemental calcium) or calcium chloride (a 10-mL vial = 273 mg of elemental calcium). Calcium chloride is sclerotic to veins and, thus, should be given via central venous access, unless patients are in an emergency situation.[31] Oral calcium repletion can be given to patients with asymptomatic or mild hypocalcemia. Vitamin D supplementation might be required to increase calcium absorption. Patients taking loop diuretics may need to be changed to thiazide diuretics to decrease urinary calcium excretion. For effective correction of hypocalcemia, concomitant hypomagnesemia should be treated.

MAGNESIUM ABNORMALITIES
Hypermagnesemia

Definition and classification

Normal magnesium concentration is 1.7 to 2.0 mg/dL. Hypermagnesemia is defined as a serum magnesium concentration greater than 2.0 mg/dL.

Cause

Hypermagnesemia is rare because of the kidney's ability to rapidly reduce its tubular reabsorption to almost negligible amounts. Renal failure is the most common cause of hypermagnesemia. Other causes include lithium therapy; hypothyroidism; Addison disease; and excessive tissue breakdown, as associated with sepsis and large burns. Hypermagnesemia is induced as treatment of eclampsia.[10,11,31,32]

Signs and symptoms

Symptoms of hypermagnesemia are not usually apparent until the serum magnesium level is more than 4.8 mg/dL. Concomitant hypocalcemia, hyperkalemia, or uremia exaggerates the symptoms. Neuromuscular symptoms are the most common. One of the earliest symptoms of hypermagnesemia is attenuation of deep tendon reflexes

Box 4
Causes of hypophosphatemia

- Alcoholism
- Aminoglycosides
- Anorexia
- Antacids
- Antineoplastic drugs
- Antiretrovirals
- Anxiety
- Asthma
- β-Agonists
- Bulimia
- Burns
- Catecholamines
- Chronic obstructive pulmonary disease
- Diarrhea
- Diuretics
- Diabetic ketoacidosis
- Dopamine
- Gastric suctioning
- Glucagon
- Glucocorticoids
- Glucose
- Hungry bone syndrome
- Hyperparathyroidism
- Hypothermia
- Inflammation
- Insulin
- Legionella
- Liver disease
- Low phosphorus diet
- Malignancy
- Malnutrition
- Metabolic acidosis
- Methylxanthines
- Phosphate binders
- Postoperative state
- Refeeding syndrome
- Respiratory alkalosis
- Salicylates

- Sepsis
- Total parenteral nutrition
- Trauma
- Vomiting

followed by facial paresthesia. Muscle weakness can progress to flaccid muscle paralysis, depressed respiration, and apnea.[32]

Hypermagnesemia depresses cardiac conduction and sympathetic ganglia. Severe hypermagnesemia can produce hypotension. Extremely high serum magnesium can cause bradycardia, complete heart block, and even cardiac arrest.[32]

Hypermagnesemia can interfere with blood clotting through interference with platelet adhesiveness, thrombin generation time, and clotting time.[33] It is also associated with nausea, vomiting, and cutaneous flushing.

Management
The treatment of cardiac dysfunction related to hypermagnesemia is the administration of calcium. Cardiorespiratory support may be needed until magnesium levels are reduced.

Dialysis is the treatment of choice for severe hypermagnesemia. If renal function is normal and cardiovascular function is adequate, saline diuresis can be used to increase renal excretion until dialysis can be performed. However, diuresis can also increase calcium excretion, and the development of hypocalcemia will make signs and symptoms of hypermagnesemia worse.

Hypomagnesemia

Definition and classification
Hypomagnesemia is defined as a serum magnesium concentration less than 1.7 mg/dL.

Cause
Hypomagnesemia is far more common than hypermagnesemia. It usually results from decreased absorption or increased loss of magnesium from either the kidneys or intestines. Alcoholics and individuals on magnesium-deficient diets can become hypomagnesemic without abnormal gastrointestinal or kidney function. Increased magnesium excretion is associated with inherited renal tubular defects; hyperaldosteronism; hypoparathyroidism; hyperthyroidism; and administration of drugs, including diuretics, antimicrobials, digoxin, chemotherapeutic agents, and immunosuppressants. Magnesium can be redistributed from extracellular to intracellular fluid by insulin therapy for diabetic ketoacidosis and in catecholamine excess states.

Signs and symptoms
Hypomagnesemia is commonly associated with other electrolyte abnormalities, including hypokalemia, hyponatremia, hypocalcemia, and hypophosphatemia. The cardiovascular and central nervous systems are most commonly affected by hypomagnesemia. Neuromuscular manifestations can include muscle weakness, paresthesia, nystagmus, tremors and fasciculations, tetany, seizures, and altered mental status.[10,11,31,32] Chvostek and Trousseau signs can also be elicited. Cardiovascular manifestations include U waves, QT interval prolongation, ventricular arrhythmias, torsade de pointes, and enhanced digitalis toxicity.[32]

Table 1
Hypercalcemic pharmacologic agents

Agent	Mechanism of Action	Time of Action	Side Effects
Normal saline, 2–6 L at 200–500 mL/h	Corrects volume depletion, promotes calciuria	—	Fluid overload
Furosemide, 20–40 mg IV	Promotes calciuria	—	Dehydration, hypokalemia
Pamidronate, 60 mg IV	Prevents bone resorption	48–72 h	Nephrotoxicity, flulike symptoms, hypocalcemia
Zoledronate, 4 mg IV	Prevents bone resorption	—	Hypomagnesemia, hypophosphatemia
Calcitonin, 4 IU/kg IM or SC	Prevents bone resorption, promotes calciuria	2 h	Tachyphylaxis, nausea, flushing
Prednisone, 60 mg PO	Prevents conversion of 25-(OH)D3 to calcitriol	—	Hypokalemia, hyperglycemia, immunosuppression
Hydrocortisone, 200–300 mg IV	Prevents conversion of 25-(OH)D3 to calcitriol	—	Hypokalemia, hyperglycemia, immunosuppression
Plicamycin 25 mcg/kg IV	Inhibits osteoclast RNA synthesis	—	Hepatotoxicity, coagulopathy
Gallium nitrate, 100–200 mg/m^2 IV	Inhibits osteoclast activity	—	Nephrotoxicity
Phosphorus PO	—	—	Nephrotoxicity, hypocalcemia, seizures, diarrhea

Abbreviations: IM, intramuscularly; IV, intravenously; PO, orally; SC, subcutaneously.

Management

The severity of hypomagnesemia and the patient's clinical status determine the treatment. For severe or symptomatic hypomagnesemia, intravenous magnesium sulfate should be administered, with the goal of maintaining the serum magnesium concentration of more than 1.0 mg/dL. The serum magnesium concentration is the major regulator of renal magnesium reabsorption, so an abrupt elevation in concentration from intravenous repletion will partially remove the stimulus for magnesium retention. Up to 50% of the infused magnesium will be excreted in the urine. Thus, large magnesium depletion requires sustained correction, preferably with oral sustained-release preparations.

Patients with concomitant hypokalemia and hypocalcemia should receive potassium and calcium replacement. In the presence of hypocalcemia, if calcium is not supplemented, the administration of magnesium sulfate can acutely drop ionized calcium by complexing calcium with sulfate ions and increasing urinary excretion.

Patients who have diuretic-induced hypomagnesemia and who cannot discontinue diuretic therapy might benefit from the addition of a potassium-sparing diuretic that increases magnesium reabsorption.[34] These drugs may also be useful in patients who have Bartter and Gitelman syndrome or cisplatin nephrotoxicity.

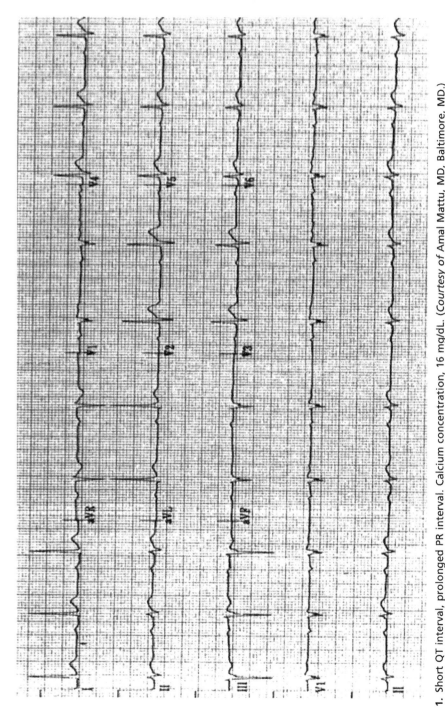

Fig. 1. Short QT interval, prolonged PR interval. Calcium concentration, 16 mg/dL. (*Courtesy of* Amal Mattu, MD, Baltimore, MD.)

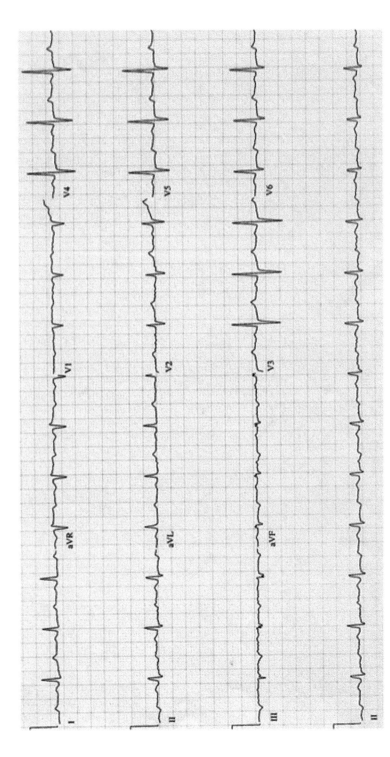

Fig. 2. Prolonged QT interval. Calcium concentration, 5.8 mg/dL. (*Courtesy of* Amal Mattu, MD, Baltimore, MD.)

PHOSPHATE ABNORMALITIES
Hyperphosphatemia

Definition and classification
Normal serum phosphate concentration is 2.5 to 4.5 mg/dL. Hyperphosphatemia is defined as a phosphate level more than than 4.5 mg/dL.

Cause
Hyperphosphatemia is caused by increased gastrointestinal absorption, decreased renal excretion, or rapid intracellular-to-extracellular shifts. Excessive phosphate intake in the presence of normal renal function is an uncommon cause of hyperphosphatemia, although the excessive use of phosphate-containing laxatives or enemas has been reported. Vitamin D intoxication can produce hyperphosphatemia as a result of excessive gastrointestinal absorption and increased renal reabsorption.

Hyperphosphatemia that persists for more than 12 hours occurs almost exclusively in the setting of acute kidney injury or chronic kidney disease.[19] Hypoparathyroidism and pseudohypoparathyroidism cause hyperphosphatemia through failure to inhibit renal phosphate reabsorption.

Increased tissue release of phosphate can be seen in patients with acute tumor lysis syndrome, rhabdomyolysis, hemolysis, hyperthermia, profound catabolic stress, and acute leukemia. These disorders can also result in acute kidney injury, which exacerbates the hyperphosphatemia.

Signs and symptoms
Acute hyperphosphatemia usually does not cause symptoms unless calcium precipitates with phosphate, leading to symptoms of hypocalcemia. A long-term complication of chronic uncontrolled hyperphosphatemia is the development of vascular and soft-tissue calcifications. Capillary and small arteriole calcifications lead to necrotic skin lesions and hemorrhagic subcutaneous lesions.[35] Cardiac depositions can disrupt the cardiac conduction system and produce significant arrhythmias. Soft-tissue deposits occur in joints, tendons, and ligaments as well as the eye.[36,37]

Management
Treatment of hyperphosphatemia targets the underlying cause, reduces absorption, and enhances excretion. Dietary restriction might be sufficient for control of hyperphosphatemia in mild renal insufficiency, but the addition of oral phosphate binders to inhibit gastrointestinal absorption is usually necessary for advanced renal insufficiency. Acute hyperphosphatemia from tumor lysis can be treated with volume expansion and forced diuresis with a loop diuretic to enhance urinary excretion. Dialysis is an effective method of eliminating phosphate.[12]

Hypophosphatemia

Definition and classification
Hypophosphatemia is defined as a phosphorus concentration less than 2.5 mg/dL. Disorders of hypophosphatemia can be classified by severity. Mild hypophosphatemia is a phosphorus level of 2.5 to 3.5 mg/dL. Moderate hypophosphatemia is a level of 1.0 to 2.4 mg/dL, and severe hypophosphatemia is a phosphorus level less than 1.0 mg/dL.

Cause
Hypophosphatemia is caused by decreased intestinal absorption, increased urinary excretion, or redistribution from an extracellular-to-intracellular shift.[13] Malabsorption, chronic diarrhea, and vitamin D deficiency all lead to decreased absorption of dietary

phosphate. Increased renal excretion of phosphate is the more common mechanism for development of hypophosphatemia.[12] Hyperparathyroidism, diuresis, and several genetic and acquired syndromes of phosphate wasting and associated skeletal abnormalities are associated with hypophosphatemia. Redistribution is an uncommon cause but can exacerbate existing hypophosphatemia produced by other causes. An extracellular-to-intracellular shift of phosphate is seen in respiratory alkalosis, treatment of diabetic ketoacidosis, refeeding syndrome, and leukemic blast crisis.[12]

Signs and symptoms

Symptoms of hypophosphatemia are usually only seen in moderate to severe disease. Acute symptoms include muscle weakness, including respiratory insufficiency and decreased myocardial contractility leading to congestive heart failure. Severe hypophosphatemia is also associated with rhabdomyolysis; hemolysis; impaired platelet and white blood cell function; and, in rare cases, neurologic disorders, such as seizures.[12,13]

Chronic hypophosphatemia results in significant bone disease and can be associated with short status and evidence of rickets.

Management

Acute treatment of hypophosphatemia is usually only necessary in patients who have moderate to severe hypophosphatemia. Oral repletion is preferable because intravenous administration of phosphate can complex calcium and lead to calcification. Intravenously, phosphate can be replaced in the form of potassium phosphate (3 mmol/mL of phosphate, 4.4 mEq/mL of potassium) or sodium phosphate (3 mmol/mL of phosphate, 4.0 mEq of sodium). The safe rate of phosphate correction ranges from 1 to 3 mmol/h. Although more rapid correction has been found to be safe, the response can be unpredictable.[12] Vitamin D supplementation is appropriate for patients with vitamin D deficiency.

SUMMARY

Disorders of calcium, magnesium, and phosphate are relatively common clinical problems, especially among critically ill patients. The disorders are associated with neuromuscular and cardiovascular symptoms given their crucial role in cellular physiology. Significant derangements of these electrolytes increase the risk of death. Treatment of these disorders should be directed at the underlying cause.

ACKNOWLEDGMENTS

The authors thank Linda Kesselring for assisting in the preparation of this article.

REFERENCES

1. Tentori F, Blayney MJ, Albert JM, et al. Mortality risk for dialysis patients with different levels of serum calcium, phosphorus, and PTH: the Dialysis Outcomes and Practice Patterns Study (DOPPS). Am J Kidney Dis 2008;52:519–30.
2. Hästbacka J, Pettilä V. Prevalence and predictive value of ionized hypocalcemia among critically ill patients. Acta Anaesthesiol Scand 2003;47:1264–9.
3. Liamis G, Rodenburg EM, Hofman A, et al. Electrolyte disorders in community subjects: prevalence and risk factors. Am J Med 2013;126:256–63.
4. Stewart AF. Hypercalcemia associated with cancer. N Engl J Med 2005;352:373–9.

5. McCurdy MT, Shanholtz CB. Oncologic emergencies. Crit Care Med 2012;40(7): 2212–22.
6. Zivin JR, Gooley T, Zager RA, et al. Hypocalcemia: a pervasive metabolic abnormality in the critically ill. Am J Kidney Dis 2001;4:689–98.
7. Guerrera MP, Volpe SL, Mao JJ. Therapeutic uses of magnesium. Am Fam Physician 2009;80:157–62.
8. Liao F, Folsom AR, Brancati FL. Is low magnesium concentration a risk factor for coronary heart disease? The Atherosclerosis Risk in Communities (ARIC) Study. Am Heart J 1998;136:480–90.
9. Fawcett WJ, Haxby EJ, Male DA. Magnesium: physiology and pharmacology. Br J Anaesth 1999;83:302–20.
10. Limaye C, Londhey V, Nadkart M, et al. Hypomagnesemia in critically ill medical patients. J Assoc Physicians India 2011;59:3–8.
11. Martin KJ, González EA, Slatopolsky E. Clinical consequences and management of hypomagnesemia. J Am Soc Nephrol 2009;20:2291–5.
12. Shiber JR, Mattu A. Serum phosphate abnormalities in the emergency department. J Emerg Med 2002;23:395–400.
13. Geerse DA, Bindels AJ, Kuiper MA, et al. Treatment of hypophosphatemia in the intensive care unit: a review. Crit Care 2010;14:R147.
14. Hruska KA, Mathew S, Lund R, et al. Hyperphosphatemia of chronic kidney disease. Kidney Int 2008;74(2):148–57.
15. Connolly GM, Cunningham R, McNamee PT, et al. Elevated serum phosphate predicts mortality in renal transplant recipients. Transplantation 2009;87:1040–4.
16. Tonelli M, Sacks F, Pfeffer M, et al. Relation between serum phosphate level and cardiovascular event rate in people with coronary disease. Circulation 2005;112: 2627–33.
17. Bringhurst F. Hormones and disorders of mineral metabolism. In: Melmed S, Polonsky KS, Larsen PR, et al, editors. Williams textbook of endocrinology. 12th edition. Philadelphia: Saunders; 2011.
18. Jahnen-Dechent W, Ketteler M. Magnesium basics. Clin Kidney J 2012;5(Suppl 1):i3–14.
19. Moe SM. Disorders involving calcium, phosphorus, and magnesium. Prim Care 2008;35:215–37.
20. Hofbauer LC, Heufelder AE. Role of receptor activator of nuclear factor-κB ligand and osteoprotegerin in bone cell biology. J Mol Med 2001;79:243–53.
21. Mayer GP, Hurst JG. Sigmoidal relationship between parathyroid hormone secretion rate and plasma calcium concentration in calves. Endocrinology 1978;102: 1036–42.
22. Carpinteri R, Porcelli T, Mejia C, et al. Glucocorticoid-induced osteoporosis and parathyroid hormone. J Endocrinol Invest 2010;33(Suppl 7):16–21.
23. Silverberg SJ, Walker MD, Bilezikian JP. Asymptomatic primary hyperparathyroidism. J Clin Densitom 2013;16:14–21.
24. Seymour JF, Gagel RF. Calcitriol: the major humoral mediator of hypercalcemia in Hodgkin's disease and non-Hodgkin's lymphomas. Blood 1993;82:1383–94.
25. Pitt SC, Sippel RS, Chen H. Secondary and tertiary hyperparathyroidism, state of the art surgical management. Surg Clin North Am 2009;89:1227–39.
26. National Cancer Institute. Hypercalcemia (PDQ). 2010. p. 1–25. Available at: http://cancer.gov/cancertopics/pdq/supportivecare/hypercalcemia/HealthProfessional. Accessed October 28, 2013.
27. Pecherstorfer M, Brenner K, Zojer N. Current management strategies for hypercalcemia. Treat Endocrinol 2003;2:273–92.

28. Fong J, Khan A. Hypocalcemia: updates in diagnosis and management for primary care. Can Fam Physician 2012;58:158–62.
29. Steele T, Kolamunnage-Dona R, Downey C, et al. Assessment and clinical course of hypocalcemia in critical illness. Crit Care 2013;17:R106.
30. Hurley K, Baggs D. Hypocalcemic cardiac failure in the emergency department. J Emerg Med 2005;28:155–9.
31. Lee JW. Fluid and electrolyte disturbances in critically ill patients. Electrolyte Blood Press 2010;8:72–81.
32. Rude RK. Magnesium depletion and hypermagnesemia. In: Rosen CJ, Compston JE, Lian JB, editors. Primer on the metabolic bone diseases and disorders of mineral metabolism. Hoboken (NJ): John Wiley & Sons, Inc; 2009. p. 325–8.
33. Ravn HB. Pharmacological effects of magnesium on arterial thrombosis–mechanisms of action? Magnes Res 1999;12:191–9.
34. Dai L-J, Raymond L, Friedman PA, et al. Mechanisms of amiloride stimulation of Mg2 + uptake in immortalized mouse distal convoluted tubule cells. Am J Physiol 1997;272(2 Pt 2):F249–56.
35. Janigan D, Hirsch D, Klassen G, et al. Calcified subcutaneous arterioles with infarcts of the subcutis and skin ("calciphylaxis") in chronic renal failure. Am J Kidney Dis 2000;35:588–97.
36. Delmez J, Slatopolsky E. Hyperphosphatemia - its consequences and treatment in patients with chronic renal disease. Am J Kidney Dis 1992;19:303–17.
37. Hamada J, Tamai K, Ono W, et al. Uremic tumoral calcinosis in hemodialysis patients: clinicopathological findings and identification of calcific deposits. J Rheumatol 2006;33:119–26.

Altered Mental Status and Endocrine Diseases

Elizabeth Park, MD[a], Michael K. Abraham, MD, MS[b],*

KEYWORDS

- Altered mental status • Diabetic ketoacidosis • Thyroid storm • Myxedema coma
- Pheochromocytoma • Addison disease

KEY POINTS

- Although altered mental status is a common presentation in the emergency department, altered mental status caused by endocrine emergencies is rare.
- The differential diagnosis for altered mental status is always varied and it is sometimes difficult to uncover the ultimate cause in the emergency department.
- When considering the differential diagnosis of an altered patient, clinicians must consider the age and sex of the patient, prior medical history, medications, and risk factors for developing endocrinopathies.

INTRODUCTION

The chief complaint of altered mental status represents up to 10% of all emergency department (ED) visits, and 5% of these are ultimately diagnosed with endocrine causes.[1] Being altered is a term that includes a spectrum of presentations including being comatose, combative, confused, having personality changes, or being difficult to arouse. It could pose a challenge to diagnose a patient with altered mental status secondary to an endocrine disorder, especially if a prior history of an endocrine disease is unknown. The diagnosis of these diseases requires a high clinical suspicion, and information gleaned from the history, physical examination findings, and laboratory studies. When considering the differential diagnosis of an altered patient, clinicians must consider the age and sex of the patient, prior medical history, medications, and risk factors for developing endocrinopathies. The cause of the endocrine disease and the precipitating factor for the diseases commonly have similar presentations, which causes increasing complexity in the diagnosis of these diseases.

The authors have nothing to disclose.

[a] Department of Emergency Medicine, Baylor College of Medicine, 1504 Taub Loop Road, Houston, TX 77030, USA; [b] Department of Emergency Medicine, University of Maryland School of Medicine, 110 South Paca Street, 6th Floor Suite 200, Baltimore, MD 21201, USA
* Corresponding author.
E-mail address: mabra003@umaryland.edu

Emerg Med Clin N Am 32 (2014) 367–378
http://dx.doi.org/10.1016/j.emc.2013.12.007
0733-8627/14/$ – see front matter © 2014 Elsevier Inc. All rights reserved.

EVALUATION AND TREATMENT OF THE PATIENT
History

All patients who present to the ED should be approached with a stepwise algorithm. As with any patient who presents to the ED, a thorough assessment of the ABCs (airway, breathing, and circulation) is required. After the patient's airway and circulatory status are assessed and stabilized, the cause of the presentation can be sought. The act of taking the history may prove difficult depending on the patient's mental status. The emergency physician may develop a plausible differential diagnosis primarily from speaking with the patient, or this may necessitate involvement of family members or caretakers. Because of the wide variety of presentations, from the subtle alterations of sensorium to a floridly psychotic state, eliciting a history that suggests an endocrinopathy as the cause of the mental status change can be difficult. Any information could be vital to diagnosing and treating the patient appropriately.

The history should begin with an adequate understanding of baseline mental status, and any reports of bizarre behavior need to be supported with specific examples. The history should focus on the onset of the symptoms and variability of the symptoms through time. Emergency physicians should not hesitate to call those who can provide the most accurate information, such as the nursing home staff, family and friends, or other health care providers who may have information about the patient. To the extent that it is possible, the history should also include a thorough medical history, and this may require a review of the patient's medical records, if available. The pertinent aspects of the medical history include any new or changed medications, substance abuse, and any antecedent illnesses.

Part of the difficulty in diagnosing endocrinopathies is that they can be exacerbated, or masked, by other processes. A thorough review of the history is necessary to evaluate the possibility of other processes, which include infection, polysubstance abuse, cerebrovascular accidents, psychiatric illness, dementia, or head trauma.

Physical Examination

The physical examination should always begin with an overview of the vital signs, which may provide an initial clue to the underlying cause. Examples of vital sign abnormalities associated with endocrinopathies are listed in **Table 1**.

After an assessment of the vital signs, a thorough head-to-toe physical examination should be performed. The examination should start with a general overview of the patient's appearance because this may give clues to the cause of their presentation. As with any patient who presents with a change in mental status, a complete neurologic examination is warranted. The neurologic examination should begin with an assessment of mental status; a commonly used tool is the mini-mental screening examination (MMSE). A quick MMSE allows the practitioner to easily and reliably determine the patient's cognitive ability. Next, the assessment should include a neurologic examination with focus on the cranial nerves to evaluate for a possible cerebrovascular accident. Other crucial components of the neurologic examination include examination of muscle tone, strength, and reflexes. Although an extensive examination of the integumentary system is rarely performed, this can be beneficial in the obtunded patient. For example, abnormalities of the skin and hair can give clues to previous hypothyroidism. **Table 2** shows other endocrinopathies and examples of pertinent physical examination findings that can be associated with them.

Table 1
Abnormal vital signs indicating possible endocrine emergencies

Hyperthermia	Thyroid storm
Hypothermia	Myxedema coma
Hypertension	Thyroid storm, pheochromocytoma
Hypotension	Adrenal crisis, DKA/HHNK (if dehydrated)
Tachycardia	Thyroid storm, pheochromocytoma, adrenal crisis (if patient is dehydrated), DKA/HHNK
Bradycardia	Myxedema coma, adrenal crisis
Tachypnea	DKA
Bradypnea	Myxedema coma

Abbreviations: DKA, diabetic ketoacidosis; HHNK, hyperglycemic hyperosmolar nonketotic.

GLUCOSE-RELATED CAUSES OF ALTERED MENTAL STATUS
Hypoglycemia

Because the endocrine system is a highly regulated series of interconnected glands that control most aspects of metabolism and homeostasis, disorders can negatively affect glucose levels. Because glucose is the primary and preferred energy source for the central nervous system, this causes alterations in mental status. The most obvious organ that may contribute to this is the insulin-producing pancreas, but almost every endocrine gland and its associated maladies can have an effect on glucose metabolism. The hypothalamic-pituitary-adrenal axis is responsible for the control of cortisol and epinephrine, among other hormones, which are crucial in the production and use of glucose by the body. Hypoglycemia is most likely seen in diabetics, but can also be seen in thyrotoxicosis, myxedema coma, pheochromocytoma, and adrenal crisis.

The main clinical differentiation that needs to be made is to determine whether the hypoglycemia is causing the patients' clinical presentation or whether is a result of another process that is causing the hypoglycemia. Simple hypoglycemia as a cause of altered mental status should show resolution of symptoms once normoglycemia has been achieved.[2] However, if the neurologic impairment remains, other causes should be considered. Just as a patient with severe sepsis can have concomitant

Table 2
Physical examination findings suggesting endocrine emergencies

Disorder	Physical Examination Findings
DKA	Kussmaul respirations, signs of dehydration, decline in mental status, fruity odor of ketones
Myxedema coma	Patient has severe decline in mental status, hypothermia, delayed deep tendon reflexes, dry skin and hair, pretibial myxedema, macroglossia, signs of heart failure
Thyroid storm	Proptosis, goiter, diaphoresis, tremors, thin hair, hyperreflexia, fever, wide pulse pressures, signs of CHF, atrial fibrillation
Adrenal crisis	Orthostatic hypotension, nausea, vomiting, darkened skin
Pheochromocytoma	Vacillating blood pressure/heart rate/temperature, diaphoresis, tremor, pallor secondary to vasoconstriction

Abbreviation: CHF, congestive heart failure.

hypoglycemia from several causes, so can the patient with an endocrinopathy. For example, the patient in myxedema coma may have hypoglycemia, and this could be caused by the infection that exacerbated the endocrine disorder, the dysfunction of the thyroid gland causing abnormal metabolism, or a combination of both. In addition to a dysfunctional endocrine gland causing problems, the use of medications can also cause hypoglycemia. Insulin is the most frequent cause in hypoglycemia, but oral antidiabetic medications, especially sulfonylureas, can also cause prolonged and severe hypoglycemia.[3] **Box 1** lists possible causes, including medication, for hypoglycemia.

Box 1
Causes of hypoglycemia

Diabetic medications
  Insulin
  Sulfonylureas
  Meglitinides
Antidiabetic medications
  β-Blockers
  Angiotensin-converting enzyme inhibitors
  Pentamidine
  Fluoroquinolones
Organ dysfunction
  Liver failure (decreased gluconeogenesis and glycogenolysis)
  Kidney failure (decreased insulin clearance)
Stress states
  Infection and sepsis
  Burns
Malnutrition
  Alcohol abuse
  Eating disorder
  Malabsorption states
Endocrinopathies
  Adrenal insufficiency
  Hypothyroidism
Neoplastic disease (rare)
  Insulinoma
  Liver metastases
Psychiatric
  Surreptitious insulin use
  Overdose

Modified from Alsahli M, Gerich JE. Acute and chronic complications of diabetes hypoglycemia. Endocrinol Metabol Clin 2013;42(4):657–76.

Common presenting symptoms for hypoglycemia include diaphoresis, irritability, and tremors. As the serum glucose gets lower, neurologic and cognitive signs begin to show, such as cognitive impairment, paralysis, and eventually seizures and coma.[2] As with any patient presenting with an alteration in mental status, whether obvious or subtle, the first test that should be obtained is a bedside glucose. An aspect of hypoglycemia that is clinically relevant is that the level of hypoglycemia may not relate to the clinical presentation. For example, a diabetic patient who regularly has difficulty controlling blood glucose may be tolerant to the effects of hypoglycemia. In addition, hypoglycemia can unmask previous clinical manifestations of cerebrovascular accident that had been clinically silent. In short, hypoglycemia can be caused by, or associated with, many endocrine disorders, and a quick bedside determination of glucose status is crucial to the approach to a patient with altered mental status.

Hypoglycemia in patients with altered mental status should be diagnosed and treated promptly. Prolonged severe hypoglycemia has been shown to be associated with brain injury and can lead to permanent neurocognitive impairment.[4] Initial stabilization is often done in the prehospital setting. Alert hypoglycemic patients should be given oral glucose, which can be in the form of glucose tablets or a high-carbohydrate juice such as orange juice. In a hypoglycemic patient who is obtunded or comatose, parenteral agents should be used. Intravenous (IV) 50% dextrose solutions should be first-line treatment. If IV access is not established, intramuscular glucagon can be administered, but this has a slower onset of action. Octreotide is another medication that has been used for refractory hypoglycemia caused by sulfonylurea overdose with good results.[5]

Frequent monitoring of glucose levels is necessary to avoid recurrent hypoglycemia. Patients may require subsequent dextrose boluses, and some patients may even require a constant infusion of dextrose to maintain normoglycemia. Once a patient is able to safely tolerate food, the patient should eat a meal that includes both easily digested carbohydrates and protein, for example a turkey sandwich on white bread. After the blood sugar is stabilized, the provider should then explore what precipitated the hypoglycemic episode.

Diabetic Ketoacidosis/Hyperglycemic Hyperosmolar Syndrome

Although thyroid and adrenal emergencies are rarer phenomena encountered in the ED, diabetes-related complications are commonplace in comparison. In hyperglycemic patients, diabetic ketoacidosis (DKA) and hyperosmolar hyperglycemic state (HHS) should be considered as possible causes of a patient having altered mental status. Even with minor derangements in laboratory tests, patients can be considered in DKA if their blood glucose is more than 250 mg/dL, they have an anion gap greater than 10, and pH less than 7.3. The severity of the altered sensorium correlates more with the serum osmolarity (>320 mOsm/L) than other laboratory findings such as the degree of hyperglycemia or the acidosis.[6] The presence of acidosis is the main differentiation between DKA and HHS. However, the altered sensorium associated with their clinical presentations can be similar, mainly because of the hyperosmolarity.[7]

Patients may have classic complaints of hyperglycemia, such as excessive thirst and frequent urination, or they may complain of nausea and vomiting. Findings on physical examination for a patient in DKA include signs of dehydration such as dry mucous membranes, tachycardia, hypotension, Kussmaul respirations, and abdominal tenderness. Mental status changes do not have to occur in every patient in DKA, but, if they do, patients can have a varying presentation from lethargy to coma.

Patients with HHS have some element of neurologic dysfunction ranging from hemiparesis and partial seizures to stupor and frank coma.[7,8]

One of the most serious complications of DKA, especially for pediatric patients, is cerebral edema. Cerebral edema occurs in about 1% of pediatric patients in DKA and should be a consideration when the patient undergoing treatment of DKA experiences a sudden change in mental status or shows signs of increased ICP.[9,10] In general, this complication is only seen in pediatric patients and although the pathophysiology is not clear, the cause centers on the inadequate increase in serum sodium levels in conjunction with the high osmolarity of the serum, high blood urea nitrogen levels, and hypocapnia.[9,10] The initial glucose or sodium levels on presentation do not affect the patient's chances of developing cerebral edema.[9] **Box 2** lists clinical as well as diagnostic results that are risk factors for patients to develop cerebral edema.

THYROID-RELATED CAUSES OF ALTERED MENTAL STATUS
Myxedema Coma

Although the prevalence of hypothyroidism is not rare, the severe form of the disease, myxedema coma, is infrequently seen in the ED. The usual description of a patient's sensorium includes a precipitous decline from the patient's baseline and presentation may range from lethargy to coma. The patient's baseline mental status is likely to encompass some findings of hypothyroidism such as amnesia, depression, or slow cognitive processing. The textbook clinical scenario of a patient in myxedema coma is an elderly woman with a history of hypothyroidism who presents in stupor after exposure to cold weather.[11,12] The severity of the hypothermia correlates with the prognosis, with the more severe the hypothermia, the worse the prognosis for the patient.[11] The overall mortality is approximately 25% for patients in myxedema coma despite appropriate medical intervention.[11–14]

If available, a history of hypothyroidism may be obtained from the family, previous medical records, or medication bottles brought in by emergency medical service providers. A thyroidectomy scar may be present on the neck. Other possible pertinent physical examination findings include hypothermia; depressed deep tendon

---

Box 2
Risk factors for pediatric DKA-induced cerebral edema

New-onset diabetes

Younger age

Longer duration of DKA symptoms

Degree of acidosis at presentation (pH<7.1)

Greater hypocapnia (Pco_2<20 mm Hg)

Greater initial rate of fluid resuscitation for treatment of severe DKA (>50 mL/kg in the first 4 hours)

Administration of insulin during the first hour of fluid resuscitation

Slower increase in measured serum sodium concentration during treatment

Bicarbonate treatment

From Olivieri L, Chasm R. Diabetic ketoacidosis in the pediatric emergency department. Emerg Med Clin North Am 2013;31(3):755–73.

reflexes; dry, doughlike skin and hair; pretibial myxedema; macroglossia; and signs of heart failure. As with any disease, the physical examination findings are on a spectrum, and the more severe the myxedema the higher the severity of the presenting signs and symptoms. Hypoglycemia is frequently present in these patients, because patients in myxedema coma have impaired glucose metabolism and retain free water. The decline in mental status can occur abruptly and usually has a trigger that causes a metabolic stress and thus the rapid decline.[15] Most commonly the onset of an infection, trauma, or a myocardial infarction starts the deterioration into myxedema coma.[14] Exogenous or iatrogenic factors, such as cold exposure, and medications that decrease central processes, such as antiepileptics, β-blockers, or sedatives, can also exacerbate the symptoms.[14] In the process of working up a patient in myxedema coma, the practitioner should entertain a broad differential diagnosis including cardiac and infectious causes while simultaneously investigating medication changes or other recent physiologic stresses. Patients with myxedema coma may present with seizures, further complicating the clinical presentation. One-quarter of the patients with myxedema coma develop seizures secondary to hyponatremia, hypoglycemia, or decreased oxygenation of the cerebral vasculature.[11] In such cases, it is important to first stabilize the patient with first-line seizure therapy and then, once the patient is stabilized, the cause can be investigated.

There should be a low threshold to intubate the patient with myxedema coma because mental status can continue to decline in the department while work-up and treatment are ongoing. It is prudent to prepare for a difficult airway in these patients secondary to an edematous pharynx and possibly even angioedema.[16]

If myxedema coma is suspected based on the initial inspection of the patient, a full thyroid panel and cortisol levels should be sent. Treatment should not wait until the laboratory values return.[12,14] Few clinicians find fault in studies associated with a general altered mental status work-up such as computed tomography head, lumbar puncture, urine drug screen, levels of medications that the patient was taking, alcohol level, ammonia level, and possibly an arterial blood gas. In small number of studies, most patients in myxedema had increased cerebrospinal fluid pressure and total protein content, likely secondary to the increased vascular permeability of the meninges.[15] A bedside echocardiogram might reveal a pericardial effusion as well. Treatment consists of airway management, thyroid repletion, and stress dose steroids. Patients in myxedema coma often have concomitant adrenal insufficiency. Once thyroid hormone is administered, there is a subsequent increase in metabolism, which requires more cortisol.[14]

Thyroid Storm

Although patients with hyperthyroidism may present with mild agitation, patients with thyroid storm can have varied presentations. Early in the progression of the disease the patient usually presents with signs and symptoms of a hypermetabolic state.[17] The clues to diagnosis can be found in the physical examination findings such as fever, tachycardia, hypertension, tremors, and agitation. Some other neurologic findings include hyperreflexia, muscle weakness, ataxia, and even myopathy.[12,18,19] The patient may also have gastrointestinal (GI) symptoms including vomiting and diarrhea. As the disease progresses the patient can present with psychosis and then enter a comatose state as the disease becomes fulminant. The overall prevalence of thyroid storm is 1% to 2% of those diagnosed with hyperthyroidism, with mortality between 20% and 50%.[18,20]

As with any endocrine disease that causes altered mental status, clinicians must first consider the diagnosis before it can be made. It is fortunate if a history of hyperthyroidism is uncovered on a review of the patient's past medical history. The diagnosis of thyroid storm is usually made on clinical grounds alone because laboratory studies can have prolonged turnaround times causing delays in management. Left untreated, the patient rapidly decompensates, shows signs of heart failure and hypotension, and succumbs to respiratory failure. With such a wide array of presentations, clinicians may decide to rule out other conditions such as meningitis, cerebrovascular accident, heat stroke, alcohol withdrawal, drug overdose, neuroleptic malignant syndrome, and diabetic ketoacidosis. Laboratory studies can be markedly abnormal but do not help distinguish between many diseases. The patient often has a concomitant process that has precipitated the thyroid storm. Treatment involves blocking thyroid hormone production with antithyroid medication and then iodine, blocking systemic effects with beta-blockade and corticosteroids, and treating the precipitating event.[12,19]

ADRENAL-RELATED CAUSES OF ALTERED MENTAL STATUS
Adrenal Insufficiency

Adrenal emergencies, similar to thyroid emergencies, can manifest either as minor mental status changes like depression or severe diseases like frank psychosis or coma. Adrenal insufficiency may have many underlying causes, including autoimmune, iatrogenic, and infectious processes. Like most endocrine diseases, adrenal insufficiency can have primary or secondary causes. Primary adrenal insufficiency is most commonly caused by autoimmune adrenalitis in Western countries such as the United States.[21] Tuberculosis should be considered in areas that are endemic or in patients who have traveled to or lived in those endemic areas because tuberculosis remains the most common infectious cause.[21,22] Human Immunodeficiency virus (HIV) is also a common infectious cause of adrenal destruction, and the clinician must be cognizant with patients known to be HIV seropositive.[23] Secondary adrenal insufficiency is caused by disorders of the hypothalamic pituitary axis, like pituitary apoplexy or tumors. Whether the patient has primary or secondary adrenal insufficiency, the patient presents similarly when in adrenal crisis.

There is a history of chronic adrenal insufficiency, especially in primary adrenal insufficiency, which can include symptoms of salt craving; hyperpigmentation of skin; GI distress such as nausea, vomiting, and diarrhea; and generalized muscle wasting and fatigue. In the acute setting, it manifests as a sudden worsening of these symptoms along with hemodynamic instability as shown by the body's inability to support the additional stress of a medical crisis such as an infection, trauma, or surgical procedure. When a patient requires a sudden increase of stress hormones or exogenous hormones are removed, the patient manifests a profound inability to maintain adequate amounts of glucocorticoids and mineralocorticoids, resulting in mental status changes, tenuous vital signs, and multiple laboratory derangements. With circulatory collapse, the patient can present as being less responsive, delirious, or in coma as the brain is hypoperfused.[22]

Primary adrenal insufficiency can produce marked hyponatremia, hypoglycemia, hypercalcemia, hyperkalemia, and possibly metabolic acidosis from inadequate organ perfusion manifested by an increased lactic acid level. Beginning the inpatient workup by sending random cortisol and adrenocorticotropic hormone levels is warranted if there are standard findings of hypovolemia or hemodynamic instability that cannot be explained otherwise, especially if the hemodynamic instability is refractory to standard therapies.[21,24] A cosyntropin stimulation test can be performed for confirmation of the diagnosis of adrenal insufficiency, but should not delay treatment.

Box 3
Causes of adrenal insufficiency

Primary

  Vascular

    Adrenal infarction, hemorrhage (lupus anticoagulant or HIIT)

  Infiltrative

    Lymphoproliferative disorder, metastatic disease, granulomatous disease (eg, sarcoidosis)

  Autoimmune

    Autoimmune adrenalitis, polyglandular autoimmune syndrome I and II

  Traumatic

    Abdominal blunt trauma or back trauma

  Drugs

    Ketoconazole (especially in patients with acquired immunodeficiency syndrome), etomidate

  Congenital

    Adrenoleukodystrophy, adrenal enzyme deficiencies

Secondary

  Vascular

    Pituitary infarction (Sheehan syndrome)

  Neoplasm

    Pituitary adenoma, metastasis

  Infective

    Tuberculosis, HIV, and fungal infection

  Infiltrative

    Granulomatous disease (sarcoidosis, histiocytosis), hemochromatosis

  Inflammatory

    Lymphocytic hypophysitis

  Traumatic

    Brain injury

  Radiation

    After pituitary radiation

  Drugs

    Patient cessation of prolonged glucocorticoid therapy (including inhaled glucocorticoid)

  Critical illness

    Relative glucocorticoid deficiency

  Others

    ACTH deficiency

Data from Adler S, Wartofsky L. Myxedema coma. In: Berghe GV, editor. Acute endocrinology: from case to consequence. New York: Humana Press; 2008. p. 29–44.

Treatment involves fluid resuscitation, repletion of electrolyte deficiencies (especially glucose), and steroid replacement therapy. Stress dose steroids given as hydrocortisone 100 mg IV as a bolus every 8 hours is sufficient for patients with adrenal insufficiency.[21] Hydrocortisone contains glucocorticoid and mineralocorticoid and sufficiently replaces both. As an alternative, dexamethasone 4 mg is also an acceptable treatment. Dexamethasone treatment has the advantage of not affecting the cosyntropin stimulation test should the provider desire to perform it, whereas hydrocortisone does affect the result. The disadvantage of dexamethasone is that it does not contain any mineralocorticoid and may need to be given in combination with fludrocortisone, a mineralocorticoid.[21,25] Although uncovering the cause of adrenal insufficiency may become a secondary consideration for the emergency physician when the patient is in an acutely decompensated state, **Box 3** lists the common causes to consider in the work-up and treatment when a patient is found to have adrenal insufficiency.

Pheochromocytoma

Although rare, and even more rarely diagnosed in the ED, pheochromocytomas need to remain on the differential diagnosis of any altered patient. The general findings may be similar to a patient having a panic attack, which can dangerously and easily be dismissed if not considering a broader differential. The 5 Ps represent the symptoms associated with pheochromocytomas: pressure (hypertension), pain (headache and chest pain), palpitations, perspiration, and pallor (caused by vasoconstriction).[26] Again, the difficulty in diagnosis lies in recognition because pheochromocytoma can encompass a wide spectrum of presentations.

The underlying mechanism of the symptoms is caused by the sudden release of epinephrine and norepinephrine into the blood stream by the adrenal tumor. The wave of catecholamine excess can thus cause symptoms similar to a fight-or-flight response. Mental status changes can also range from subtle to frank psychosis.[27] One case report details the diagnosis of a pheochromocytoma in a patient who continued to have what was labeled as a relapsing paranoid psychosis.[28] Other findings that suggest a pheochromocytoma include a paroxysmal increase in blood pressure, heart rate, temperature, a sudden onset of headache, dysrhythmias, acute GI distress, and refractory response to antihypertensive medications.[27] These paroxysms can be brought on by physical exertion, bowel movements, trauma, or even certain medications that may stimulate the sympathetic nervous system.[27] The differential diagnosis usually includes drug overdose, hyperthyroidism, and psychiatric disturbances, which may be the initial impression of the evaluating physician. It is important to thoroughly evaluate medical conditions that could need prompt treatment even if they have a pertinent history of drug abuse or psychiatric issues.

If the diagnosis is made and confirmed in the ED, the provider should focus on catecholamine blockade to control symptoms. Alpha-blockade with phentolamine or phenoxybenzamine is the preferred method to control symptoms. The addition of a β-blocker for selective symptoms can also be used. The pharmacologic treatment of a pheochromocytoma is solely a temporizing measure to bridge the patient until surgical removal of the gland.[28]

SUMMARY

The differential diagnosis for altered mental status is always varied and it is sometimes difficult to uncover the ultimate cause in the ED. Part of what distinguishes astute clinicians is considering the atypical diagnoses and pursuing them under reasonable suspicion. Endocrinopathies, although not common, are still fascinating and their diagnosis is laudable. Sorting through the history, physical examination, laboratory findings, and imaging can become a satisfying endeavor when arriving at an answer that will save the patient and restore their mental status to baseline. The problematic but remarkable aspect of the endocrine system is that it affects many other systems of the human body and the presentation can be perplexing. Knowledge of the endocrine emergencies and how they can present in the ED will inform the differential diagnosis of altered mental status and will possibly be called on at some point in the clinician's career for the treatment of such patients.

REFERENCES

1. Kanich W, Brady WJ, Huff JS, et al. Altered mental status: evaluation and etiology in the ED. Am J Emerg Med 2002;20(7):613–7.
2. Cryer PE, Axelrod L, Grossman AB, et al. Evaluation and management of adult hypoglycemic disorders: an Endocrine Society Clinical Practice Guideline. J Clin Endocrinol Metab 2009;94(3):709–28.
3. Alsahli M, Gerich JE. Acute and chronic complications of diabetes hypoglycemia. Endocrinol Metabol Clin 2013;42(4):657–76.
4. Witsch J, Neugebauer H, Flechsenhar J, et al. Hypoglycemic encephalopathy: a case series and literature review on outcome determination. J Neurol 2012; 259(10):2172–81.
5. Dougherty PP, Klein-Schwartz W. Octreotide's role in the management of sulfonylurea-induced hypoglycemia. J Med Toxicol 2010;6(2):199–206.
6. Gomez Diaz RA, Rivera Moscoso R, Ramos Rodriguez R, et al. Diabetic ketoacidosis in adults: clinical and laboratory features. Arch Med Res 1996;27(2): 177–81.
7. Kitabchi AE, Nyenwe EA. Hyperglycemic crises in diabetes mellitus: diabetic ketoacidosis and hyperglycemia hyperosmolar state. Endocrinol Metab Clin North Am 2006;35(4):725–51.
8. Kitabchi AE, Umpierrez GE, Murphy MB, et al. Hyperglycemic crises in adult patients with diabetes: a consensus statement from the American Diabetes Association. Diabetes Care 2006;29(12):2739–48.
9. Glaser N, Barnett P, McCaslin I, et al. Risk factors for cerebral edema in children with diabetic ketoacidosis. The Pediatric Emergency Medicine Collaborative Research Committee of the American Academy of Pediatrics. N Engl J Med 2001;344(4):264–9.
10. Olivieri L, Chasm R. Diabetic ketoacidosis in the pediatric emergency department. Emerg Med Clin North Am 2013;31(3):755–73.
11. Adler S, Wartofsky L. Myxedema coma. In: Berghe GV, editor. Acute endocrinology: from case to consequence. New York: Humana Press; 2008. p. 29–44.
12. Casaletto JJ. Is salt, vitamin, or endocrinopathy causing this encephalopathy? A review of endocrine and metabolic causes of altered level of consciousness. Emerg Med Clin North Am 2010;28(3):633–62.
13. Rodríguez I, Fluiters E, Pérez-Méndez LF, et al. Factors associated with mortality of patients with myxoedema coma: prospective study in 11 cases treated in a single institution. J Endocrinol 2004;180(2):347–50.
14. Devdhar M, Ousman YH, Burman KD, et al. Hypothyroidism. Endocrinol Metab Clin North Am 2007;36(3):595–615.
15. Sanders V. Neurologic manifestations of myxedema. N Engl J Med 1962;266: 599–603 concl.

16. Lee CH, Wira CR. Severe angioedema in myxedema coma: a difficult airway in a rare endocrine emergency. Am J Emerg Med 2009;27(8):1021.e1–2.
17. Burch HB, Wartofsky L. Life-threatening thyrotoxicosis. Thyroid storm. Endocrinol Metab Clin North Am 1993;22(2):263–77.
18. Stanzani Maserati M, Faustini Fustini M. Thyroid storm with atypical neurological signs: an unusual clinical emergence of a life-threatening event. Intern Emerg Med 2009;4(2):181–2.
19. Idrose A. Thyroid disorders: hyperthyroidism and thyroid storm. Tintinalli's emergency medicine. 7th edition. New York: McGraw Hill; 2011. p. 1447–53.
20. McKeown NJ, Tews MC, Gossain VV, et al. Hyperthyroidism. Emerg Med Clin North Am 2005;23(3):669–85.
21. Tenner AG, Halvorson KM. Endocrine causes of dangerous fever. Emerg Med Clin North Am 2013;31(4):969–86.
22. Friedman T. The adrenal gland. In: Andreoli TE, editor. Cecil essentials of medicine. 6th edition. Philadelphia: WB Saunders; 2004. p. 603–14.
23. Bons J, Moreau L, Lefebvre H. Adrenal disorders in human immunodeficiency virus (HIV) infected patients. Ann Endocrinol (Paris) 2013;74(5–6):508–14.
24. Taub YR, Wolford RW. Cancer emergencies, part I adrenal insufficiency and other adrenal oncologic emergencies. Emerg Med Clin North Am 2009;27(2):271–82.
25. Marik PE, Zaloga GP. Adrenal insufficiency in the critically ill: a new look at an old problem. Chest 2002;122(5):1784–96.
26. Horatas M. Pheochromocytoma. In: Domino F, editor. The 5-minute clinical consult 2009. 17th edition. New York: Lippincott Williams & Wilkins; 2014. Available at: http://online.statref.com.proxy-hs.researchport.umd.edu/document.aspx?DocID=1&FxId=31&SessionId=1C8FAA5XKJNRORWO#H&2&ChaptersTab&T-M72d9EX3U6NPmhQTKMBg%3d%3d&&31.
27. Srirangalingam U, Chew S. Phaeochromocytoma and other diseases of the sympathetic nervous system. In: Berghe GV, editor. Acute endocrinology: from case to consequence. New York: Humana Press; 2008. p. 85–117.
28. Wong C, Yu R. Preoperative preparation for pheochromocytoma resection: physician survey and clinical practice. Exp Clin Endocrinol Diabetes 2010;118(7): 400–4.

Disorders of Sodium and Water Balance

Theresa R. Harring, MD*, Nathan S. Deal, MD, Dick C. Kuo, MD*

KEYWORDS

- Dysnatremia • Water balance • Hyponatremia • Hypernatremia
- Fluids for resuscitation

KEY POINTS

- Correct hypovolemia before correcting sodium imbalance by giving patients boluses of isotonic intravenous fluids; reassess serum sodium after volume status normalized.
- Serum and urine electrolytes and osmolalities in patients with dysnatremias in conjunction with clinical volume assessment are especially helpful to guide management.
- If an unstable patient is hyponatremic, give 2 mL/kg of 3% normal saline (NS) up to 100 mL over 10 minutes; this may be repeated once if the patient continues to be unstable.
- If unstable hypernatremic patient, give NS with goal to decrease serum sodium by 8 to 15 mEq/L over 8 hours.
- Correct stable dysnatremias no faster than 8 mEq/L to 12 mEq/L over the first 24 hours.

INTRODUCTION

Irregularities of sodium and water balance most often occur simultaneously and are some of the most common electrolyte abnormalities encountered by emergency medicine physicians. Approximately 10% of all patients admitted from the emergency department suffer from hyponatremia and 2% suffer from hypernatremia.[1] Because of the close nature of sodium and water balance, and the relatively rigid limits placed on the central nervous system by the skull, it is not surprising that most symptoms related to disorders of sodium and water imbalance are neurologic and can, therefore, be devastating. Several important concepts are crucial to the understanding of these disorders, the least of which include body fluid compartments, regulation of osmolality, and the need for rapid identification and appropriate management.

The difference between a minor symptom and a life-threatening condition caused by a sodium imbalance is often a result of the rapidity of the change in sodium concentration, not necessarily the overall deficit; and how quickly the imbalance is recognized

The authors report no financial relationships in the production of this article.

Section of Emergency Medicine, Ben Taub General Hospital, Baylor College of Medicine, Emergency Center, 1504 Taub Loop, Room EC 61, Houston, TX 77030, USA

* Corresponding authors.

E-mail addresses: harring@bcm.edu; dckuo@bcm.edu

Emerg Med Clin N Am 32 (2014) 379–401

http://dx.doi.org/10.1016/j.emc.2014.01.001

emed.theclinics.com

and then treated by clinicians. Because emergency physicians do not always have the most complete background information on their patients in acute settings, this article delineates the types of sodium and water imbalances, the symptoms and signs the clinician encounters, pitfalls and complications of correcting these imbalances too aggressively, and how to base initial management of these patients.

- Sodium and water disorders occur simultaneously and most commonly affect the neurologic system, potentially leading to devastating outcomes.

PHYSIOLOGY

Total body water (TBW) accounts for approximately 60% of the total body weight in adults (**Fig. 1**); however, this figure changes with extremes of age, and within the sexes.[2] A more accurate picture of TBW can be calculated by (Equation 1, **Table 1**):

$$TBW = weight\ (kg) \times correction\ factor \qquad\qquad 1$$

The TBW is further divided into intracellular fluid, approximately 40% of total body weight; and extracellular fluid (ECF), approximately 20% of total body weight. Of the ECF, approximately two-thirds comprises interstitial fluid and one-third comprises intravascular fluid. The intravascular fluid is correspondingly close to 5% of the total body weight. The primary solute of the ECF is sodium, with a normal concentration of 140 mEq/L. As the concentration of sodium changes, neurologic symptoms may begin to manifest because of the confining nature of the skull. These symptoms may be minor or they can lead to life-threatening conditions.

Sodium regulation primarily occurs via 2 mechanisms: vasopressin and thirst regulation. For proper fluid balance, an average healthy adult requires an intake of approximately 1 to 3 L of water per day.[3,4] This amount of water replaces the amount of water lost from the body in insensible losses and urinary output, including approximately 500 to 700 mL/d from the respiratory tract, 250 to 350 mL/d from the skin, and 100 mL/d from the feces.[3] Additional water replacement may be necessary for other excessive losses, such as sweating caused by exercise or fevers.

Water diffuses via transport channels across cellular membranes, allowing osmolality to remain relatively constant between the spaces, but in effect changing the electrolyte concentrations of these compartments. Normal osmolality of plasma is 275 to 295 mOsm/L H_2O and can be estimated by (Equation 2):

$$Serum\ osmolality\ (mOsm/kg) = 2 \times Na + glucose\ (mg/100\ mL)/18 \\ + blood\ urea\ nitrogen\ (mg/100\ mL)/2.8 \qquad 2$$

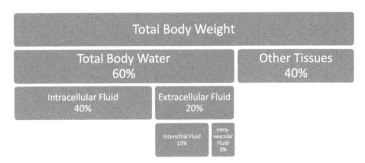

Fig. 1. Relationship of fluid compartments to total body weight. Percentages are expressed as related to total body weight.

Table 1	
Correction factors to estimate TBW volume	
Patient	**Correction Factor**
Newborn	0.8
Infant	0.7
Pediatric	0.6
Male, adult	0.6
Female, adult	0.5
Male, elderly	0.5
Female, elderly	0.45

Data from Wilson RF, Sibbald WJ. Fluid and electrolyte problems in the emergency department. JACEP 1976;5:339–46; and Kaplan LJ, Kellum JA. Fluids, pH, ions and electrolytes. Curr Opin Crit Care 2010;16:323–31.

In a healthy patient, the kidneys attempt to resorb or excrete water to preserve a normal osmolality. The primary hormone responsible for this regulation is arginine vasopressin, also referred to as antidiuretic hormone (ADH). ADH is a hormone synthesized in the posterior pituitary gland and acts on the distal convoluted tubule and the collecting duct of the nephron, resulting in increased reabsorption of free water, resulting in decreased volume of excreted urine, and concentrated urine. With this system of homeostasis, when plasma osmolality decreases, ADH is not released, water is freely excreted, and urine osmolality decreases. Conversely, when plasma osmolality increases, ADH is released, water is resorbed in the nephron, and urine osmolality increases. Plasma osmolality, with detected changes as small as 1% to 2%,[5] is the most common stimulus for ADH release; however, other factors can stimulate ADH release, including decreased intravascular volume, decreased blood pressure, pain, anxiety, nausea, pregnancy, menstruation, hypoglycemia, severe hypoxemia, hypercapnia, third spacing of fluids (eg, burns, trauma, pancreatitis), and certain drugs.[2,6,7]

The other route by which water is balanced is through the thirst mechanism. Because ADH is only able to regulate how much water the body holds onto, the thirst mechanism allows a stimulus to alter the amount of water that is consumed. Because of sensible and insensible water losses, the thirst mechanism allows the body to prevent dehydration, even under extreme water losses. Generally, the thirst mechanism determines the upper limit of the plasma osmolality, whereas the secretion of ADH determines the lower limit of the plasma osmolality.[7] If these regulation systems are functioning correctly, proper water balance is normally achieved.

HYPONATREMIA

Hyponatremia, defined as serum sodium level of less than 135 mEq/L, or severe hyponatremia as a level less than 125 mEq/L, is most commonly encountered in hospitalized patients or in patients with underlying medical diseases. The prevalence of hyponatremia is estimated to range between 3 and 6 million persons per year in the United States, and approximately one-quarter of these patients likely seek initial medical treatment in the emergency department.[8] Approximately 4% of adult medicine patients encountered in the emergency department have hyponatremia,[9] and approximately 15% of adult patients admitted to the hospital have hyponatremia.[10] Patients with hyponatremia have up to 33% higher mortality compared with normonatremic patients,[10] with an overall mortality of 3% to 29%.[11] The risk of mortality with hyponatremia may be associated with other underlying illnesses such as heart disease, pneumonia, and liver disease; but there seems to be no correlation with the severity of hyponatremia and the risk of increased mortality.[10,11] Therefore, the recognition of all patients with hyponatremia is of utmost importance to the emergency department clinician.

Signs and Symptoms

Symptoms of hyponatremia can range from mild to severe: some patients are asymptomatic, others present with seizures. The symptoms are typically related to the level and rapidity of sodium change and to the presence and degree of cerebral edema. As water moves into brain cells, the serum sodium level decreases; patients begin to have headache, nausea, vomiting, restlessness, anorexia, muscle cramps, lethargy, and confusion. The brain attempts to adapt quickly to hyponatremia by losing other intracellular solutes to decrease the chance of cerebral edema,[12] which then becomes a factor in treatment. Most patients with symptomatic hyponatremia have some sort of neurologic complaint; however, some may present with a traumatic complaint, such as after a fall.[1] If hyponatremia is not stabilized or corrected, patients can decompensate to seizures, coma, or even death.

Evaluation and Diagnosis

When the emergency physician cares for a patient with hyponatremia, the first step is to recognize the volume status of the patient and the plasma osmolality (**Fig. 2**).[3] True hyponatremia is present with low plasma osmolality; other types of hyponatremia are caused by fluid shifts resulting from osmotically active solutes, such as glucose, urea, or mannitol, or resulting from high levels of protein or lipids.[3] Patients with hyponatremia may be hypovolemic, euvolemic, or hypervolemic; the volume status of the patient often dictates different treatment strategies: fluid resuscitation versus fluid restriction. The types of hyponatremia along with the physical and laboratory signs that often accompany each type are presented in **Table 2**.

Urine electrolytes are helpful in guiding therapy before administration of medications or fluids, and these tests should be ordered in the emergency department if possible. The serum sodium deficit can be calculated using the following equation (Equation 3):

$$\text{Total body Na deficit (mEq/L)} = (\text{desired serum Na} - \text{actual serum Na}) \times \text{TBW}$$

3

However, most equations have some downfalls and do not account for the homeostatic principles governing human physiology, leading to multiple variations of these equations.[13,14] In this matter, the body is not a closed system, so although equations are useful to roughly gauge how much solution should be used initially, the clinician must continually reevaluate the patient and adjust treatment as needed.

Hypovolemic hyponatremia

Hypovolemic hyponatremia is a loss of TBW and sodium. Usually, the patient presents with signs and symptoms suggestive of dehydration, including low blood pressure, nausea, vomiting, and tachycardia. Losses of water and sodium can be caused by renal dysfunction, or renal function may be preserved. Examples of renal water losses include overzealous diuretic use, renal tubular acidosis, renal failure, and mineralocorticoid deficiency.[3] Examples of extrarenal water losses include diarrhea, vomiting, pulmonary losses, heat exposure, sweating, biliary drains, high-output gastrointestinal fistulas, third-space losses such as burns, or pancreatitis.[3,4] Patients with renal water

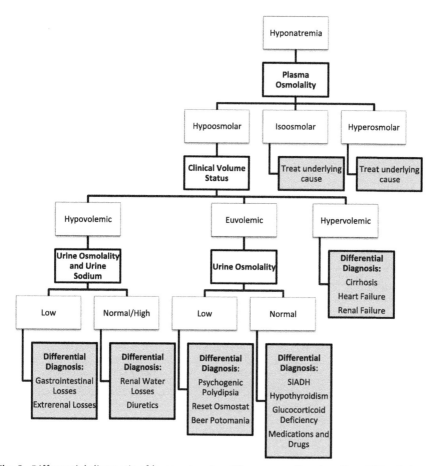

Fig. 2. Differential diagnosis of hyponatremia with serum sodium less than 135 mEq/L.

losses tend to have high urinary sodium, whereas patients with extrarenal water losses have low urinary sodium.

Hypervolemic hyponatremia

Hypervolemic hyponatremia, on the other hand, is often reflected by an increase in TBW, whereas sodium levels decrease. These patients typically present with symptoms of fluid overload, including peripheral edema, ascites, anasarca, or pulmonary edema. Commonly encountered patients with hypervolemic hyponatremia include patients with chronic renal failure, congestive heart failure, nephrotic syndrome, or cirrhosis.[3] Patients with renal failure and overload have high urinary sodium levels, whereas patients with cirrhosis, congestive heart failure, or nephrotic syndrome have low urinary sodium levels.

Euvolemic hyponatremia

Patients with euvolemic hyponatremia fall on the spectrum between hypovolemic and hypervolemic hyponatremia; they often have normal total body sodium levels, but have slightly decreased intravascular volume, without clinical signs of symptoms of dehydration.[3] The most common cause of euvolemic hyponatremia is the syndrome

Table 2
Classifications and causes of hyponatremia by volume status

Physical Signs	Laboratory Signs	Examples
Hypovolemic Hyponatremia		
Orthostasis	Low plasma osmolality	Gastrointestinal losses
Low blood pressure	Increased blood urea nitrogen level	Renal losses
Tachycardia	Hypokalemia	Diuretic use
	Low urine osmolality	Addison disease
	Low urine sodium level	Increased insensible losses
		Third-space shifts
Euvolemic Hyponatremia		
	Low plasma osmolality	Syndrome of inappropriate ADH
	High/low urine osmolality	Hypothyroidism
	High/low urine sodium level	Glucocorticoid deficiency
		Severe pain or nausea
		Trauma
		Beer potomania
		Psychogenic polydipsia
		Medications/drugs (**Table 4**)
Hypervolemic Hyponatremia		
Ascites	Low plasma osmolality	Cirrhosis
Edema	Low urine osmolality	Congestive heart failure
Anasarca	Low/high urine sodium level	Nephrotic syndrome
		Renal failure
Other Causes of Hyponatremia (Including High and Normal Plasma Osmolality Hyponatremias)		
Primary/secondary adipsia	Extreme hyperglycemia	Multiple myeloma
Hypodipsia	Hypertriglyceridemia	Hyperlipidemia
Increased urea level	Adrenal insufficiency	Mannitol

Data from Refs.[2,3,7,118]

of inappropriate ADH (SIADH). Causes of SIADH are varied, but include many central nervous system, pulmonary, and carcinoma causes (**Table 3**).[7,15–63] Euvolemic hyponatremia may also be caused by hypothyroidism, excessive pain, stress, nausea, or water intoxication caused by psychogenic polydipsia. Many types of medications can also cause euvolemic hyponatremia (see **Table 4**).

A subset of patients with euvolemic hyponatremia caused by SIADH have a phenomenon referred to as reset osmostat, the second most common form of SIADH.[16] These patients continue to regulate water excretion with ADH secretion, but their threshold is based around a lower serum osmolality set point, and release of ADH seems to be premature.[16] Patients are still able to suppress ADH and urinary dilution once they have retained sufficient free water, resulting in surpassing their set point and causing significant hyponatremia.[16] This preserved function is what separates these patients from other types of SIADH. The severity of hyponatremia in patients with reset osmostat is not based primarily on the amount of free water intake but also on the level of osmostat resetting.[7] The causes for having reset osmostat may be similar to those that predispose a person to any of the causes of SIADH: pulmonary, carcinoma, or central nervous system disease.[16] The exact mechanism by which reset osmostat occurs is still unknown, but it may be caused by interruption of the afferent limb of the baroregulatory reflex that inhibits ADH secretion.[15]

Patients who have recently ingested 3, 4-methylenedioxymethamphetamine (MDMA), also known commonly as the street drug ecstasy, may also present to the emergency department with SIADH. Previously, it was believed that excessive dancing, high amounts of sweating, and intake of large amounts of free water contributed to hyponatremia in the clubbing population, who may also be exposed to MDMA.[64–66] However, 1 high-profile case in 1995 resulting in the death of Leah Betts suggested that increased ADH production was believed to contribute to the patient's severe hyponatremia and water intoxication.[67] Previous studies with rat models have shown that MDMA causes increased levels of oxytocin and ADH,[68] but a recent study by Wolff and colleagues[63] on self-described human clubbing volunteers reported results consistent with SIADH after MDMA use. Emergency clinicians must be aware of this population, because many protocols of suspected or known drug ingestions receive large amounts of intravenous fluids during resuscitation; aggressive fluid resuscitation in these individuals exacerbates hyponatremia, possibly causing seizures, coma, or cerebral edema. If MDMA ingestion is suspected, the clinician should refrain from prophylactic intravenous fluids until serum or urine studies are available.[63,69]

- Clinicians should not reflexively administer intravenous fluids to patients after ingestion. Thoroughly evaluate the patient and decide if the patient requires fluids to increase intravascular volume.

Treatment

Unstable patients
When patients are acutely symptomatic from their hyponatremia, the physician must quickly identify and treat the sodium imbalance, because the risks of untreated hyponatremia clearly outweigh the risks of slow correction achieved with conservative measures. In a patient who is actively seizing, is neurologically compromised, or has respiratory arrest caused by hyponatremia, a bolus of hypertonic saline, given as 3% normal saline (NS) at a dose of 2 mL/kg (maximum 100 mL) should be given.[2,7,70–72] The bolus should be given over 10 to 60 minutes and can be repeated once if severe symptoms are still evident. A bolus of 2 mL/kg increases the serum sodium level by approximately 2 mEq/L. This increase in serum sodium level should stop current symptoms and prevent other severe neurologic consequences. During infusion of hypertonic saline, the patient and the serum sodium levels much be monitored closely to look for any signs of deteriorating neurologic status or symptoms of fluid overload, which may dictate further management.

- For the unstable hyponatremic patient, give 2 mL/kg of 3% NS up to 100 mL over 10 minutes; this may be repeated once if the patient continues to be unstable.

Stable patients
The treatment of hyponatremia in stable patients is otherwise based on the volume status of the patient. In patients with hypovolemic hyponatremia, intravascular repletion of volume is paramount. In patients with hypervolemic or euvolemic hyponatremia, fluid restriction or removal of excess fluid dictates care. The goals of treatment are to increase serum sodium levels and to not exceed a correction rate of 10 mEq/L to 12 mEq/L in the first 24 hours, with some experts suggesting not

to exceed 6 mEq/L in the first 24 hours. Overall, if the patient is asymptomatic, the clinician can focus on the cause of hyponatremia and direct their efforts to correcting that medical condition, rather than aggressively treating the hyponatremia.

The mainstay of treatment of hypovolemic hyponatremia is volume expansion. Intravenous fluid resuscitation must be initiated, and any underlying problem causing the hypovolemic hyponatremia must be corrected, including the removal of any medications that may be contributing. Once the patient is clinically euvolemic, the sodium level must be reassessed. If there continues to be a sodium imbalance, the clinician must then direct their attempts at correcting the sodium level as is appropriate. Often, the initial fluid used for resuscitation is 0.9% NS in the form of

Table 3 Common causes of SIADH	
Category	Cause of SIADH
Malignancy	Bladder carcinoma Duodenal carcinoma Ewing sarcoma Head or neck carcinoma Leukemia Lymphoma Mesothelioma Pancreatic carcinoma Pulmonary carcinoma Prostatic carcinoma Sarcoma Thymoma Ureteral carcinoma
Pulmonary	Acute respiratory failure Asthma Cystic fibrosis Empyema Pneumonia Pneumothorax Positive pressure ventilation Tuberculosis
Central nervous system	Acute intermittent porphyria Acute psychosis Agenesis of corpus callosum Atrophy of cerebrum or cerebellum Brain abscess Brain tumors Cavernous sinus thrombosis Cerebrovascular accidents Delirium tremens Guillain-Barré syndrome Encephalitis Head trauma Hydrocephalus Meningitis Multiple system atrophy Neonatal hypoxia Rocky Mountain spotted fever Subarachnoid hemorrhage

(continued on next page)

Table 3 (continued)	
Category	**Cause of SIADH**
Medications/drugs	Alcohol abuse and malnutrition
	Butyrophenones
	Carbamazepine
	Cisplatin
	Chlorpropamide
	Clofibrate
	Cyclophosphamide
	Cytoxan
	Desmopressin
	Ecstasy
	Interferon α and γ
	Methotrexate
	Monoamine oxidase inhibitors
	Monoclonal antibodies
	Morphine
	Nicotine
	Nonsteroidal antiinflammatory drugs
	Opiates
	Oxcarbazepine
	Oxytocin
	Phenothiazines
	Selective serotonin reuptake inhibitors
	Sodium valproate
	Thiazide diuretics
	Tricyclic antidepressants
	Vasopressin
	Vinca alkaloids
Other	AIDS
	Glucocorticoid insufficiency
	Idiopathic
	Myxedema
	Postoperative period

Data from Refs.[7,15–63]

fluid boluses. As the intravascular volume is restored, ADH is no longer secreted, renal function improves, and excess free water given during fluid resuscitation can be excreted. Because of this homeostatic balance and the changes that continue to occur, during resuscitation, sodium levels must be carefully monitored. In addition, the clinician must ensure strict monitoring of urine output; the patient may require a Foley catheter to be placed if unable to assist with this monitoring. In patients with preserved renal function, the sodium level should increase slowly but appropriately; however, if serum sodium levels begin to increase too quickly and free water is excreted, as in the patient with recovering renal function or previous renal impairment, hypotonic fluids such as 0.45% NS or even D5W (dextrose 5% in water solution) may be necessary.

Treatment of patients with hypervolemic and euvolemic hyponatremia frequently and most commonly entails sodium and water restriction, occasionally with adjunctive use of furosemide or another loop diuretic in specific situations. However, in stable patients, optimization of the underlying medical condition usually corrects the hyponatremia. Special attention must be placed on correction of hypokalemia, because repletion of potassium also increases the serum sodium level.

Table 4
Common medications or classes of medications that may cause hyponatremia

Acetaminophen	Angiotensin-Converting Enzyme Inhibitors	Antiaggregant
ADH	Barbiturates	β-Blockers
Carbamazepine	Carboplatin	Cisplatin
Clofibrate	Colchicine	Cyclophosphamide
Desmopressin	Haloperidol	Isoproterenol
Loop diuretics	Monoamine oxidase inhibitors	Morphine
Nicotine	Nonsteroidal antiinflammatory drug	Opioids
Oxcarbazepine	Oxytocin	Phenothiazines
Proton pump inhibitors	Psychotropics	Selective serotonin reuptake inhibitors
Sodium valproate	Sulfonylureas	
Thiazide diuretics	Tolbutamide	Tricyclic antidepressants
Venlafaxine	Vinca alkaloids	Vincristine

Data from Refs.[1–3,6,15]

Another treatment modality available to treat euvolemic and hypervolemic hyponatremia is the use of vaptans. Previously, these subgroups of patients with hyponatremia had to endure uncomfortable fluid restrictions, loop diuretics such as furosemide, which can cause other electrolyte imbalances, or medications that caused additional side effects such as demeclocycline, lithium, or phenytoin.[15,73] With the advent of vasopressin receptor antagonists, also known as vaptans, patients with chronic euvolemic or hypervolemic hyponatremia have another option for treatment. Vaptans bind to vasopressin type 1 (V1) or type 2 (V2) receptors; V2 receptors are expressed in the renal collecting duct cells. Vaptans block the binding of ADH onto V2 receptors, preventing free water reabsorption and causing increased urine volume.[73] The diuresis caused by vaptans is similar in quantity to the diuresis induced by furosemide, but there is not an increase in excretion of electrolytes.[73] This diuresis of water with relative sparing of electrolytes by vaptans is termed aquaresis; aquaresis decreases urine osmolality and causes an increase in serum sodium.[73] Two options are available in the United States: an intravenous preparation, conivaptan, and an oral preparation, tolvaptan.[72] Conivaptan is a combined vasopressin receptor antagonist to V1 and V2 receptors and is indicated for short-term treatment of hospitalized patients.[72] Tolvaptan is a selective V2 receptor antagonist, but per the US Food and Drug Administration should not be used for longer than 30 days.[72] Side effects include dry mouth, thirst, and increased urination. Both of these vaptans have the possibility of causing hepatic injury, and caution should be used when administering the medication to patients with known liver disease.[72] Frequent monitoring of liver enzymes is warranted in all patients receiving the medications, and total therapy length should be limited in patients with any evidence of emerging liver disease.[72]

Vaptans may play a role in the treatment of chronic euvolemic and hypervolemic hyponatremia, but there have been no studies that have evaluated their use in the setting of acute hyponatremia that is seen in the emergency department and there is no current role in the treatment of acute symptomatic hyponatremia.

- Stable patients with hyponatremia should have their serum sodium level corrected no faster than 10 mEq/L to 12 mEq/L over the first 24 hours.

Cerebral Edema

Cerebral edema through the shift of water from extracellular stores occurs to balance out the relative hyponatremia in the vascular space. Patients particularly at risk for cerebral edema include postmenopausal women, women on thiazide diuretics, children, psychiatric patients with polydipsia, and hypoxemic patients.[71] To combat this shift from causing too many homeostatic changes, the brain quickly loses solutes to try to prevent profound cerebral edema.[12] However, if the hyponatremia is corrected too quickly with these homeostatic balancing mechanisms intact, brain cells can shrink as serum sodium is repleted.[7] From multiple studies, it has been well established that correction of the sodium should not occur quicker than approximately 0.5 to 1 mEq/L/h or a total of 10 to 12 mEq/L per 24 hours,[3,70,71,74–77] again with some experts recommending not to exceed 6 mEq/L. Once a hyponatremic patient has been identified and treatment has been started, the clinician should check electrolyte levels frequently; in the most symptomatic of patients, checking levels of sodium every 2 hours is prudent and allows close guidance of medical therapy. It has been shown in case reports that if the patient's sodium level begins to correct too quickly and adjustment of the intravenous fluids is not adequate to slow the change, the hyponatremic patient may require infusion of hypotonic fluids to decrease the sodium level again.[78–80] These measures are to prevent the most dreaded complication known as osmotic demyelination syndrome.

Osmotic Demyelination Syndrome

Osmotic demyelination syndrome was first described in the medical literature in 1959[81] and is the iatrogenic irreversible clinical syndrome of neurologic symptoms that occurs after too rapid of a correction of serum sodium.[77] A subset of this syndrome is known as central pontine myelinolysis, when the effects are primarily seen from damage in the brainstem; however, many patients with the syndrome have other foci of demyelination within the central nervous system anywhere throughout the nervous system.[77,82] This severe complication is caused by exceeding generally agreed safe limits of serum sodium correction, with corrections greater than 12 mEq/L in 24 hours, 25 mEq/L in 48 hours, or inadvertent hypernatremia during correction of hyponatremia.[77,83] The nervous system damage is postulated to be caused by rapid swelling of brain and nervous system parenchyma during fluid resuscitation, because this tissue cannot adapt quick enough to the changing osmolality. Patients with chronic hyponatremia may be particularly susceptible to osmotic demyelination syndrome, especially those with underlying alcoholism, malnutrition, toxins, hypoxia, other central nervous system disease, or other metabolic syndromes.[3,7,71,74,77,81–83] Symptoms of osmotic demyelination syndrome include fluctuating levels of consciousness or confusion, behavioral changes, dysarthria, mutism, dysphagia, and seizures.[3,77,82] These symptoms may culminate in a devastating condition, including a locked-in state, in which the patients are awake but unable to move or communicate, or quadriparesis.[3,77]

Despite the severity of osmotic demyelination syndrome, and the devastating results that may ensue, the possibility of the syndrome should not prevent a clinician from aggressively treating symptomatic patients with hyponatremia. Most neurologic symptoms associated with hyponatremia are from cerebral edema and herniation,[71,84–86] so patients with symptomatic hyponatremia require immediate treatment. Without prompt treatment, patients may progress to severe seizures, coma, or death; the risk to the patient outweighs the risk of osmotic demyelination syndrome when they are severely symptomatic.

Pediatric Considerations

In general, any child who requires intravenous fluid administration should be considered to be at risk for development of hyponatremia.[87] The use of intravenous fluids in the pediatric population should be considered an invasive treatment and the same amount of care and attention should be applied as when administering any other medication.[87]

Children may be at higher risk for development of cerebral edema because of the physiologic nature of a higher ratio of brain volume to skull size.[71] The true incidence of symptomatic hyponatremia in children is not known because of lack of prospective studies.[87] However, 1 retrospective review[88] found approximately 22% of children who were admitted to the hospital had hyponatremia, and symptomatic hyponatremia was found in 10% of children younger than 2 years presenting to the emergency department with seizures.[89] Of those children with hyponatremia, 53% to 78% with serum sodium level less than 125 mEq/L developed symptomatic hyponatremia.[70,90,91] Children particularly at risk for hyponatremia include those younger than 16 years and children with hypoxia.[87] Hypoxia is the strongest predictor of mortality in pediatric patients with symptomatic hyponatremia.[92] Hyponatremia from SIADH is particularly noxious in children with neurologic injury such as encephalitis; mild hyponatremia has been associated with significant neurologic sequelae, including herniation.[93,94] Special attention and close monitoring of serum sodium level in any child at risk for hyponatremia or with any of these conditions is necessary to prevent serious neurologic complications.

Symptomatic hyponatremia should always be aggressively treated with the use of hypertonic 3% saline.[87] The serum sodium level should be increased by approximately 1 mEq/L per hour until the patient is seizure free, the serum sodium has corrected to 125 to 130 mEq/L, or the serum sodium level has increased by 20 mEq/L.[70,71,83,95,96] The optimal rate of correction of serum sodium level seems to be between 15 and 20 mEq/L over the first 48 hours, because patients with this range of correction have lower mortality and better neurologic outcome compared with those with slower correction.[83,86]

- Hypotonic fluids are no longer recommended for maintenance fluids in the pediatric population because of iatrogenic hyponatremia.

HYPERNATREMIA

Hypernatremia is defined as serum sodium level greater than 145 mEq/L and is less common than hyponatremia. Most commonly, hypernatremia occurs in hospitalized patients, but it can also occur in approximately 0.2% of patients who present to the emergency department.[97]

Hypernatremia is always associated with intracellular dehydration caused by decrease of TBW and is always associated with decreased intake of free water. As a result of losses through bowel, urine, and pulmonary losses, without adequate water intake to overcome these losses, a patient becomes more and more dehydrated and hypernatremic unless the patient ingests enough free water, even if the renal function is intact.[7] Hypernatremia commonly occurs in patients with impaired thirst mechanisms, or inability to acquire adequate free water, such as in the elderly, infants, or otherwise impaired individuals (eg, patients on a ventilator, in a coma). Excessive water loss may further contribute to hypernatremia, but again, unless the thirst mechanism or access to water is limited, the patient should be able to compensate with increased ingestion of free water.[7,98]

Signs and Symptoms

Symptoms of hypernatremia are similar to those of hyponatremia, because of effects that are again based primarily on the central nervous system.[1,99] During hypernatremia, brain cells shrink substantially as water moves into the extracellular space. This situation can cause intracerebral hemorrhage as a result of tearing of cerebral blood vessels.[3,100] Other consequences of hypernatremia include decreased left ventricular contractility, hyperventilation, impaired glucose use, muscle cramps, and rhabdomyolysis.[99] Patients may present with lethargy, weakness, or restlessness; infants may present with irritability. Neurologic examination may show increased tone, nuchal rigidity, brisk reflexes, myoclonus, asterixis, chorea, or seizures.[87] If not assessed and treated appropriately, the patient may progress to seizures, coma, or death.[3,12,101] One study[1] found that patients with hypernatremia are less likely to receive specific care for the dysnatremia, and have higher in-hospital mortality. Symptoms are again related not only to the absolute increase in serum sodium levels but also to the rapidity at which the increase occurs, because this correlates with the speed of brain cell dehydration.[7]

Evaluation and Diagnosis

The initial step in evaluating a patient with hypernatremia is to again start with the volume status of the patient. The volume status then helps guide the clinician to specific treatments (**Fig. 3**).

Hypovolemic hypernatremia

Hypovolemic hypernatremia is usually caused by an inability to detect or respond to the sensation of thirst. Primary adipsia or hypodipsia is caused by damage of the

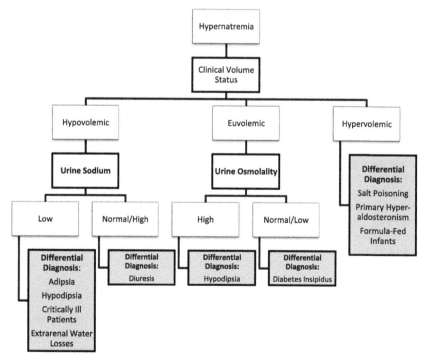

Fig. 3. Differential diagnosis of hypernatremia with serum sodium greater than 145 mEq/L.

hypothalamic osmoreceptors that cause the thirst mechanism when plasma osmolality begins to increase.[102,103] This situation typically occurs in alert and awake patients without neurologic defects and without limited access to free water. The cause of hypernatremia in these patients tends to be the limited ingestion of free water. Critically ill patients are at a high risk for the development of hypernatremia. In these patients, careful monitoring of serum sodium and water intake and output is necessary to prevent unwanted neurologic consequences.[104]

Another cause of hypovolemic hypernatremia is from secondary adipsia or hypodipsia resulting from lesions that spare the hypothalamic osmoreceptors but affect consciousness, speech, physical ability, or prevent absorption of water from the gastrointestinal tract.[7] Most commonly, these patients are obtunded because of medical conditions such as hyperglycemia, or patients who have suffered strokes, or postoperative patients with increased renal or extrarenal losses along with decreased mentation or limited water intake.[7]

- Critically ill patients and those patients at risk for developing decreased water intake should have electrolytes monitored frequently to ensure that serum sodium levels are not increasing.

Hypervolemic hypernatremia

Hypervolemic hypernatremia is almost never sporadic, but usually is the result of iatrogenic complications, or accidental or intentional poisoning. Examples of hypervolemic hypernatremia include the administration of sodium bicarbonate during cardiac arrest or during the treatment of acidosis, the previous use of hypertonic saline during therapeutic abortions, and the improper preparation of solutions for enteral or parenteral feedings, or peritoneal dialysis.[3,105–107] Infants seem to be the population most at risk for hypervolemic hypernatremia, because they are less able to excrete a high sodium load, and they are unable to ask for or acquire water. In addition, infants who are fed formula may accidently ingest a hyperosmolal solution as a result of an improperly prepared solution. Primary hyperaldosteronism can also lead to hypervolemic hypernatremia; however, the level of hypernatremia is typically milder and does not lead to neurologic symptoms.

- Formula-fed infants with neurologic changes should have serum sodium levels checked, and caregivers should be questioned about how they prepare formula.

Euvolemic hypernatremia

Euvolemic hypernatremia is most often caused by diabetes insipidus. In this disease, the body does not respond to ADH, either peripherally or centrally. Because of the lack of ADH response, the patient continues to make maximally dilute urine with low urine osmolality. Sodium excretion in the urine continues, but is less than the overall amount of water excreted, thus resulting in hypernatremia. Causes of diabetes insipidus are divided into 2 categories: central and nephrogenic. Common causes of central diabetes insipidus are trauma, pituitary surgery, and malignancies.[3] Common causes of nephrogenic diabetes insipidus include renal disease, medications, and genetic disorders.[3]

Treatment

Unstable patients

Acute hypernatremia carries mortality between 28% and 70%.[1,3,7] Symptoms most often are caused by the rapidity of change of sodium level, not necessarily the overall deficit; therefore, sodium correction should occur over roughly the same time period that it occurred. The fear of cerebral edema should be displaced by the clinician when treating the patient with acute hypernatremia; idiogenic osmoles, organic molecules that attempt to maintain brain cell hydration, have not had time to appear in brain cells, and the risk of cerebral edema with fast correction is minimal compared with the mortality and morbidity associated with acute hypernatremia.[3,12] Correction of hypernatremia should be initiated with isotonic fluids and should occur over a minimum of 48 hours. The serum sodium level should not decrease by more than 8 to 15 mEq/L in any 8-hour period if the patient is symptomatic.[4,100,108,109] Overly rapid correction of hypernatremia with the use of hypotonic fluids may lead to seizures, permanent brain damage, or death.[7,100,108,110]

If the patient with hypernatremia shows evidence of dehydration, fluid resuscitation should take first priority, and the patient should be provided with adequate amounts of intravenous fluid to restore plasma volumes. Isotonic solutions should be used in these situations, because the patient normally has hypernatremia as a result of hypovolemia and isotonic solutions are likely still relatively hypotonic compared with the patient's serum. However, the serum sodium must be closely monitored to prevent correction from happening too quickly and leading to additional neurologic problems.[7] Approximately half of the water deficit should be provided in the first 12 to 24 hours, and the other half should be provided over the next 24 hours.[4] The free water deficit in adults can be calculated by the following equation (Equation 4):

$$\text{Water deficit (L)} = [(\text{measured Na/normal Na}) - 1] \qquad\qquad 4$$

Again, frequent measurements of serum sodium to allow quick tailoring of therapy are necessary, because patients often do not precisely follow the guidelines used by the clinician. If correction occurs too rapidly, or if the patient begins to show symptoms of cerebral edema or hyponatremia, the clinician should immediately stop treatment of hypernatremia, and treat the patient as if they have hyponatremia with fluid restriction or addition of electrolytes/saline to the fluid infusion.

- Unstable patients with hypernatremia should receive isotonic fluids, with a goal to lower the serum sodium by 8 mEq/L to 15 mEq/L over the first 8 hours.

Stable patients

Chronic or slowly occurring hypernatremia does not cause as many symptoms and does not carry as high mortality, because of the presence of idiogenic osmoles.[3,12] Because of the brain's self-preservation strategy by production of idiogenic osmoles that allows relative maintenance of brain cell hydration,[3,12] rapid restoration of serum sodium levels to normal in patients with chronic hypernatremia may cause further complications because of resultant cerebral edema caused by these organic molecules. In the asymptomatic patient, correction of the serum sodium level should occur slowly, at a rate no greater than 0.5 mEq/L/h and no more than 8 mEq/L to 15 mEq/L per day.[3,4,99,100]

The specific causes of hypernatremia also have specific treatments tailored to the nature of the serum sodium excess. In cases of accidental excess sodium excretion, removal of sodium is the goal of treatment. If the patient is asymptomatic and has normal renal function, then the clinician may wait for natural excretion, which should not cause large shifts in brain cell hydration status. If renal function is impaired, then excess sodium needs to be removed through phlebotomy or dialysis. In patients with adipsia or hypodipsia, whether primary or secondary, patient, family, and caregiver education is paramount. The patient, family, or caregiver needs explanation about sensible and insensible water losses, the need for replacement daily of these losses, and how to monitor and accurately adjust water needs on a day-to-day basis.

With adequate education and frequent follow-up visits assessing hydration and serum sodium levels, these patients may remain eunatremic and euvolemic.

- Stable patients with hypernatremia should have serum sodium corrected by 8 mEq/L to 15 mEq/L per day until the sodium has normalized.

Pediatric Considerations

Hypernatremia in pediatric populations is rare outside other medical problems. Hypernatremia was found to occur in approximately only 0.004% of newborns and accounts for only approximately 0.04% of pediatric hospital admissions.[111] However, hypernatremia is associated with mortality of 15% in children,[18] and when encountered by the clinician, it should be taken seriously. Mild hypernatremia should not be considered benign, but rather should prompt further investigation and prompt attention to free-water administration.[87] Children that have particularly high mortality and morbidity associated with hypernatremia are infants with hypernatremic dehydration and children with end-stage liver disease.[111–114]

The outpatient pediatric group at highest risk of developing hypernatremia is breast-fed infants.[115] Infants that are primarily breast-fed and have more than 7% weight loss or who have jaundice should undergo prompt evaluation for hypernatremia.[87] Dehydration caused by diarrhea is another cause of acute hypernatremia[111]; however, because of the widespread availability of oral rehydration solutions, clinicians are seeing these patients less commonly.[87]

Pediatric patients with hypernatremia often have hypovolemia, and attention must first focus on correction of volume status. Once oral hydration can be tolerated, it should be used because oral hydration allows acute hypernatremia to be corrected faster, and leads to fewer seizures.[116]

- Breast-fed infants are one of the highest-risk groups for developing hypernatremia caused by dehydration; when possible, oral rehydration is preferred, because of decreased risk of complications.

FLUIDS USED FOR RESUSCITATION

In most cases of sodium imbalance, intravascular volume is depleted. The first priority of management in a patient with dysnatremia when associated with hypovolemia is restoration of the intravascular space. Infusion of isotonic 0.9% NS is the best initial fluid choice. In patients with preserved renal function, the patient excretes either excess sodium or water through the urine.[2,7] Even if the patient does not have normal renal function, intravascular volume takes priority over sodium balance.

The clinician should be aware of the fluids available for treatment (**Table 5**), should recognize the importance of the composition of each of the different types of fluids, and should treat intravenous fluids as any other medication prescribed to the patient.[4] Many complications can occur in electrolyte and water balance if a patient receives all of their fluids intravenously,[4] and the clinician should be aware of these possible complications.

Normotonic or isotonic fluids, such as 0.9% NS and lactated Ringer solution, are so named because they have an osmolality similar to that of plasma, approximately 275 to 295 mOsm/L H_2O. Because of the risk of osmotic demyelination syndrome associated with overly rapid correction of hyponatremia,[77] hypertonic saline greater than 3% NS is rarely used for correction. Some recommend initial intravascular volume repletion with solution closer to the electrolyte balance of plasma such as

Table 5
Sodium concentrations in fluid compartments and commonly used intravenous fluids

Fluid	Sodium Concentration (mEq/L)
Plasma	140
0.9% NS	154
0.45% NS	77
3% NS	513
Lactated Ringer solution	130
D5W	0
0.45% NS + 75 mEq sodium bicarbonate	152

lactated Ringer solution,[2] but most use 0.9% NS as the primary resuscitation fluid.[7] D5W, 0.45% NS, or any other hypotonic fluids should not be used as primary resuscitation fluids, because these fluids can lead to osmotic diuresis; instead, they should be preserved for maintenance fluids only.[4]

The clinician must seriously consider the amount and type of intravenous fluid used in treatment of pediatric patients. Hypotonic fluids, once routinely recommended for use in pediatric patients,[117] have been linked to more than 50 deaths or neurologic injuries in children after resultant hyponatremia.[87] Recommendations now exist that hypotonic fluids should be avoided in the pediatric population unless there is a well-established free-water deficit, hypernatremia, or ongoing water losses.[87,88] Most children evaluated in the emergency department and found to be in need of intravenous fluids have some signs of volume depletion.[87] Current recommendations state that these children should receive isotonic intravenous fluids, similar to the recommendations in adults.[87,88] Isotonic fluid administration in children, as in adults, should not result in hypernatremia or fluid overload unless there is a defect in excretion of excess sodium or free water.[87]

SUMMARY

Disorders of sodium and water occur simultaneously. The emergency physician must be aware of these disorders to quickly and accurately identify them in life-threatening situations. Often, disorders of sodium and water are chronic, but acute cases require rapid intervention. Before evaluation or possible correction of a sodium imbalance, the clinician must correct any intravascular volume losses. This correction is best achieved by infusion of isotonic NS. If depleted intravascular volume is the main cause of the sodium imbalance and renal function remains normal, the sodium imbalance should autocorrect without any neurologic side effects.

Overall, hyponatremia is often caused by a defect in water excretion, whereas hypernatremia is often caused by a defect in thirst regulation or water acquisition. Because of dreaded neurologic complications, the imbalance in the serum sodium should be corrected in approximately the same time frame as it initially occurred. Overly rapid correction may cause osmotic demyelination syndrome in patients with hyponatremia, or cerebral edema in patients with hypernatremia. Narrow control of the disorder of sodium balance should be the goal of the clinician. Emergency physicians should be aware that these imbalances of water and sodium are frequently encountered in the emergency department and should be aware of the pathophysiology that regulates them and the appropriate treatments based on patient symptoms and the underlying cause of the dysnatremia.

REFERENCES

1. Arampatzis S, Frauchiger B, Fiedler GM, et al. Characteristics, symptoms, and outcome of severe dysnatremias present on hospital admission. Am J Med 2012;125:1125.e1–7.
2. Wilson RF, Sibbald WJ. Fluid and electrolyte problems in the emergency department. JACEP 1976;5:339–46.
3. Kelen G, Hsu E. Fluids and electrolytes. In: Tintinalli J, editor. Tintinalli's emergency medicine: a comprehensive study guide. 7th edition. New York: McGraw Hill Medical; 2011. p. 117–21.
4. Kaplan LJ, Kellum JA. Fluids, pH, ions and electrolytes. Curr Opin Crit Care 2010;16:323–31.
5. Verney EB. Absorption and excretion of water; the antidiuretic hormone. Lancet 1946;2:739, 781.
6. Liamis G, Milionis H, Elisaf M. A review of drug-induced hyponatremia. Am J Kidney Dis 2008;52:144–53.
7. Kovacs L, Robertson GL. Disorders of water balance–hyponatraemia and hypernatraemia. Baillieres Clin Endocrinol Metab 1992;6:107–27.
8. Boscoe A, Paramore C, Verbalis JG. Cost of illness of hyponatremia in the United States. Cost Eff Resour Alloc 2006;4:10.
9. Lee CT, Guo HR, Chen JB. Hyponatremia in the emergency department. Am J Emerg Med 2000;18:264–8.
10. Waikar SS, Mount DB, Curhan GC. Mortality after hospitalization with mild, moderate, and severe hyponatremia. Am J Emerg Med 2009;122:857–65.
11. Hoorn EJ, Zietse R. Hyponatremia and mortality: moving beyond associations. Am J Kidney Dis 2013;62(1):139–49.
12. Arieff AI, Guisado R. Effects on the central nervous system of hypernatremic and hyponatremic states. Kidney Int 1976;10:104–16.
13. Adrogue HJ, Madias NE. Hyponatremia. N Engl J Med 2000;342:1581–9.
14. Tzamaloukas AH, Malhotra D, Rosen BH, et al. Principles of management of severe hyponatremia. J Am Heart Assoc 2013;2:e005199.
15. Baylis PH. The syndrome of inappropriate antidiuretic hormone secretion. Int J Biochem Cell Biol 2003;35:1495–9.
16. Zerbe R, Stropes L, Robertson G. Vasopressin function in the syndrome of inappropriate antidiuresis. Annu Rev Med 1980;31:315–27.
17. DeFronzo RA, Goldberg M, Agus ZS. Normal diluting capacity in hyponatremic patients. Reset osmostat or a variant of the syndrome of inappropriate antidiuretic hormone secretion. Ann Intern Med 1976;84:538–42.
18. Moritz ML, Ayus JC. The changing pattern of hypernatremia in hospitalized children. Pediatrics 1999;104:435–9.
19. Luzecky MH, Burman KD, Schultz ER. The syndrome of inappropriate secretion of antidiuretic hormone associated with amitriptyline administration. South Med J 1974;67:495–7.
20. ten Holt WL, van Iperen CE, Schrijver G, et al. Severe hyponatremia during therapy with fluoxetine. Arch Intern Med 1996;156:681–2.
21. Jackson C, Carson W, Markowitz J, et al. SIADH associated with fluoxetine and sertraline therapy. Am J Psychiatry 1995;152:809–10.
22. Liu BA, Mittmann N, Knowles SR, et al. Hyponatremia and the syndrome of inappropriate secretion of antidiuretic hormone associated with the use of selective serotonin reuptake inhibitors: a review of spontaneous reports. CMAJ 1996;155:519–27.

23. Jacob S, Spinler SA. Hyponatremia associated with selective serotonin-reuptake inhibitors in older adults. Ann Pharmacother 2006;40:1618–22.
24. Movig KL, Leufkens HG, Lenderink AW, et al. Association between antidepressant drug use and hyponatraemia: a case-control study. Br J Clin Pharmacol 2002;53:363–9.
25. Peterson JC, Pollack RW, Mahoney JJ, et al. Inappropriate antidiuretic hormone secondary to a monamine oxidase inhibitor. JAMA 1978;239:1422–3.
26. Vincent FM, Emery S. Antidiuretic hormone syndrome and thioridazine. Ann Intern Med 1978;89:147–8.
27. Rao KJ, Miller M, Moses A. Water intoxication and thioridazine (Mellaril). Ann Intern Med 1975;82:61.
28. Peck V, Shenkman L. Haloperidol-induced syndrome of inappropriate secretion of antidiuretic hormone. Clin Pharmacol Ther 1979;26:442–4.
29. Meinders AE, Cejka V, Robertson GL. The antidiuretic action of carbamazepine in man. Clin Sci Mol Med 1974;47:289–99.
30. Gold PW, Robertson GL, Ballenger JC, et al. Carbamazepine diminishes the sensitivity of the plasma arginine vasopressin response to osmotic stimulation. J Clin Endocrinol Metab 1983;57:952–7.
31. Flegel KM, Cole CH. Inappropriate antidiuresis during carbamazepine treatment. Ann Intern Med 1977;87:722–3.
32. Van Amelsvoort T, Bakshi R, Devaux CB, et al. Hyponatremia associated with carbamazepine and oxcarbazepine therapy: a review. Epilepsia 1994;35:181–8.
33. Kuz GM, Manssourian A. Carbamazepine-induced hyponatremia: assessment of risk factors. Ann Pharmacother 2005;39:1943–6.
34. Holtschmidt-Taschner B, Soyka M. Hyponatremia-induced seizure during carbamazepine treatment. World J Biol Psychiatry 2007;8:51–3.
35. Dong X, Leppik IE, White J, et al. Hyponatremia from oxcarbazepine and carbamazepine. Neurology 2005;65:1976–8.
36. Nielsen OA, Johannessen AC, Bardrum B. Oxcarbazepine-induced hyponatremia, a cross-sectional study. Epilepsy Res 1988;2:269–71.
37. Ikeda K, Moriyasu H, Yasaka M, et al. Valproate related syndrome of inappropriate secretion of antidiuretic hormone (SIADH)–a case report. Rinsho Shinkeigaku 1994;34:911–3.
38. Robertson GL, Bhoopalam N, Zelkowitz LJ. Vincristine neurotoxicity and abnormal secretion of antidiuretic hormone. Arch Intern Med 1973;132:717–20.
39. Ravikumar TS, Grage TB. The syndrome of inappropriate ADH secretion secondary to vinblastine-bleomycin therapy. J Surg Oncol 1983;24:242–5.
40. Raftopoulos H. Diagnosis and management of hyponatremia in cancer patients. Support Care Cancer 2007;15:1341–7.
41. Berghmans T. Hyponatremia related to medical anticancer treatment. Support Care Cancer 1996;4:341–50.
42. Lee YK, Shin DM. Renal salt wasting in patients treated with high-dose cisplatin, etoposide, and mitomycin in patients with advanced non-small cell lung cancer. Korean J Intern Med 1992;7:118–21.
43. Giaccone G, Donadio M, Ferrati P, et al. Disorders of serum electrolytes and renal function in patients treated with cis-platinum on an outpatient basis. Eur J Cancer Clin Oncol 1985;21:433–7.
44. DeFronzo RA, Braine H, Colvin M, et al. Water intoxication in man after cyclophosphamide therapy. Time course and relation to drug activation. Ann Intern Med 1973;78:861–9.

45. Bressler RB, Huston DP. Water intoxication following moderate-dose intravenous cyclophosphamide. Arch Intern Med 1985;145:548–9.
46. Harlow PJ, DeClerck YA, Shore NA, et al. A fatal case of inappropriate ADH secretion induced by cyclophosphamide therapy. Cancer 1979;44:896–8.
47. Frahm H, von Hulst M. Increased secretion of vasopressin and edema formation in high dosage methotrexate therapy. Z Gesamte Inn Med 1988;43:411–4.
48. Langfeldt LA, Cooley ME. Syndrome of inappropriate antidiuretic hormone secretion in malignancy: review and implications for nursing management. Clin J Oncol Nurs 2003;7:425–30.
49. Johnson BE, Chute JP, Rushin J, et al. A prospective study of patients with lung cancer and hyponatremia of malignancy. Am J Respir Crit Care Med 1997;156:1669–78.
50. Sorensen JB, Andersen MK, Hansen HH. Syndrome of inappropriate secretion of antidiuretic hormone (SIADH) in malignant disease. J Intern Med 1995;238:97–110.
51. Klein LA, Rabson AS, Worksman J. In vitro synthesis of vasopressin by lung tumor cells. Surg Forum 1969;20:231–3.
52. Talmi YP, Hoffman HT, McCabe BF. Syndrome of inappropriate secretion of arginine vasopressin in patients with cancer of the head and neck. Ann Otol Rhinol Laryngol 1992;101:946–9.
53. Cullen MJ, Cusack DA, O'Briain DS, et al. Neurosecretion of arginine vasopressin by an olfactory neuroblastoma causing reversible syndrome of antidiuresis. Am J Med 1986;81:911–6.
54. Marks LJ, Berde B, Klein LA, et al. Inappropriate vasopressin secretion and carcinoma of the pancreas. Am J Med 1968;45:967–74.
55. Eliakim R, Vertman E, Shinhar E. Syndrome of inappropriate secretion of antidiuretic hormone in Hodgkin's disease. Am J Med Sci 1986;291:126–7.
56. Belton K, Thomas SH. Drug-induced syndrome of inappropriate antidiuretic hormone secretion. Postgrad Med J 1999;75:509–10.
57. Cusick JF, Hagen TC, Findling JW. Inappropriate secretion of antidiuretic hormone after transsphenoidal surgery for pituitary tumors. N Engl J Med 1984;311:36–8.
58. Anderson RJ, Pluss RG, Berns AS, et al. Mechanism of effect of hypoxia on renal water excretion. J Clin Invest 1978;62:769–77.
59. Fabian TJ, Amico JA, Kroboth PD, et al. Paroxetine-induced hyponatremia in the elderly due to the syndrome of inappropriate secretion of antidiuretic hormone (SIADH). J Geriatr Psychiatry Neurol 2003;16:160–4.
60. Kimelman N, Albert SG. Phenothiazine-induced hyponatremia in the elderly. Gerontology 1984;30:132–6.
61. Ishii K, Aoki Y, Sasaki M, et al. Syndrome of inappropriate secretion of antidiuretic hormone induced by intraarterial cisplatin chemotherapy. Gynecol Oncol 2002;87:150–1.
62. Kadowaki T, Hagura R, Kajinuma H, et al. Chlorpropamide-induced hyponatremia: incidence and risk factors. Diabetes Care 1983;6:468–71.
63. Wolff K, Tsapakis EM, Winstock AR, et al. Vasopressin and oxytocin secretion in response to the consumption of ecstasy in a clubbing population. J Psychopharmacol 2006;20:400–10.
64. McCann UD, Eligulashvili V, Ricaurte GA. (+/-)3,4-Methylenedioxymethamphetamine ('ecstasy')-induced serotonin neurotoxicity: clinical studies. Neuropsychobiology 2000;42:11–6.

65. Kalant H. The pharmacology and toxicology of "ecstasy" (MDMA) and related drugs. CMAJ 2001;165:917–28.
66. Matthai SM, Davidson DC, Sills JA, et al. Cerebral oedema after ingestion of MDMA ("ecstasy") and unrestricted intake of water. BMJ 1996;312:1359.
67. Laurence J. Ecstasy: safety report. The Times 1995.
68. Forsling ML, Fallon JK, Shah D, et al. The effect of 3,4-methylenedioxymetham-phetamine (MDMA, 'ecstasy') and its metabolites on neurohypophysial hormone release from the isolated rat hypothalamus. Br J Pharmacol 2002;135:649–56.
69. Farah R. Ecstasy (3,4-methylenedioxymethamphetamine)-induced inappropriate antidiuretic hormone secretion. Pediatr Emerg Care 2008;24:615–7.
70. Sarnaik AP, Meert K, Hackbarth R, et al. Management of hyponatremic seizures in children with hypertonic saline: a safe and effective strategy. Crit Care Med 1991;19:758–62.
71. Lauriat SM, Berl T. The hyponatremic patient: practical focus on therapy. J Am Soc Nephrol 1997;8:1599–607.
72. Lehrich RW, Ortiz-Melo DI, Patel MB, et al. Role of vaptans in the management of hyponatremia. Am J Kidney Dis 2013;62:364–76.
73. Peri A. The use of vaptans in clinical endocrinology. J Clin Endocrinol Metab 2013;98:1321–32.
74. Cluitmans FH, Meinders AE. Management of severe hyponatremia: rapid or slow correction? Am J Med 1990;88:161–6.
75. Gross P, Reimann D, Neidel J, et al. The treatment of severe hyponatremia. Kidney Int Suppl 1998;64:S6–11.
76. Lien YH, Shapiro JI. Hyponatremia: clinical diagnosis and management. Am J Med 2007;120:653–8.
77. Sterns RH, Riggs JE, Schochet SS Jr. Osmotic demyelination syndrome following correction of hyponatremia. N Engl J Med 1986;314:1535–42.
78. Soupart A, Ngassa M, Decaux G. Therapeutic relowering of the serum sodium in a patient after excessive correction of hyponatremia. Clin Nephrol 1999;51:383–6.
79. Yamada H, Takano K, Ayuzawa N, et al. Relowering of serum Na for osmotic demyelinating syndrome. Case Rep Neurol Med 2012;2012:704639.
80. Oya S, Tsutsumi K, Ueki K, et al. Reinduction of hyponatremia to treat central pontine myelinolysis. Neurology 2001;57:1931–2.
81. Adams RD, Victor M, Mancall EL. Central pontine myelinolysis: a hitherto undescribed disease occurring in alcoholic and malnourished patients. AMA Arch Neurol Psychiatry 1959;81:154–72.
82. Wright DG, Laureno R, Victor M. Pontine and extrapontine myelinolysis. Brain 1979;102:361–85.
83. Ayus JC, Krothapalli RK, Arieff AI. Treatment of symptomatic hyponatremia and its relation to brain damage. A prospective study. N Engl J Med 1987;317:1190–5.
84. Ellis SJ. Severe hyponatraemia: complications and treatment. QJM 1995;88:905–9.
85. Ayus JC, Olivero JJ, Frommer JP. Rapid correction of severe hyponatremia with intravenous hypertonic saline solution. Am J Med 1982;72:43–8.
86. Ayus JC, Arieff AI. Chronic hyponatremic encephalopathy in postmenopausal women: association of therapies with morbidity and mortality. JAMA 1999;281:2299–304.
87. Moritz ML, Ayus JC. Preventing neurological complications from dysnatremias in children. Pediatr Nephrol 2005;20:1687–700.

88. Hoorn EJ, Geary D, Robb M, et al. Acute hyponatremia related to intravenous fluid administration in hospitalized children: an observational study. Pediatrics 2004;113:1279–84.

89. Farrar HC, Chande VT, Fitzpatrick DF, et al. Hyponatremia as the cause of seizures in infants: a retrospective analysis of incidence, severity, and clinical predictors. Ann Emerg Med 1995;26:42–8.

90. Wattad A, Chiang ML, Hill LL. Hyponatremia in hospitalized children. Clin Pediatr 1992;31:153–7.

91. Halberthal M, Halperin ML, Bohn D. Lesson of the week: acute hyponatraemia in children admitted to hospital: retrospective analysis of factors contributing to its development and resolution. BMJ 2001;322:780–2.

92. Nzerue CM, Baffoe-Bonnie H, You W, et al. Predictors of outcome in hospitalized patients with severe hyponatremia. J Natl Med Assoc 2003;95:335–43.

93. Moritz ML, Ayus JC. La Crosse encephalitis in children. N Engl J Med 2001;345:148–9.

94. McJunkin JE, de los Reyes EC, Irazuzta JE, et al. La Crosse encephalitis in children. N Engl J Med 2001;344:801–7.

95. Verbalis JG. Adaptation to acute and chronic hyponatremia: implications for symptomatology, diagnosis, and therapy. Semin Nephrol 1998;18:3–19.

96. Fraser CL, Arieff AI. Epidemiology, pathophysiology, and management of hyponatremic encephalopathy. Am J Med 1997;102:67–77.

97. Palevsky PM, Bhagrath R, Greenberg A. Hypernatremia in hospitalized patients. Ann Intern Med 1996;124:197–203.

98. Robertson GL, Aycinena P, Zerbe RL. Neurogenic disorders of osmoregulation. Am J Med 1982;72:339–53.

99. Lindner G, Funk GC. Hypernatremia in critically ill patients. J Crit Care 2013;28:216.e11–20.

100. Adrogue HJ, Madias NE. Hypernatremia. N Engl J Med 2000;342:1493–9.

101. Finberg L. Pathogenesis of lesions in the nervous system in hypernatremic states. I. Clinical observations of infants. Pediatrics 1959;23:40–5.

102. DeRubertis FR, Michelis MF, Davis BB. "Essential" hypernatremia. Report of three cases and review of the literature. Arch Intern Med 1974;134:889–95.

103. Halter JB, Goldberg AP, Robertson GL, et al. Selective osmoreceptor dysfunction in the syndrome of chronic hypernatremia. J Clin Endocrinol Metab 1977;44:609–16.

104. Lindner G, Kneidinger N, Holzinger U, et al. Tonicity balance in patients with hypernatremia acquired in the intensive care unit. Am J Kidney Dis 2009;54:674–9.

105. Finberg L, Kiley J, Luttrell CN. Mass accidental salt poisoning in infancy. A study of a hospital disaster. JAMA 1963;184:187–90.

106. De Villota ED, Cavanilles JM, Stein L, et al. Hyperosmolal crisis following infusion of hypertonic sodium chloride for purposes of therapeutic abortion. Am J Med 1973;55:116–22.

107. Mattar JA, Weil MH, Shubin H, et al. Cardiac arrest in the critically ill. II. Hyperosmolal states following cardiac arrest. Am J Med 1974;56:162–8.

108. Finberg L. Hypernatremic (hypertonic) dehydration in infants. N Engl J Med 1973;289:196–8.

109. Ross EJ, Christie SB. Hypernatremia. Medicine 1969;48:441–73.

110. Bruck E, Abal G, Aceto T Jr. Pathogenesis and pathophysiology of hypertonic dehydration with diarrhea. A clinical study of 59 infants with observations of respiratory and renal water metabolism. Am J Dis Child 1968;115:122–44.

111. Forman S, Crofton P, Huang H, et al. The epidemiology of hypernatraemia in hospitalised children in Lothian: a 10-year study showing differences between dehydration, osmoregulatory dysfunction and salt poisoning. Arch Dis Child 2012;97:502–7.
112. Morris-Jones PH, Houston IB, Evans RC. Prognosis of the neurological complications of acute hypernatraemia. Lancet 1967;2:1385–9.
113. Fraser CL, Arieff AI. Hepatic encephalopathy. N Engl J Med 1985;313:865–73.
114. Warren SE, Mitas JA 2nd, Swerdlin AH. Hypernatremia in hepatic failure. JAMA 1980;243:1257–60.
115. Manganaro R, Mami C, Marrone T, et al. Incidence of dehydration and hypernatremia in exclusively breast-fed infants. J Pediatr 2001;139:673–5.
116. Pizarro D, Posada G, Villavicencio N, et al. Oral rehydration in hypernatremic and hyponatremic diarrheal dehydration. Am J Dis Child 1983;137:730–4.
117. Holliday MA, Segar WE. The maintenance need for water in parenteral fluid therapy. Pediatrics 1957;19:823–32.
118. Lin M, Liu SJ, Lim IT. Disorders of water imbalance. Emerg Med Clin North Am 2005;23:749–70, ix.

Approach to Metabolic Acidosis in the Emergency Department

Mike Rice, MD, Bashar Ismail, MD, M. Tyson Pillow, MD, MEd*

KEYWORDS

- Metabolic acidosis • Acid-base disorders • Anion gap • Non-anion gap

KEY POINTS

- The approach that encompasses all acid-base derangements is to think of these disorders as a process, treat the underlying cause, and treat the patient, not the numbers.
- In thinking of acid-base disorders as a process, it is important to understand normal acid-base regulation in the body.
- Many different acids, pathologic abnormalities, and metabolic processes can contribute to the metabolic component of acid-base alterations.

INTRODUCTION

Several obstacles make it difficult to understand acid-base disorders in the emergency department (ED): (1) understanding of basic principles, which is frequently obscured by rote memorization of equations; (2) the perceived requirement to know intermediary metabolism; (3) the arbitrary and interchangeable use of "CO_2" to mean bicarbonate and/or P_{CO_2}; (4) the fact that patients rarely present with the primary complaint of "I have acidosis." It is also easy to get the impression that all laboratory tests will give exact, unwavering answers, and that calculations using these results will yield precise numbers that lead to the only correct answer.[1] Rather than thinking about acid-base disorders as numbers and arrows on a chart, each disturbance should be thought of as a *process*. The goal, with few exceptions, is therefore to identify and treat the underlying cause, not just the numbers.

In thinking of acid-base disorders as a process, it is important to understand the normal process of acid-base regulation in the body. Put simply, the body's goal is to eliminate the large burden of acid generated in the creation and storage of energy required for cellular metabolism. The pH is maintained between 7.35 and 7.45 by several intricate processes between the renal and respiratory systems (**Box 1**).

Baylor College of Medicine, Houston, TX, USA
* Corresponding author. Section of Emergency Medicine, Ben Taub General Hospital, Baylor College of Medicine, 1504 Taub Loop, Houston, TX 77030.
E-mail address: tysonpillow@gmail.com

Emerg Med Clin N Am 32 (2014) 403–420
http://dx.doi.org/10.1016/j.emc.2014.01.002
0733-8627/14/$ – see front matter © 2014 Elsevier Inc. All rights reserved.

> **Box 1**
> **The carbonic acid buffer system**
>
> $$\underset{\text{Proton}}{H^+} + \underset{\text{Bicarbonate Ion}}{HCO_3^-} \leftrightarrow \underset{\text{Carbonic Acid}}{H_2CO_3} \leftrightarrow \underset{\text{Water}}{H_2O} + \underset{\text{Carbon Dioxide}}{CO_2}$$
>
> If the concentration of each component remains unchanged, then simple calculations will tell you the ratios of one component to another, based on the pKa. From this, one can easily calculate the pH. If the concentration of any component changes, a new and different equilibrium will be reached, along with a different pH.

Respiratory Physiology

The lung expels 15,000 mmol of CO_2 per day in the healthy state. This rate is approximately 150 times more than the amount of acid excreted by the kidneys. Ventilation, therefore, serves as a primary compensatory mechanism.

Renal Physiology

The kidneys play an integral role in several other vital aspects of acid-base balance. Intricate biochemical reactions in the nephron facilitate the following: (1) maintenance of buffer capacity in blood; (2) excretion of inorganic acids, which the respiratory system is incapable of handling; (3) regeneration of lost bicarbonate ion; (4) the ability to increase H^+ excretion on a long-term basis, thereby giving the kidneys the ability to repair nonrenal causes of metabolic acidosis; (5) free proton excretion, although very limited in amount, which occurs only in the kidneys.

Pathophysiology

Metabolic acidosis is perhaps the most common derangement in acid-base encountered in the ED. It is a metabolic disturbance producing an increase in $[H^+]$ or a decrease in $[HCO_3^-]$. Although they are often used interchangeably, "acidosis" is separate from "acidemia," which is a serum pH lower than 7.35 (**Box 2**).

Metabolic acidosis can be produced by 3 major mechanisms:

1. Increased acid formation
2. Decreased acid excretion
3. Loss of bicarbonate

Box 3 shows a list of common diagnoses based on these mechanisms. Most commonly, however, the diagnoses are grouped in terms of those that create elevated anion gaps (AG) and those that do not.

APPROACH TO ACID-BASE DISORDERS

It is again important to emphasize that interpretation of acid-base status must be done in the context of the patient.[2] Another first step is to confirm the consistency of the

> **Box 2**
> **Definition of pH (with Henderson-Hasselbalch equation)**
>
> $$pH = -\log[H+] = pK_a + \log_{10}([A^-]/[HA])$$

| Box 3 |
| Causes of metabolic acidosis |

Increased acid production

- Lactic acidosis
- Ketoacidosis
- Ingestions
- Drug infusions

Loss of bicarbonate

- Diarrhea (severe)
- Ureterostomy
- Proximal renal tubular acidosis (type 2)

Diminished acid excretion

- Renal failure
- Distal renal tubular acidosis (type 1)
- Hyporeninemic hyperaldosteronism renal tubular acidosis (type 4)

arterial blood gas to the electrolyte panel by comparing the $[HCO_3^-]$ (should be no more than 2 mmol/L difference).

Once a metabolic acidosis is confirmed, it is useful to have a standard approach to interpretation. One such approach can be seen in **Fig. 1**.

Respiratory Compensation

In an isolated metabolic acidosis, the degree of acute respiratory compensation can be predicted based on the Winter formula (**Box 4**). This calculation is not applicable in chronic disease processes, because the kidneys compensate by increased reabsorption of bicarbonate.

Serum Anion Gap

There is not an actual anion gap, because plasma and urine are electrically neutral. There is only a gap between the most commonly measured cations and anions.[3,4] Originally, this was defined as: $AG = (Na^+ + K^+) - (Cl^- + HCO_3^-)$. In the United States, potassium is commonly excluded because it is relatively low compared with the other ions, leaving the equation: $AG = Na^+ - (Cl^- + HCO_3^-)$. Without potassium, normal anion gap is 8 ± 4 mmol/L. Newer autoanalyzes are even more specific with the normal anion gap being 7.2 ± 2 (range 3–11 mmol/L).[5,6]

Decreases in albumin are very common and can affect the anion gap. In patients with chronic illness, starvation, cancer, and so on, it is useful to correct the anion gap according to the Figge equation (**Box 5**).

Delta Gap/Ratio

This calculation simply compares the change in the anion gap to the change in the bicarbonate concentration.[4] Has the bicarbonate ion concentration decreased more than is explained by the increase in the AG gap, or decreased less than is predicted by the increase in the AG? This analysis is used to ascertain the presence of other concomitant acid-base disorders (**Table 1**).

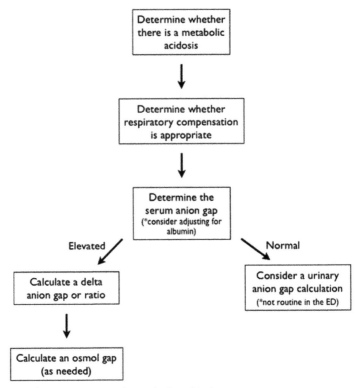

Fig. 1. Approach to assessment of metabolic acidosis.

Osmol Gap

This calculation is useful in acid-base disturbances with a high AG, because it can help in determining the presence of methanol or ethylene glycol intoxication. For purposes in the ED, the calculated serum osmolality is

$$Osms\ (calc.) = 2 \times Na^+ + glucose/18 + BUN/2.8 + EtOH/4.6$$

Urinary Anion Gap

Although not commonly used in the ED, this analysis is useful for differentiating causes of normal AG acidosis, specifically between gastrointestinal (GI) causes and renal causes (**Box 6**). The goal is to determine if the kidneys are responding normally to an acid load. If so, then the cause of metabolic acidosis is not renal. The normal urine anion gap is positive. Increased ammonium excretion by the renal tubules is the appropriate compensatory response to nonrenal causes of metabolic acidosis. Thus a negative anion gap in the urine indicates a nonrenal cause for normal AG acidosis.

Box 4
Winter formula

Winter formula : $pCO_2 = 1.5 \times HCO_3^- + 8(+/-2)$

Box 5
Anion gap corrected for albumin (normal albumin assumed to be 4.4 g/dL)
Corrected AG = AG + 2.5 × (4.4 − observed serum albumin)

ELEVATED ANION GAP ACIDOSES

The anion gap becomes elevated whenever an acid accumulates (organic, inorganic, or exogenous) and is not buffered by bicarbonate. The most common causes can be remembered with the mnemonic CAT MUD PILES (**Box 7**).

A subset of these acidoses is referred to as high anion gap acidosis. They are lactic acidosis, ketoacidosis, ingested toxins, and renal failure. They are defined by an elevated anion gap and a decreased level of bicarbonate.

Carbon Monoxide

Carbon monoxide (CO) results from incomplete oxidation of almost any carbon-containing material and is generated whenever combustion occurs in low oxygen environments. It is extremely harmful, primarily because it impairs oxygen delivery. The heme iron in hemoglobin has 200 to 250 times greater affinity for CO than for O_2. The result is decreased O_2 carrying capacity of blood, which may be severe depending on the extent of exposure. Routine blood gas analysis will not reveal the presence of CO. If CO poisoning is a clinical possibility, then direct measurement of the COHb level is mandatory.

Surprisingly, metabolic alterations may be a more sensitive indicator of the toxic effects of CO poisoning than any particular COHb level, although no acid-base state specifically predicts the presence of CO.[7] There are several mechanisms by which CO affects the pH. First, minimal toxicity can provoke a respiratory alkalosis in response to decreased oxygenation. Second and most obvious, lactic acidosis can occur from tissue hypoxia, leading to an increased AG acidosis. It turns out that the pH, reflective of increased [H^+], is a better predictor than COHb of poor outcomes. Unfortunately overall, the pH has so far not been a good predictor of the need for hyperbaric oxygen (HBO) therapy. Third, CO interferes with the cytochrome electron transport system, specifically mitochondrial cytochrome oxidase. Interference with oxidative phosphorylation will also generate lactic acidosis, but interference in the electron transport chain may result in more subtle damages, mediated by nitric oxide.

Table 1			
Use of the delta gap and ratio			
Event	**Delta Gap (ΔAG/ΔHCO$_3^-$)**	**Delta Ratio**	**Coexisting Acid-Base Disorders**
Bicarbonate decrease ≈ AG increase	0 ± 6	0.8–1.2	Anion gap acidosis only
Bicarbonate decreases more than increase in AG	<−6	0.3–0.7	1. Non-AG metabolic acidosis 2. Respiratory alkalosis
Bicarbonate decreases less than increase in AG	>6	>1.2	1. Metabolic alkalosis 2. Respiratory acidosis

---
Box 6
Urinary anion gap

$$UAG = Na^+_{(urine)} + K^+_{(urine)} - Cl^-_{(urine)}$$

Cyanide

Fire smoke is the leading cause of cyanide exposure in the western world. It is certainly the leading cause of fire-related deaths in the western world, and thermal burns account for a rather small percentage of the total. Residential fires account for two-thirds of lives lost from fires in the United States. There are several mechanisms by which fire smoke causes morbidity and mortality: direct thermal injury of the upper airway, poisoning by CO, and poisoning by cyanide. It is becoming more apparent that all fires have the potential to generate HCN as well as CO.[8,9] Unfortunately the treatment of CO and HCN have different goals, and these goals conflict with one another.

HCN is generated by the combustion of nitrogen-containing compounds, including synthetic materials such as plastics, paints, nylon, acrylics, and polyurethane foam. However, production is not limited to synthetics, as combustion of wool, silk, cotton, paper, and wood also generate HCN. Given the wide variety of materials that produce HCN on combustion, its presence should be suspected in any fire, commercial or residential.

Worldwide, the careless preparation and consumption of improperly processed cassava is the leading cause of potential exposure to cyanide, but accurate statistics are hard to come by because this population is extremely poor, rural, and medically underserved.[10] Toxicity occurs from linamarin, a cyanogenic glycoside. At present more than 500 million people in Africa and South America rely on cassava as a food source. Tropical ataxic neuropathy is the most common and well-studied manifestation of chronic exposure to cyanogenic glycosides.[11,12]

Unfortunately rapid determination of the presence of HCN in blood is not available to us. There seems to be little direct correlation of CO and HCN levels so that carboxyhemoglobin concentration cannot be used as a proxy for HCN. There is, however, a

---
Box 7
Differential diagnosis of elevated gap acidosis (CAT MUD PILES)

C – Carbon monoxide, cyanide

A – Alcoholic ketoacidosis (starvation ketoacidosis)

T – Toluene*

M – Methanol, metformin

U – Uremia

D – Diabetic ketoacidosis

P – Propylene glycol, paraldehyde, phenformin

I – Isoniazid, iron

L – Lactic acidosis

E – Ethylene glycol, ethanol

S – Salicylates

* Can cause both a normal AG and elevated AG acidosis.

---

fairly high degree of correlation between HCN and lactate, a plasma lactate concentration greater than 10 mEq/L being a sensitive indicator for the presence of HCN toxicity.[13] Whole blood cyanide levels will only be useful on a post-hoc basis. If ordered, the test should be drawn and sent to the laboratory as soon as possible because HCN has a very short half-life.

Alcoholic Ketoacidosis (and Starvation Ketoacidosis)

This condition only occurs in chronic alcoholics, particularly those that have no glycogen stores and get most of their caloric intake from ethanol. Binge drinking is a common precedent to the development of alcoholic ketoacidosis (AKA), but in the "classic" presentation ethanol consumption has ceased 1 to 3 days before admission due to severe abdominal pain and vomiting. Although this time period is often quoted, the truth is that AKA may appear while drinking continues up to 7 days after cessation. Despite complaints of severe abdominal pain, the examination may be surprisingly benign, showing only diffuse tenderness without guarding or rebound. As in diabetic ketoacidosis (DKA) (see section on diabetic ketoacidosis below), ketoacidosis results from elevated glucagon levels caused by insufficient intracellular glucose. However, in contrast to DKA, serum glucose is normal or low. Also, the ratio of β-hydroxybutyrate to acetoacetate is 7:1 in AKA versus 3:1 in DKA. Commonly, the threshold of the nitroprusside test (which detects acetoacetate) is not reached and returns as negative.[14,15]

Starvation ketoacidosis is, by far, the most common of the 3 causes of ketoacidosis, occurring in every ED several times a day. It is also by far the most benign. Ketoacidosis is typically not very severe. As in AKA, serum glucose is normal or low and there is a predominance of β-hydroxybutyrate.[16]

Toluene

Toluene is an aromatic hydrocarbon commonly used in the manufacture of many commercial products, including carburetor cleaner, oil paints and stains, spray paints, glues, paint thinners, lacquers and varnishes, and in the past, transmission fluid. All of these products are easily obtained because automobile supply shops, paint stores, hardware stores, and arts and crafts shops are near to most people. Most of these products are also volatile, meaning they vaporize at relatively low temperatures. Because toluene can produce a state of euphoria, is cheap and readily available, is easily inhaled, and is not illegal to possess, it has become a drug of abuse. It has been a problem not only in the United States, but also worldwide.[17]

Metabolism is accomplished via exhalation (less than 20% of the total as unchanged toluene) and hepatic metabolism by the cytochrome p450 system (CYP2E1) to benzoic acid (accounting for 80% of the total). Benzoic acid, a carboxylic acid, is conjugated to glycine to form hippuric acid, along the way generating a free proton and the potential for developing metabolic acidosis.[18] Glucuronidation also occurs, producing benzoyl glucuronide. Finally, these conjugates are excreted in the urine.

Toluene has been associated with normal AG and increased AG metabolic acidosis. The earliest case reports documented a normal anion gap acidosis, frequently with profound hypokalemia, K^+ as low as 1.4 mEq/L, and suggested this was from development of a type I (distal) renal tubular acidosis (RTA).[19] Other studies have documented an increased anion gap acidosis from hippuric acid or benzoic acid, or both.[20,21] The important point is that in individual cases one may find either a normal or an elevated AG acidosis, or sometimes both. One of the more interesting ideas is that even in patients with normal AG acidosis the pathophysiology is not that of a type 1 RTA, but rather the production and rapid excretion of hippuric acid associated with volume depletion.[22] Hippuric acid production increases rapidly after toluene inhalation, and it is cleared rapidly by the kidney; this is unmatched by excretion of a proton, as NH_4^+. Therefore Na^+ or K^+ or both must be excreted, leading to volume depletion and hypokalemia. The anion gap remains normal because the anion of the offending acid is not retained.

Toluene has many adverse effects. In the central nervous system, it may acutely cause intoxication, bizarre behavior, or hallucinations. Most often these are transient, resolving with cessation of drug use, and are not associated with abnormalities on the computed tomographic (CT) scan. However chronic abuse can lead to significant long-term neurologic disability, including ataxia, a Parkinson-like syndrome, and eye movement disorders.[17] Associated with the long-term effects are a wide variety of changes seen on CT or MRI. Toxicity affecting other organs includes prolongation of the QT interval, syncope, dilated cardiomyopathy, elevated liver enzymes, hepatomegaly, rhabdomyolysis, which may be severe, and hypophosphatemia.[17]

Methanol

Methanol can be found in paints, solvents, antifreeze, and as a fuel source for outdoor stoves and torches. In the body, it is converted to formaldehyde and then formic acid (formate), leading to its toxic effects and elevated anion gap acidosis. The classic ophthalmologic complaints have been reported to occur with all patients who have acidemia.[23] Methanol also elevates the osmolal gap, but may present with a "false normal" gap.

Clinically, methanol levels can be measured, but are not very useful in the acute stabilization phase due to a delay in getting results. Signs and symptoms of methanol poisoning include agitation, psychosis, altered level of consciousness, seizures, visual symptoms (blurry vision, visual impairment, photophobia), retinal edema, and nausea and vomiting. Head CT may reveal cerebral edema or basal ganglia hemorrhage or infarcts.[24,25]

Uremia

As renal failure progresses and glomerular filtration rate (GFR) decreases to less than 50 mL/min, there is a build-up of inorganic and organic acids that causes an elevated gap acidosis.[26] In addition, NH_4 production is decreased, leaving the kidney unable to buffer the increased acid load. [HCO_3^-] levels rarely decrease to less than 15 mmol/L, and the anion gap is usually less than 20 mmol/L.[27]

Clinically, uremia can have a variety of signs and symptoms. Commonly, these patients may present with drowsiness, lethargy, anorexia, nausea and vomiting, pruritus, alterations in skin pigmentation, anemia, platelet dysfunction, chest pain (pericarditis), and endocrine effects as well.[27]

Diabetic Ketoacidosis

Historically DKA occurred almost solely in type 1 diabetics, typically young and thin, and whose pancreatic islet cells had stopped producing insulin altogether. Today, patients with type 2 diabetes frequently present with DKA as well.[28] The unifying pathophysiology is still hyperglycemia, ketonemia, and acidemia induced by insufficient levels of insulin and increased levels of glucagon. Ultimately, glucagon leads to oxidation of free fatty acids producing β-hydroxybutyrate and acetoacetate.

Clinically, the classic symptoms of DKA include nausea, vomiting, polyuria, polydipsia, polyphagia, and sometimes abdominal pain. Physical examination will also reveal diffuse abdominal pain and dehydration. Kussmaul respirations are another classic sign of DKA. It is important to remember, however, that as early DKA has become easier to recognize, the full spectrum of symptoms may not be present in every patient. A previous study noted a mean serum glucose of 675 mg/dL and mean bicarbonate of 6 mmol/L in a series of patients with nonfatal DKA.[28,29] Ketonuria is a defining sign of DKA as the β-hydroxybutyrate to acetoacetate ratio is approximately 3:1, making the nitroprusside test useful in this setting.

Propylene Glycol, Paraldehyde

Propylene glycol is a delivery vehicle for many commonly used drug infusions in the ED and intensive care unit setting. These drug infusions include lorazepam, diazepam, phenytoin, etomidate, nitroglycerin, and esmolol. The amount of propylene glycol delivered depends on the concentration in each particular solution as well as the rate of delivery, and cumulative doses appear to be important. Therefore, this is usually a problem discovered in the inpatient setting, not the ED. The cause of the acidosis remains unclear, although toxicity is frequently associated with elevated lactate levels. To make the diagnosis, one needs the following: (1) knowledge of the existence of this clinical entity and its presentation and (2) an elevated anion gap acidosis and an elevated osmolal gap, or (3) readily obtainable propylene glycol levels. Treatment consists of changing to a drug formulation containing little or no propylene glycol, such as midazolam, and hemodialysis if acidosis is severe and the patient has deteriorated clinically.[30,31]

Paraldehyde was once used commonly for alcohol withdrawal. It is rarely, if ever, used today, but continues to be included in the "P" of the mnemonic. Ingestion leads to the formation of acetic and chloracetic acids, leading to metabolic acidosis.[32]

Isoniazid, Iron

The incidence of tuberculosis is at its lowest rate ever in the United States.[33] However, isoniazid continues to be an incredibly important drug in the treatment of tuberculosis as both prophylaxis and treatment. Isoniazid (INH) exerts its most significant toxic effects through interference with pyridoxine (Vitamin B_6). γ-Aminobutyric acid is the primary inhibitory neurotransmitter in the central nervous system. Decreased levels of γ-aminobutyric acid are thought to be the primary pathologic event in INH neurotoxicity, leading directly to seizures and lactic acidosis because of the lack of neuronal inhibition.[34] INH inhibits lactate clearance and decreases the metabolism of β-hydroxybutyrate as well, leading to further acidosis.

Seizures, profound metabolic acidosis, and coma are noted in almost all articles to be the hallmarks of INH toxicity, and seizures, including status epilepticus, are frequently the presenting event.

Metabolic acidosis with a high anion gap is a frequent accompaniment of seizures. Most of the time, this is due to lactate, as one would expect with seizures. There does not seem to be anything special about the acidosis that would lead to predicting INH. In the literature, there is no incidence of significant metabolic acidosis from INH ingestion that was not related directly to seizures.

Iron toxicity leads to metabolic acidosis in several different ways.[35,36] First, it uncouples mitochondrial oxidative phosphorylation, affecting ATP synthesis. Second, it forms free radicals, damaging cell membranes. Third, it has direct GI and cardiovascular toxicity, including GI hemorrhage and myocardial suppression. These effects culminate into elevated lactate production from the combination of cardiogenic shock, hemorrhagic shock, anaerobic metabolism, and unbuffered protons.

Lactic Acidosis

Lactic acidosis is an extremely common occurrence, especially in the ED. A lactate level greater than 4 mEq/L with acidemia is a common definition of lactic acidosis across the literature. There are 3 types of lactic acidosis. The L-isomer of lactate is responsible for types A and B lactic acidosis. The D-isomer is responsible for the third type.[14,37]

Type A lactic acidosis represents most lactic acidoses and is defined by tissue hypoxia. In general, there are 2 mechanisms responsible: inadequate oxygen delivery and increased oxygen requirements. The most common cause in this category is shock, but also includes pulmonary disease, toxins, other causes of severe hypoxemia, anemia, and thromboembolic events.[32]

Type B lactic acidosis is a less-well understood entity whereby there is an increased lactate level with preserved oxygen delivery to tissues. Causes of type B acidosis include diabetes mellitus, glycogen storage diseases, ethanol, hepatic failure, malignancy, and drugs. Some of the most notable causes include metformin, antiretroviral medications, propofol infusions, and Hodgkin lymphoma.[32]

D-Lactic acidosis is a rare cause of lactic acidosis. The common presentation occurs in a patient with previous small bowel resection, short bowel syndrome, or a blind loop. Intestinal bacteria form the D-isomer of lactate after a large carbohydrate load.[38] Because it cannot be metabolized by the body, D-lactic acid accumulates. Neurologic dysfunction manifested as confusion, slurred speech, and ataxia presents in association with a high AG acidosis for which no clear cause can be found, unless one is aware of this illness.

Ethylene Glycol, Ethanol

Ethylene glycol is found in antifreeze, deicing solutions, and brake fluids because it lowers the freezing point of water. In the body, it is converted into glycolic acid (as well as glyoxylic acid and oxalic acid), which is the primary cause of the elevated anion gap.[39] Ethylene glycol creates an elevated osmolal gap, but toxicity can present with a "false-normal" osmolal gap. Differentiating toxic alcohol ingestions is aided by the fact that neither methanol nor ethylene glycol produce ketones.

Clinically, ingestion should be suspected based on history. Other clues to the diagnosis may be crystalluria (caused by calcium oxalate monohydrate or dihydrate), fluorescence of urine or vomitus, prolonged QT on electrocardiogram (secondary to hypocalcemia), and CT scan of the head showing cerebral edema.[40,41]

Acute ethanol intoxication can also produce an elevated anion gap acidosis by a different mechanism than that of AKA. There are 4 proposed mechanisms for increased lactate levels in the context of ethanol intoxication[42,43]: (1) Ethanol is normally oxidized to acetaldehyde and then acetic acid. Oxidation of one molecule produces reduction of another in any redox reaction. Therefore metabolism of ethanol produces acetate and an increased number of reducing equivalents, promoting the reduction of NAD^+ to NADH. A high $NADH:NAD^+$ favors reduction of pyruvate to lactate; therefore lactate levels increase. (2) Ethanol impairs the use of lactate in the Cori cycle (gluconeogenesis from lactate in the liver and kidney). Because excess lactate is not used for glucose production, the serum levels increase. (3) Thiamine deficiency leading to an increase in lactate production. (4) Impaired liver function leading to a decrease in lactate clearance. This increase in lactate applies only to patients with severe liver disease and occurs because more than half of the lactate normally produced is metabolized in the liver. Decreased metabolic consumption by the liver leads to increased serum lactate levels.

Clinically it is most important to be able to recognize AKA. There are several studies in volunteers and patients documenting elevations of lactate in acute ethanol intoxication, but in most, the elevations are minimal, rarely going higher than 3 mEq/L.

Salicylates

Salicylates are often recognized as being an ingredient in pain medications and cold medicines, but may also be present in some skin or teething ointments and antidiarrheals. Toxicity may be acute or chronic in nature. They create a mixed acid-base disturbance that can be incredibly complex.[37] Salicylates directly stimulate the respiratory center in the medulla, leading to a respiratory alkalosis, and uncouple oxidative phosphorylation, leading to a metabolic acidosis. In addition, renal bicarbonate excretion is increased in response to the hyperventilation: keto acids are produced by inhibition of the Krebs cycle; lactic acid accumulates from mitochondrial impairment; and free salicylic acid also accumulates.

Clinically, salicylate toxicity presents with altered mental status, tachypnea, hyperthermia, pulmonary edema, and shock. Tinnitus is an important clue to the presence of toxicity, but it may be difficult to elicit this history from the altered patient.

NORMAL ANION GAP (HYPERCHLOREMIC) ACIDOSES

Normal anion gap or hyperchloremic acidosis is caused by an inability to excrete $[H^+]$, or the loss of $[HCO_3^-]$. In normal anion gap acidosis there is no disruption of intermediary metabolism producing organic acids, and no addition of organic acids from an exogenous source. The mnemonic HARD UP is commonly used to remember the causes of normal anion gap acidosis (**Box 8**).

As mentioned above, the urinary anion gap can be used to help distinguish renal versus nonrenal causes of the acidosis (see **Box 6**). It is also useful to think of normal anion gap acidosis in terms of the observed effect on serum potassium (**Table 2**). However, this article focuses on the most common differentials.

Hyperalimentation

Essentially, hyperalimentation may result in a normal anion gap acidosis if sufficient amounts of bicarbonate (or solutes such as lactate or acetate) are not included in the solutions. Metabolism of the amino acids leads to the release of protons without bicarbonate to buffer them.[44]

Acetazolamide

Acetazolamide is the representative drug of carbonic anhydrase inhibitors. They work on the proximal tubules to block the dehydration of luminal carbonic acid, preventing

---

Box 8
Differential diagnosis of normal anion gap acidosis (HARD UP)

H – Hyperalimentation

A – Acetazolamide (carbonic anhydrase inhibitors)

R – Renal tubular acidosis, renal failure (early)

D – Diarrhea, diuretics, dilutional acidosis

U – Ureteroenterostomy

P – Pancreatic fistula

Table 2
Differential diagnosis of normal anion gap acidosis (expanded)

Normal Anion Gap Acidosis		
Low Potassium	**Normal or High Potassium**	**Other**
Renal tubular acidosis • Distal (type 1) • Proximal (type 2)	Renal tubular acidosis • Type 4	Expansion acidosis
Carbonic anhydrase inhibitors	Early renal failure • GFR 20–50 mL/min	Cation exchange resin
Ureteral diversions	Hydronephrosis	
Diarrhea	Low aldosterone • Hyporeninemic hypoaldosteronism	
Surgical drainage or fistula	Drug induced • Potassium-sparing • Others	
Posthypocapneic acidosis	Addition of inorganic acid	
	Sulfur toxicity	
	Cholestyramine	

the proximal reabsorption of sodium bicarbonate. The acidosis it causes is usually not severe because of the kidney's compensation mechanisms, including bicarbonate reabsorption in the distal nephron and decreased filtration of bicarbonate.[45]

Topiramate (Topamax) is an underrecognized cause of normal anion gap acidosis.[46] It has been approved since 1996 as a second-line antiepileptic, but also has US Food and Drug Administration approval for migraine prophylaxis, and most recently with phentermine as a weight-loss drug. It has several common off-label uses as well, including treatment of essential tremor and neuropathic pain. It has carbonic anhydrase-like effects, effectively producing a type 4 RTA (see section of renal tubular acidosis below for further discussion). Mild decreases in $[HCO_3^-]$ (approximately 4 mEq/L) are common, and in both children and adults, there are case reports of $[HCO_3^-]$ as low as 10 mEq/L.

Renal Tubular Acidosis

RTA is a disorder characterized by defects in the ability of the renal tubules to maintain normal acid-base status.[47,48] Despite this defect, glomerular filtration rate is usually preserved. Along with diarrhea, it is a major cause of normal anion gap acidosis. **Table 3** summarizes the key differences between the 3 major types of RTAs.

Type 1 RTA (also referred to as distal, classic, or gradient-limited) is characterized by a defect in distal tubular secretion of protons, loss of ≈3% of the filtered load of bicarbonate, and a complete inability to acidify the urine. As expected, urinary ammonium levels are low. Sodium and potassium are also lost in the urine, leading to mild volume depletion and potentially severe hypokalemia. Although the pH can be quite low, hypokalemia is the most important feature for the emergency physician. It can be profound and life-threatening, leading to severe muscle weakness and myocardial irritability, requiring aggressive treatment. Type 1 RTAs most commonly occur with systemic inflammatory diseases, but can also be genetic, drug-induced, or secondary to transplant rejection.[50] Drug causes include toluene, lithium, pentamidine, rifampin, and amphotericin B (which produces an effect similar to type 1 RTA by altering the distal nephron and causing a leakage of $[H^+]$).[43] Although less relevant, type 1 RTA produces nephrocalcinosis and nephrolithiasis but type 2 does not.

Table 3			
Characteristics of the types of renal tubular acidosis			
	Type 1 (Distal)	Type 2 (Proximal)	Type 4 (Hypoaldosteronism)
Defect	Distal acidification	Proximal bicarbonate reabsorption	Decrease in or resistance to aldosterone
Serum bicarbonate	<10 mEq/L (varies)	~12–20 mEq/L	>17 mEq/L (varies)
Serum potassium	Reduced[a]	Reduced	Increased
Urine pH	>5.3	Can be <5.3	Can be <5.3

[a] May also be hyperkalemic.[49]

Type 2 RTA (also referred to as proximal or quantity-limited) is a defect in bicarbonate reabsorption leading to increased delivery to the distal tubule. Normally, 85% of filtered bicarbonate is reabsorbed in the proximal tubule. In type 2 RTA, there is limited ability to augment bicarbonate reclamation. As one might expect, bicarbonate loss is much greater in type II RTA (see **Table 3**). This disorder is usually found in children, or in association with multiple myelomas in adults.

Fanconi syndrome refers to type 2 RTAs in which there is a greater defect than just impaired bicarbonate reabsorption in renal tubular function. Hyperaminoaciduria, glycosuria, hyperphosphaturia, and uric acid loss also occur. Some causes of type 2 RTA result only in bicarbonate loss and some result in the Fanconi syndrome.

Type 4 RTA results from decreased sodium absorption, [H^+] secretion, and potassium secretion in the distal tubule. It occurs in 50% of patients with hyporeninemic hypoaldosteronism and typically occurs in older diabetic patients with mild to moderate renal impairment, ± with or without concurrent congestive heart failure.[32] It leads to normal anion gap acidosis, lowered sodium, elevated potassium, and low levels of urinary ammonium ion. Type 4 RTA also occurs in obstructive uropathy and chronic tubulointerstitial diseases. Diuretics such as spironolactone, amiloride, triamterene (see section on diarrhea/diurectics below) produce a similar clinical syndrome.

Renal Failure

Although renal failure (GFR <20 mL/min) occurs prominently on any list of increased anion gap acidosis, it may also cause a normal anion gap acidosis (20 mL/min < GFR < 50 mL/min). Sometimes failure to maintain net acid excretion occurs before organic anions build up causing the increased gap acidosis. Chloride is retained instead, to maintain appropriate electrical gradients, and a normal anion gap acidosis occurs. Interstitial renal disease is a prime example, as defects in proton excretion occur with relatively high GFRs, before retention of organic acid anions.

Diarrhea/Diuretics

Diarrheal illness is the most common cause of normal anion gap acidosis. Diarrheal stools contain sodium, potassium, and bicarbonate, but little chloride. Therefore volume depletion, hypokalemia, and metabolic acidosis characterize this illness. Associated with this is increased chloride reabsorption in the distal nephron and contraction of volume around a fixed concentration of chloride. Because there is no acid with an associated unmeasured anion, the anion gap remains unchanged. As the bicarbonate concentration decreases, the chloride concentration increases. In addition to direct potassium loss in the stool, volume contraction triggers the release of aldosterone, leading directly to distal tubular reabsorption of sodium in exchange for potassium, thereby promoting volume expansion at the cost of hypokalemia.

Diuretics (such as spironolactone and amiloride) result in decreased sodium reabsorptions, [H$^+$] secretion, and potassium secretion at the distal tubule, causing a hyperkalemic, hyperchloremic metabolic acidosis similar to type 4 RTA (see above).

Dilutional (or Volume Expansion) Acidosis

Dilutional (or volume expansion) acidosis is a very common cause of normal AG acidosis and typically occurs during large-volume resuscitation with normal saline. Even though it occurs frequently, there have been no studies demonstrating harmful effects from its presence. Although several potential mechanisms exist, historically the pathophysiology was thought to be that the addition of large volumes of a pH neutral fluid to the plasma would dilute the [HCO$_3^-$]. More recent theories include the kidney's inability to handle the increased chloride load, leading to bicarbonate loss to maintain neutrality.[51]

Ureteroenterostomy

Injury to the bladder sometimes necessitates surgical diversion of the ureters to the sigmoid colon, adding excretion of urine to the function of the sigmoid and rectum. However the bowel mucosa has an ion transporter in place for reabsorption of chloride in exchange for bicarbonate. Because urine has a high chloride concentration and remains in contact with the sigmoid mucosa for a prolonged time, this exchange takes place, serum chloride increases, and serum bicarbonate decreases, causing a normal AG acidosis. Although this is now a rare procedure, up to 80% of patients with ureterosigmoidostomies suffer this complication.

An ileal conduit (or bladder) is formed by diverting urine flow from the kidneys into a reservoir created from the ilium. This conduit is drained through a stoma created in the abdominal wall, into a collecting bag. Although the same chloride/bicarbonate exchange process exists in the ileum, urine does not remain in contact with ileal mucosa long enough for metabolic acidosis to develop unless there is an outflow obstruction.[52]

Pancreatic Fistula

Pancreatic fistulas (both external and internal) are [HCO$_3^-$] rich and divert fluid away from the normal reabsorption that occurs in the bowel.[53] Other types of fistulas, tubes placed for drainage, and ostomies can produce similar effects due to the loss of [HCO$_3^-$].

TREATMENT OF ACIDOSIS

Therapy is almost always directed at treating the underlying condition, independent of the pH.[54] There are a few exceptions to this rule, but they are rare. The primary problem with acidosis is myocardial suppression. Alkali therapy would seem to be an obvious choice for the management of acidosis, but has limited value and potential harm. First, it is not an effective buffer in the normal range of serum pH. At normal pH, it serves more as a transport role for the carbon dioxide in the blood. Second, bicarbonate therapy can be harmful. It has a very high ability to generate CO$_2$ and lower the serum and cerebrospinal fluid pH, making the acidosis worse.[54] Finally, it may lead to calcium and potassium shifts, predisposing the heart to arrhythmias, as well as hypernatremia and volume expansion.[55]

In severe cases of acidosis (pH<7.0) where the normal compensation mechanisms are overwhelmed, leading to cardiovascular instability, bicarbonate therapy can be attempted.[54,55]

SUMMARY

Acid-base disorders should be thought of as a *process*. The history, physical examination, review of medications, suspicion for toxic substances, and an inquiring mind will determine the presence and likely causes of most disturbances in acid-base balance, particularly when there is only one aberration in pH physiology (ie, the simple acid-base disorders). Using the available tools of diagnosis (calculating anion gap, delta gap, urinary gap) can be useful in the differential diagnosis, but is certainly not foolproof given the wide range of normal values in laboratory testing and the standard deviation of these values. Mnemonics (HARD UP, CAT MUD PILES) help to recall the most common derangements, but a differential diagnosis based on all clinical information.

When interpreting acid-base disorders, it is important to remember that there can be only one primary respiratory disturbance at any time. There is either alveolar hyperventilation (indicating a primary respiratory alkalosis) or alveolar hypoventilation (indicating a primary respiratory acidosis). However, one patient may have several disparate and opposite metabolic disturbances at the same time. There may be several mechanisms producing metabolic acidosis at the same time, as well as different processes producing metabolic alkalosis. There is certainly no special limit to the number of metabolic disturbances one particular patient may have. Many different acids, pathologic abnormalities, and metabolic processes can contribute to the metabolic component of acid-base alterations.

Ultimately, the approach that encompasses all acid-base derangements is to think of these disorders as a process, treat the underlying cause, and treat the patient, not the numbers.

REFERENCES

1. Berend K. Acid-base pathophysiology after 130 years: confusing, irrational, and controversial. J Nephrol 2013;26(2):254–65.
2. Morris C, Low J. Metabolic acidosis in the critically ill: part 1. Classification and pathophysiology. Anaesthesia 2008;63(3):294–301.
3. Aiken C. History of the medical understanding and misunderstanding of acid base balance. J Clin Diagn Res 2013;7(9):2038–41.
4. Reddy P, Mooradian A. Clinical utility of anion gap in deciphering acid-base disorders. Int J Clin Pract 2009;63(10):1516–25.
5. Kraut J, Nagami G. The serum anion gap in the evaluation of acid-based disorders: what are the limitations and can its effectiveness be improved? Clin J Am Soc Nephrol 2013;8(11):2018–24.
6. Sadjadi S, Manalo R, Jaipaul N, et al. Ion-selective electrode and anion gap range: what should the anion gap be? Int J Nephrol Renovasc Dis 2013;6: 101–5.
7. Tomaszewski C. Carbon monoxide. In: Nelson L, Lewin N, Howland M, et al, editors. Goldfrank's toxicologic emergencies. 9th edition. New York: McGraw-Hill; 2011. p. 1658–70.
8. O'Brien D, Walsh D, Terriff C, et al. Empiric management of cyanide toxicity associated with smoke inhalation. Prehosp Disaster Med 2011;26(5): 374–82.

9. Anseeuw K, Delvau N, Burillo-Putze G, et al. Cyanide poisoning by fire smoke inhalation: a European expert consensus. Eur J Emerg Med 2013;20(1):2–9.

10. Dhas P, Chitra P, Jayakumar S, et al. Study of the effects of hydrogen cyanide exposure in Cassava workers. Indian J Occup Environ Med 2011;15(3):133–6.

11. Teles F. Chronic poisoning by hydrogen cyanide in cassava and its prevention in Africa and Latin America. Food Nutr Bull 2002;23(4):407–12.

12. Adamolekun B. Neurological disorders associated with cassava diet: a review of putative etiological mechanisms. Metab Brain Dis 2011;26(1):79–85.

13. Holstege C, Isom G, Kirk M. Cyanide and hydrogen sulfide. In: Nelson L, Lewin N, Howland M, et al, editors. Goldfrank's toxicologic emergencies. 9th edition. New York: McGraw-Hill; 2011. p. 1678–88.

14. DuBose T. Acidosis and alkalosis. In: Longo D, Fauci A, Kasper D, et al, editors. Harrison's principles of internal medicine. 18th edition. New York: McGraw-Hill; 2012.

15. Umpierrez G, DiGirolamo M, Tuvlin J, et al. Differences in metabolic and hormonal milieu in diabetic- and alcohol-induced ketoacidosis. J Crit Care 2000; 15(2):52–9.

16. Cartwright M, Hajja W, Al-Khatib S, et al. Toxigenic and metabolic causes of ketosis and ketoacidotic syndromes. Crit Care Clin 2012;28(4):601–31.

17. Long H. Inhalants. In: Nelson L, Lewin N, Howland M, et al, editors. Goldfrank's toxicologic emergencies. 9th edition. New York: McGraw-Hill; 2011. p. 1157–65.

18. Fischman C, Oster J. Toxic effects of toluene: a new cause of high anion gap metabolic acidosis. JAMA 1979;241(16):1713–5.

19. Taher S, Anderson R, McCartney R, et al. Renal tubular acidosis associated with toluene "sniffing". N Engl J Med 1974;290(14):765–8.

20. Baskerville J, Tichenor G, Rosen P. Toluene induced hypokalemia: case report and literature review. Emerg Med J 2001;18(6):514–6.

21. Camara-Lemarroy C, Gonzalez-Moreno E, Rodriguez-Gutierrez R, et al. Clinical presentation and management in acute toluene intoxication: a case series. Inhal Toxicol 2012;24(7):434–8.

22. Dickson R, Luks A. Toluene toxicity as a cause of elevated anion gap metabolic acidosis. Respir Care 2009;54(8):1115–7.

23. Dethlefs R, Naraqi S. Ocular manifestations and complications of acute methyl alcohol intoxication. Med J Aust 1978;2(10):483–5.

24. Aquilonius S, Askmark H, Enoksson P, et al. Computerized tomography in severe methanol intoxication. BMJ 1978;2(6142):929–30.

25. Phang P, Passerini L, Mielke B, et al. Brain hemorrhage associated with methanol poisoning. Crit Care Med 1988;16(2):137–40.

26. Bargman J, Skorecki K. Chronic kidney disease. In: Longo D, Fauci A, Kasper D, et al, editors. Harrison's principles of internal medicine. 18th edition. New York: McGraw-Hill; 2012.

27. Meyer T, Hostetter T. The pathophysiology of uremia. In: Taal M, Chertow G, Marsden P, et al, editors. The kidney. 9th edition. Philadelphia: Elsevier; 2012. p. 2000–20.

28. Powers A. Diabetes mellitus. In: Longo D, Fauci A, Kasper D, et al, editors. Harrison's principles of internal medicine. 18th edition. New York: McGraw-Hill; 2012.

29. Beigelman P. Severe diabetic ketoacidosis. 482 episodes in 257 patients; experience of three years. Diabetes 1971;20(7):490–500.

30. Bania T. Intravenous fat emulsions. In: Nelson L, Lewin N, Howland M, et al, editors. Goldfrank's toxicologic emergencies. 9th edition. New York: McGraw-Hill; 2011. p. 976–81.

31. Zosel A, Egelhoff E, Heard K. Severe lactic acidosis after an iatrogenic propylene glycol overdose. Pharmacotherapy 2010;30(2):219.
32. Casaletto J. Differential diagnosis of metabolic acidosis. Emerg Med Clin North Am 2005;23:771–87.
33. Centers for Disease Control. Reported tuberculosis in the United States. Available at: http://www.cdc.gov/tb/. Accessed December 9, 2013.
34. Hernon C, Boyer E. Antituberculous medications. In: Nelson L, Lewin N, Howland M, et al, editors. Goldfrank's toxicologic emergencies. 9th edition. New York: McGraw-Hill; 2011. p. 834–44.
35. Mills K, Curry S. Acute iron poisoning. Emerg Med Clin North Am 1994;12(2): 397–413.
36. Perrone J. Iron. In: Nelson L, Lewin N, Howland M, et al, editors. Goldfrank's toxicologic emergencies. 9th edition. New York: McGraw-Hill; 2011. p. 596–603.
37. Wiener S. Toxicologic acid-base disorders. Emerg Med Clin North Am 2014;32: 149–65.
38. Uribiarri J, Oh M, Carroll H. D-lactic acidosis: a review of clinical presentation, biochemical features, and pathophysiologic mechanisms. Medicine 1998; 77(2):73–82.
39. Wiener S. Toxic alcohols. In: Nelson L, Lewin N, Howland M, et al, editors. Goldfrank's toxicologic emergencies. 9th edition. New York: McGraw-Hill; 2011. p. 1400–11.
40. Zeiss J, Velasco ME, McCann KM, et al. Cerebral CT of lethal ethylene glycol intoxication with pathologic correlation. AJNR Am J Neuroradiol 1989;10(2): 440–2.
41. Morgan B, Ford MD, Follmer R. Ethylene glycol ingestion resulting in brainstem and midbrain dysfunction. J Toxicol Clin Toxicol 2000;38(4):445–51.
42. MacDonald L, Kruse J, Levy D, et al. Lactic acidosis and acute ethanol intoxication. Am J Emerg Med 1994;12(1):32–5.
43. Shull P, Rapoport J. Life-threatening reversible acidosis caused by alcohol abuse. Nat Rev Nephrol 2010;6(9):555–9.
44. Kato K, Sugiura S, Yano K, et al. The latent risk of acidosis in commercially available total parenteral nutrition products: a randomized clinical trial in postoperative patients. J Clin Biochem Nutr 2009;45(1):68–73.
45. Liamis G, Millionis H, Elisaf M. Pharmacologically-induced metabolic acidosis: a review. Drug Saf 2010;33(5):371–91.
46. Mirza N, Alfirevic A, Jorgensen A, et al. Metabolic acidosis with topiramate and zonisamide: an assessment of its severity and predictors. Pharmacogenet Genomics 2011;21(5):297–302.
47. Rodriguez S. Renal tubular acidosis: the clinical entity. J Am Soc Nephrol 2002; 13(8):2160.
48. Reddy P. Clinical approach to renal tubular acidosis in adult patients. Int J Clin Pract 2011;65(3):350–60.
49. Hass C, Pohlenz I, Lindher U, et al. Renal tubular acidosis type IV in hyperkalemic patients—a fairy tale or reality? Clin Endocrinol (Oxf) 2013;78(5):706–11.
50. Kocyigit I, Unal A, Kavuncuoglu F, et al. Renal tubular acidosis in renal transplantation recipients. Ren Fail 2010;32(6):687–90.
51. Wolf M. Whole body acid-base and fluid-electrolyte balance: a mathematical model. Am J Physiol Renal Physiol 2013;305(8):F1118–31.
52. Weise W, Serrano F, Fought J, et al. Acute electrolyte and acid-base disorders in patients with ileostomies: a case series. Am J Kidney Dis 2008;52(3): 494–500.

53. Eovaldi B, Zanetti C. Non-anion gap metabolic acidosis in a patient with a pancreaticopleural fistula. J Am Osteopath Assoc 2011;111(5):344–5.
54. Morris C, Low J. Metabolic acidosis in the critically ill: part 2. Causes and treatment. Anaesthesia 2008;63(4):396–411.
55. Sabatini S, Kurtzman N. Bicarbonate therapy in severe metabolic acidosis. J Am Soc Nephrol 2009;20(4):692–5.

Neonatal Endocrine Emergencies
A Primer for the Emergency Physician

Elizabeth Park, MD[a], Nadia M. Pearson, DO[b],
M. Tyson Pillow, MD, MEd[a],*, Alexander Toledo, DO, PharmD[a]

KEYWORDS

- Neonatal emergencies • Hypothyrodism • Congenital adrenal hyperplasia
- Hypoglycemia • Jaundice • Hyponatremia • Hypocalcemia

KEY POINTS

- Neonatal endocrine emergencies are uncommon and may present a particular challenge for diagnosis in the emergency department.
- The overlap between endocrine and metabolic emergencies in neonates is significant.
- The resuscitation principles for neonates remain the same in any neonatal emergency, such as securing the airway and stabilizing hemodynamics.
- Implementing screening programs more broadly worldwide and improving the current tests remains the challenge for future health care providers and those practicing abroad.

INTRODUCTION

Neonates have a tendency of presenting discreetly. Neonatal endocrine emergencies are uncommon and may present a particular challenge for diagnosis in the emergency department. In the United States, newborn screening tests are used for early detection and treatment. Each state has a different panel of required screening tests for genetic, metabolic, and congenital issues, some of which are discussed in this article. Most of the screening tests are not immediately available to the emergency care provider. Although many cases are discovered postpartum in the nursery or neonatal intensive care unit, any health care provider who may deal with deliveries and the care of neonates needs to develop an astute sense for these emergencies and the rapid intervention required to offset any permanent neurologic damage from delayed diagnosis. The overlap between endocrine and metabolic emergencies in neonates is significant, but is beyond the scope of this article. This article focuses on the most common and most

Disclosures: None.
[a] Section of Emergency Medicine, Baylor College of Medicine, 1504 Taub Loop Road, Houston, TX 77030, USA; [b] Department of Emergency Medicine, San Antonio Military Medical Center, 3551 Roger Brooke Drive, San Antonio, TX 78234, USA
* Corresponding author.
E-mail address: tysonpillow@gmail.com

critical endocrine emergencies encountered in the first 4 weeks of life, including hypoglycemia, jaundice, hypothyroidism, congenital adrenal hyperplasia, inborn errors of metabolism, and common electrolyte disorders.

HYPOGLYCEMIA

Hypoglycemia continues to be the most frequently encountered endocrine abnormality in neonates. Diagnosis of the hypoglycemic newborn based on physical examination alone is difficult. Findings can be subtle and nonspecific. Clinical signs of hypoglycemic include respiratory distress, apnea, lethargy, hypotonia, seizures, jitteriness, myoclonus, temperature instability, weak or high-pitched cry, and difficulty with feeding. These signs could also be the presentation for a multitude of other conditions such as sepsis, congenital heart disease, prematurity, other metabolic diseases, drug withdrawal, or increased intracranial pressure.[1]

A neonate can have transiently low glucose levels that resolve without intervention. It is part of the normal physiologic process for glucose levels to dip after the first few hours after birth. Although the mechanism is not completely understood, it is likely caused by the combination of an abrupt cessation of maternal glucose supply through the placenta and transition to gluconeogenesis and glycogenolysis. More specifically, glucagon and cortisol regulate low blood sugar levels by increasing these processes, which requires some time to take full effect in the neonate.[2] The glycemic nadir (as low as 30 mg/dL) occurs at 1 to 2 hours after birth and slowly rises, reaching adult levels at 3 to 4 days of age.[3,4]

Routine screening and monitoring of blood glucose concentration is not needed in healthy term newborn infants after a normal pregnancy and delivery.[4] The typical heel-prick neonatal screening tests are obtained after 24 hours of life. In contrast, the authors recommend that bedside glucose testing be performed for any patients with complications of delivery, vital sign instability, neurologic findings, maternal history of endocrine disorders, or any other sign of concern. If there is concern that the neonate is hypoglycemic before the 24-hour screening tests are drawn, then it should be obtained immediately. Point-of-care test strip glucose analyzers may vary by 10 to 20 mg/dL especially at the lowest concentrations, therefore laboratory evaluation is recommended.[4] There is no universally accepted definition of hypoglycemia in a neonate who is otherwise healthy with no risk factors.[4,5] An accepted numerical value of less than 47 mg/dL is often cited in the literature. Hypoglycemia in otherwise healthy neonates is generally corrected by initiating feedings.[2]

Risk factors for prolonged hypoglycemia include having a diabetic mother, the infant being small for gestational age (SGA) or large for gestational age (LGA), initial respiratory distress, or prematurity.[2,3] Without the presence of these risk factors, otherwise healthy singleton pregnancies produce more cases of hypoglycemia when the mother spiked a fever during labor, the neonates' family had public rather than private insurance, and if the patient was born earlier while still remaining in the context of being full term.[6] In neonates who are premature or have increased rates of insulin production baseline secondary to being exposed to high levels of blood glucose during gestation within a diabetic mother, the episode of hypoglycemia can be more profound.[2] Newborn hypoglycemia is most common in an infant born to a diabetic mother (either type I or II diabetes mellitus [DM], or gestationally induced DM), wherein the infant was constantly exposed to increased glucose levels from the mother's blood.[2,7] As a compensation response, the fetus' beta cells of the pancreas remain in a state of overproduction. When the placental supply is abruptly cut off, it can take hours to days for the neonatal insulin drive to downregulate.[1] During this time, feedings often suffice.

However, intravenous dextrose infusions or further treatment options as discussed later may need to be initiated if an inadequate response is obtained or if the neonate is not able to tolerate oral feeds. In a study done with mothers with type 2 diabetes and gestational diabetes, the neonates whose mothers needed treatment with glyburide or insulin during pregnancy had a higher incidence of hypoglycemia within the first hour of birth.[8] Those women who were treated with diet alone for their diabetes did not produce neonates with hypoglycemia as frequently.[8]

If the blood glucose continues to remain low despite feedings and intravenous dextrose administration, congenital hyperinsulinemia, glycogen storage diseases, disorders of fat oxidation, hypopituitarism, and genetic issues such as Beckwith-Wiedemann, Costello, and mosaic Turner syndrome should be considered and investigated.[1,2] In such cases, a detailed obstetric and family history along with the ethnic origins of the parents need clarification. Certain obstetric elements may signal that the infant has an inborn error of metabolism, which occurs in 1:1500 births. For example, HELLP (hemolysis, elevated liver enzymes, low platelet count) syndrome or acute fatty liver of pregnancy could signal an underlying fatty acid oxidation disorder in the fetus.[1] Any step of carbohydrate or fatty acid metabolism can be affected with an enzyme deficiency and subsequent buildup of substrates that can cause metabolic derangements.[7] Certain ethnic groups to question more extensively for family congenital disorders include Ashkenazi Jews, Old Order Mennonites, Mediterranean races, French Canadians, and Africans.[1]

In terms of the acute setting, diagnosing the exact reason for the hypoglycemia is not as critical as normalizing the value to prevent irreversible neurologic damage. In general, the first line of treatment is initiating breast or bottle feedings. There is currently no evidence that hypoglycemia with no clinical signs harms the neonate or produces lasting neurologic sequelae.[9] However, if clinical signs of hypoglycemia are present and laboratory values confirm the abnormality, then neonates require regular glucose checks and should be transferred to the neonatal intensive care unit for further evaluation and monitoring.[4,9] Neonates of insulin-dependent mothers need glucose level checks at 1, 2, 3, 6, and 12 hours post partum for normalization.[9] Other tests that concurrently should be checked in these patients include bilirubin levels, hematocrit, and calcium levels.[9] There are no exact guidelines of when a sick-appearing neonate needs tests for investigation into whether hypoglycemia is the primary or secondary cause of the presentation. However, a consideration of risk factors such as maternal comorbidities, the physical examination, and lack of clinical improvement with treatment should trigger the clinician to start the work-up.

There is ongoing debate about when to intervene with asymptomatic hypoglycemic patients and whether or not to start dextrose infusions. Those infants whose blood sugars continue to be less than 50 mg/dL even with oral feedings and have risk factors for remaining in a hyperinsulinemic state should likely be started on dextrose infusions.[9] Target glucose levels are not established as a standard of treatment because the goal is to prevent adverse neurologic outcomes. Dextrose infusions generally start at a bolus of 2 to 3 mL/kg of 10% dextrose solution followed by a drip at 80 to 100 mL/kg/d.[2,4] If the levels do not respond, then gradual escalation to 30 mg/kg/min has been documented.[2] With concentrations higher than 12.5% dextrose, a central line must be inserted into the patient for protection of peripheral vasculature.

There are a variety of reasons why the neonate may fail to maintain adequate glucose levels. Further treatment options that can be explored include glucagon, steroids, diazoxide, and octreotide depending on the presumed cause of the hypoglycemia. Sometimes surgical management is required for certain types of insulin-secreting adenomas, whereas others can be medically managed.[1,10] Diazoxide works at the level of the beta islet cells to close the channels that regulate insulin secretion.[2] Diazoxide is a benzothiazine derivative and works within 1 hour of administration. Dosages start at 10 to 15 mg/kg/d and are given for about 5 to 8 days. If diazoxide fails to achieve normalization of levels, then octreotide, a somatostatin analogue, is initiated. Octreotide inhibits the secretion of insulin in a more direct fashion but also has a shorter duration of action.[2] If hypoglycemia is not caused by hyperinsulinemia, then glucagon is usually introduced. Intravenous dosing starts from 3 µg/kg to 20 µg/kg and is given continuously for 1 day.[2] Other treatments that may be attempted but are not proved to show dependable results include glucocorticoids and nifedipine.[2]

It is important to note the outcomes of neonates who receive a delayed diagnosis and initiation of treatment of hypoglycemia. In one study that performed magnetic resonance imaging (MRI) scans of babies at least 18 months after symptomatic neonatal hypoglycemia, 95% had signs of white matter damage and, of those, 43% had severe signs.[11] Other findings discovered on MRI included evidence of stroke and hemorrhage. In another study, 30% of the patients with congenital hyperinsulinemia who received medical therapy did not achieve milestones of development appropriately.[2] Those who failed medical therapy and needed surgical intervention fared worse.

In hypoglycemia of the newborn or older infant, consideration of other causes and differential diagnoses is of the utmost importance. In the approach to a generalized work-up for hypoglycemia in an older child or adult, inadequate intake, poor absorption, increased usage, disordered processing, or usage of glucose still applies. Considering sepsis and initiating appropriate work-up are important in the setting of maternal fever during delivery, neonate with sick contacts, febrile neonate, neonate with altered mental status, and neonate with neurologic changes, in addition to the signs and symptoms listed previously for hypoglycemia. It is important to ensure careful maternal history of a breastfeeding mother to include medications and or drug use that also may cause hypoglycemia in an infant less than 30 days of age. This history elicited to search for causes of inadequate intake should include how often and how long the infant is feeding on each breast, appropriate latch, maternal assessment of milk production, and growth of infant from birth weight. If the infant is formula fed, appropriate mixing of the formula is important in this assessment because inappropriate mixing can also lead to other electrolyte derangements. Poor absorption in an infant with hypoglycemia may manifest with a history of inadequate weight gain despite adequate feeding, or excessive loss such as diarrhea. According to the American Academy of Pediatrics, an infant can lose up to 10% of body weight after birth, but should recover by about a week of age. Assessing these historical facts helps guide the work-up of an infant with a presentation of frank hypoglycemia.

HYPOTHYROIDISM

The second most common endocrine emergency in neonates after hypoglycemia is hypothyroidism, which is another disorder that requires prompt diagnosis and treatment to improve prognosis and reduce the chances of developmental delay.[1] Although the incidence of neonatal hypothyroidism varies by country, congenital hypothyroidism in the United States occurs in 1 in 2000 to 1 in 4000 live births.[12] Congenital hypothyroidism is classified into primary and secondary as well as permanent and transient cases. Thyroid dysgenesis accounts for 85% of permanent primary congenital hypothyroidism, whereas inborn errors of thyroid hormone biosynthesis account for 10% to 15% of cases.[12] Secondary cases are often associated with congenital hypopituitarism rather than isolated thyroid-stimulating hormone (TSH) deficiency. As with hypoglycemia, there can be multiple causes, but, in the acute care setting, identifying the abnormality and initiating treatment is of critical importance.

Screening methods were introduced because hypothyroid neonates are largely asymptomatic at birth. Screening for hypothyroidism, which began in the early 1970s, has reduced cases of mental retardation. When signs and symptoms do present, usually around 6 weeks of age, they can include poor feeding, constipation, an increased need for sleep, greater than average weight, and jaundice. On physical examination, some findings signaling the need for further evaluation include large, puffy facies; macroglossia; hypotonia; or a distended abdomen, sometimes with an umbilical hernia.[12,13] The mother's history may also provide clues to further investigate the neonate for hypothyroidism. A maternal history of taking antithyroid medications, autoimmune disorders, or residing in a country with high incidence of iodine deficiency is helpful in diagnosing the neonate.[14,15] There may also be a history of thyroid problems in the family, such as thyroid dysgenesis, for which a genetic linkage has been shown.[14] Central hypopituitarism is often associated with congenital midline defects such as cleft palate.

In neonatal hypothyroidism, there are special considerations that need to be factored into the clinician's interpretation of results and diagnosis of the disorder. In normal neonatal physiology, thyroid hormone levels do not remain constant during the infants' first days of life and these levels depend on the gestational age of the patient.[14] In a healthy full-term infant the TSH is increased for the first few days of life, which is when the thyroid screening tests are obtained.[12] The levels normalize within the first month of life, which is when a patient is brought in for retest to confirm the diagnosis or to determine whether it was a transiently high level.[12] In premature neonates, the TSH is increased compared with that of full-term babies and must be interpreted in relation to reference ranges according to their gestational age.

There has been much research into the timing and the type of screening test for hypothyroidism. Debate as to whether to use only TSH or a combination of TSH and T4 for screening and when the levels should be drawn and the cutoff levels for treatment have been ongoing.[12–14] The most recent research suggests that checking TSH levels with the rest of the screening tests after birth and again within the first 30 days of life detects the greatest number of hypothyroidism cases.[13,14] When the patient is discharged before a second screen can be done, the caretaker needs to follow up for a retest. This method achieved the highest rates for identifying hypothyroid cases, at 2.6 per 1000 births.[14] By using only the first screening test, only half of the cases would be identified. For very low birth weight patients, most cases were detected with this screening method.

It may be impossible to determine whether a persistently increased TSH level is transient, but because the effects to the development of the infant of withholding treatment can be so severe, the standard is to treat the patient for hypothyroidism for the first 3 years of life after a positive screening.[13] Treatment starts immediately with levothyroxine 10 to 15 μg/kg/d. In the acute setting, the levothyroxine needs to be uptitrated as soon as possible until T4 levels are more than 130 mmol/L (10 μg/dL) and TSH levels are also within the reference range.[12] After this initial stabilization of levels, they may rechecked every month for the first 6 months of life to ensure adequate dosing.[12]

The prognosis of those infants who are started on therapy within the first 30 days of life is good. Studies have shown that they perform similarly to their peers on cognitive tests in grade school.[14] Factors that may influence this outcome depend on the severity of the hypothyroidism and the time of initiating treatment (after 30 days of life) as well as not starting the dose of medications at a high enough level.[13,14] Before screening tests were routine in developed countries, congenital hypothyroidism was the most common cause of mental retardation. Only about 25% of the world has mandatory newborn screening programs and a world health initiative may be underway to increase the screening in other countries, especially in those areas with endemic iodine deficiency.[16]

HYPERBILIRUBINEMIA

Emergency department (ED) physicians are certain to encounter infants presenting with jaundice, because 60% of newborns have some degree of jaundice.[17] Infants often even present to the emergency setting for a routine postnatal bilirubin check because the primary care providers and/or laboratories are unavailable. Bilirubin is produced by the breakdown of hemoglobin. In its unconjugated state, it can be bound to albumin in the blood, or in a free, water-insoluble state. When unconjugated, it is difficult to excrete and can cause central nervous system toxicity. This toxicity is still commonly referred to as kernicterus, but more recently has been termed bilirubin-induced neurologic dysfunction.[18] As bilirubin passes through the liver, it is conjugated to a water-soluble form that may be easily excreted. This process is the same in newborns as in adults; however, lower enzyme levels and lower amounts of binding substrate predispose them to jaundice more easily. Determining the type of hyperbilirubinemia is the first step in the diagnosis and management in these infants.

Unconjugated Hyperbilirubinemia

The diagnosis of unconjugated hyperbilirubinemia can range from normal physiologic processes to rare, life-threatening diseases. Even physiologic processes may, rarely, precipitate toxic levels of hyperbilirubinemia. Risk factors for more serious causes of jaundice include prematurity, jaundice within the first 24 hours of life, rapid rate of increase of bilirubin (>0.5 mg/dL/h), anemia, or hepatosplenomegaly.[19,20] The ED physician must realize that it is important to correlate levels with the clinical presentation.

Physiologic jaundice occurs when normal bilirubin released by the breakdown of hemoglobin transiently overwhelms the neonate's ability to conjugate and excrete it. Levels are usually around 12 mg/dL in a term infant at 72 hours.[19] This type of jaundice usually occurs at about 1 to 2 weeks of life. Two other presentations that should be distinguished are breast feeding failure jaundice (caused by dehydration) and so-called breast milk jaundice (a poorly understood phenomenon seen with breast milk). Breast feeding jaundice is caused by inadequate feeding and therefore inadequate excretion of bound bilirubin through the gastrointestinal tract. Breast milk jaundice is a diagnosis of exclusion, can be familial, and can last longer (months).

During the work-up of a jaundiced infant, physiologic jaundice remains a diagnosis of exclusion. In the neonate, jaundice may be secondary to another disease process or a part of a more complicated disease process. Significant dehydration, cephalohematomas, hemolysis, and sepsis may be causative factors of the jaundice. Other causes include inborn errors of metabolism, congenital hyperthyroidism, and Crigler-Najjar syndrome. **Table 1** lists potential causes of unconjugated hyperbilirubinemia.

The work-up of the jaundiced infant begins with a thorough history and physical examination. **Box 1** lists risk factors for severe hyperbilirubinemia. In the well-appearing infant, bilirubin and hemoglobin may be checked. The indirect bilirubin level is plotted on a nomogram and risk of disease is based on the level versus the age of the infant in hours. There are many different calculators that can also be used. One of the common Internet-based calculators is www.bilitool.org. Given a normal hemoglobin and no other worrisome history or symptoms of other acute illness, follow-up can be arranged

Table 1
Causes of unconjugated hyperbilirubinemia

Common causes	Physiologic jaundice
	Breast feeding failure jaundice
	Breast milk jaundice
	Cephalohematomas
Rare causes	Sepsis
	Hemolysis
	Maternal diabetes
	Intestinal obstruction
	Hereditary spherocytosis/elliptocytosis
	Congenital hyperthyroidism
	Inborn errors of metabolism
	Gilbert syndrome
	Crigler-Najjar syndrome
	Lucey-Driscoll syndrome
	Down syndrome

From Claudius I, Fluharty C, Boles R. The emergency department approach to newborn and childhood metabolic crisis. Emerg Med Clin North Am 2005;23:843–83.

based on the infant's risk of developing worsening hyperbilirubinemia. Breast feeding is generally continued unless breast milk jaundice is the suspected cause of hyperbilirubinemia. In this case, feedings may be discontinued transiently if bilirubin levels are greater than 17 to 20 mg/dL, in conjunction with admission for phototherapy. However, a full work-up should ensue because discontinuation of breastfeeding is usually not necessary. For patients with indirect bilirubin levels that require treatment, the mainstay is phototherapy and ensuring adequate hydration. A patient may, rarely,

Box 1
Risk factors for severe hyperbilirubinemia

Major risk factors

- Jaundice in the first 24 hours
- Blood group incompatibility or other known hemolytic disease
- Gestational age less than 37 weeks
- Previous sibling received phototherapy
- Cephalohematoma or significant bruising
- Exclusive breastfeeding

Minor risk factors

- Gestational age 37 to 38 weeks
- Jaundice before discharge
- Previous sibling with jaundice
- Macrosomic infant of diabetic mother
- Maternal age greater than or equal to 25 years
- Male gender

Data from Subcommittee on Hyperbilirubinemia. Management of hyperbilirubinemia in the newborn infant 35 or more weeks of gestation. Pediatrics 2004;114:29.

fail to respond to phototherapy, and exchange transfusion with or without intensive phototherapy can be considered.

If the patient is toxic or ill appearing, then the treatment priority is given to the potential underlying disease. Most commonly, these patients undergo a sepsis work-up and other studies as appropriate in addition to phototherapy. These patients may get a complete blood count with peripheral smear, Coombs test, analysis of maternal and fetal blood types, and urine analysis and culture. Glucose-6-phosphate dehydrogenase levels should be checked if the patient does not respond to phototherapy or is suspected based on background.

Conjugated Hyperbilirubinemia

Conjugated hyperbilirubinemia does not carry the neurologic risk of unconjugated hyperbilirubinemia, but is a herald of serious disorders. As such, the work-up is directed at identifying and treating underlying disorders. **Table 2** lists the differential diagnoses, most notably sepsis, inborn errors of metabolism, and biliary disorders. Therefore, the work-up commonly includes a full septic work-up (including a TORCH [toxoplasmosis, other (syphilis, varicella, parvovirus B19), rubella, cytomegalovirus, herpes] panel), blood gas, lactate, complete liver function panel, ammonia, electrolytes, blood urea nitrogen, and creatinine. In certain cases, it may expand to include urine for reducing substances, alpha1-antitrypsin, sweat chloride, abdominal imaging, and other tests as needed. Treatment and prognosis depend on the underlying diagnosis.

ELECTROLYTES

There are a few electrolyte disturbances that, in addition to hypoglycemia, need to be considered as potential causes of seizure presentation in the neonate. Both calcium and sodium derangements can be the causative disturbance for a variety of underlying reasons.

Hyponatremia

Hyponatremia (serum sodium <130 mEq/L) is second only to febrile seizure as a cause for first-time seizure in an infant.[21] The incidence of symptomatic hyponatremia in

Table 2 Causes of conjugated hyperbilirubinemia	
Common causes	Sepsis TORCH infections: • Toxoplasmosis • Other (syphilis, varicella, parvovirus B19) • Rubella • Cytomegalovirus • Herpes
Rare causes	Biliary atresia Inborn errors of metabolism Cystic fibrosis Alpha1-antitrypsin deficiency Neonatal iron storage diseases Alagille syndrome Hepatic infarction Byler disease

From Claudius I, Fluharty C, Boles R. The emergency department approach to newborn and childhood metabolic crisis. Emerg Med Clin North Am 2005;23:843–83.

children is not known because of a lack of prospective studies.[22] However, one retrospective review found that approximately 22% of children who were admitted to the hospital had hyponatremia, and symptomatic hyponatremia was found in 10% of children less than 2 years of age presenting to the ED with seizures.[23,24] During infancy, common presentations to the ED include gastrointestinal losses and water intoxication. Neonates (who lacks the ability to concentrate their urine) frequently receive free water or inappropriately diluted formula from their parents, leading to hyponatremia. Symptoms include not only seizure but also lethargy, muscle cramping, decreased reflexes, and acute respiratory failure.[25] They may also have hypothermia and hyperglycemia.[24–28]

Pediatric hyponatremia, as in adults, is classified based on total body water content. In general, significant symptoms do not appear until the sodium is less than 120 mEq/L, but may be present with rapid decreases in the normal range. Of those children with hyponatremia, 53% to 78% with serum sodium less than 125 mEq/L developed symptomatic hyponatremia.[29,30] As mentioned earlier, receiving free water from parents is a common cause, and bottle-fed infants are at increased risk.[25,27,28,31] Other causes include syndrome of inappropriate antidiuretic hormone (SIADH), congenital adrenal hyperplasia, congestive heart failure, cirrhosis, and nephrosis. Special attention to, and close monitoring of, serum sodium level in any child at risk for hyponatremia or with any of the conditions discussed earlier is necessary to prevent serious neurologic complications.

In general, use of intravenous fluids in the pediatric population should be considered an invasive treatment, and should have the same amount of care and attention applied as when administering any other medication.[22] Children may be at higher risk for development of cerebral edema because of the physiologic nature of a higher ratio of brain volume to skull size.[32]

Symptomatic hyponatremia (seizure, coma, or signs of herniation) should always be aggressively treated with the use of hypertonic 3% saline.[22] The serum sodium level should be increased by approximately 1 mEq/L per hour until the patient is seizure free, the serum sodium has corrected to 125 to 130 mEq/L, or the serum sodium level has increased by 10 mEq/L.[29,32–35] In infants, this can be accomplished by the following equation: volume of 3% saline = 10 mEq/L × body weight (kg) × 0.6 (extracellular fluid space). Another common regimen for a bolus is 3 to 5 mL/kg of 3% saline solution run over 30 to 60 minutes. The optimal rate of correction of serum sodium seems to be between 15 and 20 mEq/L over the first 48 hours, because patients with this range of correction have lower rates of mortality and better neurologic outcome compared with those with slower correction.[33–35] In less symptomatic patients, water restriction treats hyponatremia caused by water intoxication and SIADH. In hypovolemia, resuscitation fluids should be carefully calculated to increase the serum sodium appropriately while replacing volume. Diuretics may be necessary in hypervolemic hyponatremic states.

Hypocalcemia

Serum levels of calcium usually decline in the postnatal time period, but there are 2 noted time frames for clinically significant hypocalcemia: early postnatal (within a few days) and late postnatal (5–10 days after birth).[36] In a recent study, Thomas and colleagues[37] reported a retrospective chart review of infants presenting to 2 large medical centers in Texas with the diagnosis of moderate to severe hypocalcemia. The definition used for severe hypocalcemia was an ionized calcium of less than 4 mg/dL with the leading presentation of seizures consistent with tetany in all but 2 of the included infants. Infants excluded from the sample had hypocalcemia associated with other entities such as prematurity, congenital heart disease, DiGeorge syndrome, sepsis, renal disease, or other neurologic or gastrointestinal manifestation. In this group it was also noted that several subjects had low levels of magnesium as well as phosphorus that needed to be corrected as well. Initial management of seizure with known calcium levels less than 7 mg/dL can be treated with 100 to 300 mg/kg of calcium gluconate given intravenously.[36] Further evaluation as an inpatient in addition to broad emergent work-up should specifically include levels of 25-hydroxy-vitamin D as well as intact parathyroid hormone levels.

CONGENITAL ADRENAL HYPERPLASIA

Although congenital adrenal hyperplasia (CAH) is not a common neonatal endocrine disorder, it is still screened for in the United States and other countries. Obvious physical examination findings on birth are helpful in diagnosing this rare and potentially fatal disorder but are not always present. Patients are subdivided into classic and nonclassic types, which present with obvious versus more subtle clinical findings, respectively. Classic CAH is more severe. The classic presentation is a neonate, usually 2 weeks after birth, who is atypically somnolent, vomiting, feeding poorly, and showing signs of dehydration such as a depressed fontanel and decreased skin turgor.[38] This presentation, as is often the case with neonates, still raises a broad differential diagnosis. However, in the critically ill neonate, a basic metabolic panel to check for the typical electrolyte abnormalities of hyponatremia and hyperkalemia is warranted. On physical examination of the female neonate, ambiguous genitalia may include a sizable clitoris and fused labia majora.[39–41] Intact uterus and fallopian tubes with no anatomic abnormalities are evident on subsequent ultrasonography. With severe cases of CAH, girls may initially be assigned as boys immediately after birth because the genitalia may be more similar to those of a boy. True male babies appear normal at birth with no signs of ambiguous genitalia, but may have some enlargement of the penis and testes along with skin hyperpigmentation. The nonclassic form of CAH does not produce high enough levels of androgens to virilize girls, therefore findings on physical examination may be absent.[40]

The classic form occurs in about 1 in 16,000 births worldwide, whereas the incidence of the nonclassic form may vary according to the population.[40,42] For instance, in the United States, the nonclassic form was positively screened for in 1 in 130,000 births.[40] The incidence of the disease is closer to 1 in 2000, so the screening test does not pick up all forms of the mild disease.[36] However, in other white populations in eastern Europe, for example, it may be more common, affecting up to 1% to 2% of the population because of the carrier population.[40] Certain other groups such as the Yupic Eskimos in Alaska, Philippinos, Brazilians, and those living on an island in France called La Reunion are known to have the most cases.

In the steroid synthesis pathway, which occurs within the adrenal cortex, cholesterol is converted to many intermediates with the sex hormones, cortisol, and aldosterone being the desired products in normal physiology. CAH is an autosomal recessive disorder in which one of the 5 enzymes in the pathway to create cortisol is defective with a buildup of undesired products that can cause side effects such as virilization in female neonates, hemodynamic instability, and electrolyte abnormalities. The common pathophysiology that occurs with this group of enzyme deficiencies is a deficiency in aldosterone. Sodium channels cannot regulate fluid balance properly, thus leading to hypotension.[40] Certain intermediates that build up can even serve as antagonists to aldosterone, exacerbating the state. Sodium cannot get into the intravascular space effectively without aldosterone regulation.[40] Potassium, also part of the exchange process in sodium channels, cannot be excreted, leading to hyperkalemia. These neonates are also deficient in cortisol, which is integral for the regulation of blood pressure, fluid status, and glucose levels. Renin levels increase in an attempt to compensate.[40] The most common enzyme deficiency in this group of disorders is the 21-hydroxylase deficiency, which comprises 90% of cases.[39] This enzyme converts 17-hydroxyprogesterone (17-OHP) to 11-deoxycortisol, which is eventually converted to cortisol and another precursor that is converted to aldosterone.[40] Without the proper levels of cortisol and aldosterone, these patients present with symptoms of adrenal insufficiency and metabolic derangements: hypotension, hyponatremia, hyperkalemia, and altered mental status. If not detected early these patients often present in florid shock.

In the United States, along with many other countries, CAH is tested for in the panel of newborn screening tests. It has been used as part of the screening tests since 1977.[40] Once the newborn screen returns with an abnormal result, the health care provider must decide whether patients have CAH if they are not showing symptoms of salt wasting. Subsequent laboratory tests for 17-OHP levels, the intermediate that would be increased in 21-hydroxylase deficiency, are sent. The test is done either as an enzyme-linked immunosorbent assay (ELISA) or by mass spectrometry, which is more accurate and reduces the rate false-positives compared with ELISA.[40] Diagnosis is more difficult in premature neonates and those with other comorbidities because stress hormones may be high, which can cause a transient increase in this screening test.[40] The diagnosis is further complicated because levels of 17-OHP are increased in the first few days of life. Because many healthy babies are discharged from the hospital within this time, if a newborn screen is drawn early, then there is a greater chance for false-positives. Studies show that, for every case of CAH identified through screening tests, another 200 babies undergo further testing, ultimately not being true-positives.[40] The current methods of screening for CAH show a poor positive predictive value at 0.53% to 1%.[40,42] A method to improve the screening accuracy is by correlating the levels according to gestational age.[42] If the initial level is increased, then it is repeated. If this repeat is still increased, then the patient can be diagnosed by a pediatric endocrinologist with a cosyntropin stimulation test, which must be done after the first 24 hours of life. If there is clinical suspicion that the patient has CAH, then health care providers can go straight to the stimulation test without another repeat level. False-negative cases also occur. About 10% of classic CAH cases have low initial levels of 17-OHP.

The decision to treat a patient for CAH depends on the suspicion that the patient has the condition. Treatment is not benign and patients may develop side effects from steroids such as Cushing syndrome, hyperglycemia, or cataracts. The consensus is that, if the patient has physical signs of CAH and is unstable, then it is reasonable to start intravenous normal saline infusion and steroid therapy for adrenal insufficiency.[40] Once diagnosis is made, treatment begins with hydrocortisone at 20 mg/m^2 daily divided into 3 equal doses per day and fludrocortisone 0.1 mg per day. If the neonate is decompensating, then additional 0.9% NaCl boluses, high doses of intravenous hydrocortisone (100 mg/m^2 daily), and fludrocortisone 0.1 mg twice a day should be started. The dose for hydrocortisone should be increased only to the point at which the patient suppresses androgen excess and can still achieve proper growth, not until the levels of 17-OHP are within normal values. Also, after the acute crisis is controlled, the patient is switched to oral fludrocortisone and oral sodium chloride supplements. In nonclassic CAH, treatment is not recommended until symptoms develop.[39,40] Other recommendations for follow-up of nonclassic CAH cases are covered in the pediatric endocrinology literature.

INBORN ERRORS OF METABOLISM

Although a full discussion of inborn errors of metabolism is beyond the scope of this article, the emergency physician should be familiar with a few key aspects of these diseases and their emergent presentations. In general, there are 3 main mechanisms of illness:

1. Accumulation of toxic small molecules
2. Energy deficiency
3. Chronic accumulation of large molecules

The common thread between these three pathways is a genetic mutation that leads to protein malfunction and a blocked metabolic pathway. Also common among each is seizures, stroke, lethargy, encephalopathy, and abnormal tone. Abnormal odors may be present in small molecule and energy metabolism, but are rare as presenting clinical symptoms.[43]

In general, the accumulation of toxic intermediates (usually acids) takes place between day 2 and 5 of life, thus a newborn appears normal and does not have signs or symptoms immediately after birth.[44] In utero, the placenta removes the toxic metabolites. Severe metabolic acidosis is a common feature in this category and can also be accompanied by hyperpnea/tachypnea, hyperammonemia, and altered mental status.[44] A more common presentation of encephalopathy associated with an undiagnosed inborn error is central apnea and respiratory distress. Sepsis in an infant with an undiagnosed inborn error of metabolism progresses to shock more rapidly and should be considered in the differential diagnosis in the setting of poor feeding, recurrent vomiting, seizures, abnormal muscle tone, lethargy, or acute life-threatening event. Untreated, accumulation of toxins with noted encephalopathy quickly leads to coma, multisystem organ failure, and death.

Mitochondrial disorders are the prototypic disorders of energy deficiency. Unlike the accumulation of toxic intermediates, the placenta is not protective, and the fetus may develop birth defects, abnormal facies, and other prenatal problems. Seizures, cardiomyopathy, and hepatocellular disease are common hallmarks leading to lactic acidosis, multisystem organ failure, and death.[44]

Accumulation of large molecules results in a chronic disease process that rarely presents emergently. Instead, the severity of disease is related to location and amount of stored material. Joint contractures, valvular disease, cataracts, and neurologic problems are common.

The work-up of potential inborn errors of metabolism is extensive and specific to the suspected disease process. Focus is placed on small toxic molecules (ammonia), and energy deficiency (hypoglycemia) because these present emergently and a prolonged state of coma caused by these entities directly correlates with nonreversible neuronal damage.[45] Screening tests may include complete blood count, electrolytes, blood urea nitrogen, creatinine, arterial or venous blood gas, ammonia, lactate, urine analysis, liver function tests, coagulation studies, and potentially creatinine kinase. An increased anion gap is the most sensitive and specific sign of an organic acidemia (>20 is highly abnormal) and increased ammonia (>150–200 μM) is the hallmark of a urea cycle defect.[45] It is always advised that early consultation with a metabolic specialist can help to determine when and whether specialty laboratory testing is indicated.

The mainstay of therapy is dextrose infusion because this provides energy and increases endogenous insulin production, thereby preventing catabolism. Consideration must also be given to the need for bicarbonate therapy; the management and further prevention of cerebral edema; and, in rare instances, simultaneous insulin and dextrose administration. In cases of significant impairment caused by hyperammonemia, hemodialysis may be considered in consultation with a nephrologist.[45] This care is beyond the scope of normal emergency medicine practice, so prompt transfer to a pediatric facility after stabilization is critical.

SUMMARY

The resuscitation principles for neonates remain the same in any neonatal emergency, such as securing the airway and stabilizing hemodynamics. However, stabilizing endocrine disorders can be challenging because they can affect several organ systems simultaneously, and have various presentations (which may or may not be subtle), making diagnosis difficult without laboratory studies and clinical acumen. Screening tests have improved significantly in the past few decades and have become standard of practice in many areas of the world. Although not all-inclusive, their implementation has significantly reduced morbidity and mortality in neonates. Implementing screening programs more broadly worldwide and improving the current tests remains the challenge for future health care providers and those practicing abroad. With further attention and study into these disorders and the best treatment practices, these patients can be given the best outcomes.

REFERENCES

1. Rios A, Adams D. Specific congenital metabolic disorders. In: McInerny TK, editor. American academy of pediatrics textbook of pediatric care. Elk Grove Village (IL): American Academy of Pediatrics; 2009. p. 970–87.
2. Sweet C, Grayson S, Polak M. Management strategies for neonatal hypoglycemia. J Pediatr Pharmacol Ther 2013;18:199–208.
3. Rozance P, Hay W. Neonatal hypoglycemia–answers, but more questions. J Pediatr 2012;161(5):775–6.
4. Committee on Fetus and Newborn, Adamkin DH. Postnatal glucose homeostasis in late-preterm and term infants. Pediatrics 2011;127:575–9. http://dx.doi.org/10.1542/peds.2010-3851.
5. Tin W. Defining neonatal hypoglycaemia: a continuing debate. Semin Fetal Neonatal Med 2013. http://dx.doi.org/10.1016/j.siny.2013.09.003.
6. DePuy A, Coassolo KM, Som DA, et al. Neonatal hypoglycemia in term, nondiabetic pregnancies. Am J Obstet Gynecol 2009;200(5):45–51.
7. de Lonlay P, Giurgea I, Touati G, et al. Neonatal hypoglycaemia: aetiologies. Semin Neonatol 2004;9:49–58.
8. Ramos G, Hanley AA, Aguayo J, et al. Neonatal chemical hypoglycemia in newborns from pregnancies complicated by type 2 and gestational diabetes mellitus-the importance of neonatal ponderal index. J Matern Fetal Neonatal Med 2012; 25(3):267–71.
9. Nafday S. Neonatal medical conditions. In: McInerny TK, editor. American academy of pediatrics textbook of pediatric care. Elk Grove Village (IL): American Academy of Pediatrics; 2009. p. 883–91.
10. Stanley C. Hypoglycemia in the neonate. Pediatr Endocrinol Rev 2006;4(Suppl 1): 76–81.
11. Burns C, Rutherford MA, Boardman JP, et al. Patterns of cerebral injury and neurodevelopmental outcomes after symptomatic neonatal hypoglycemia. Pediatrics 2008;122(1):65–74.

12. Rastogi M, LaFranchi S. Congenital hypothyroidism. Orphanet J Rare Dis 2010; 5(17).
13. Buyukgebiz A. Newborn screening for congenital hypothyroidism. J Clin Res Pediatr Endocrinol 2013;5(Suppl 1):8–12.
14. Korzeniewski S, Kleyn M, Young WI, et al. Screening for congenital hypothyroidism in newborns transferred to neonatal intensive care. Arch Dis Child Fetal Neonatal Ed 2013;98:F210–315.
15. LaFranchi S. Approach to the diagnosis and treatment of neonatal hypothyroidism. J Clin Endocrinol Metab 2011;96(10):2959–67.
16. Azar-Kolakez A, Ecosse E, Dos Santos S, et al. All-cause and disease-specific mortality and morbidity in patients with congenital hypothyroidism treated since the neonatal period: a national population-based study. J Clin Endocrinol Metab 2013;98(2):785–93.
17. American Academy of Pediatrics. Provisional Committee for Quality Improvement and Subcommittee on Hyperbilirubinemia. Practice parameter: management of hyperbilirubinemia in the healthy term newborn. Pediatrics 1994;94:558–65.
18. Johnson L, Bhutani V. The clinical syndrome of bilirubin-induced neurologic dysfunction. Semin Perinatol 2011;35(3):101–13.
19. Claudius I, Fluharty C, Boles R. The emergency department approach to newborn and childhood metabolic crisis. Emerg Med Clin North Am 2005;23: 843–83.
20. Sarici S, Serdar M, Korkmaz A, et al. Incidence, course and prediction of hyperbilirubinemia in near-term and term newborns. Pediatrics 2004;113(4):775–80.
21. Cornelli H, Gormley C, Baker R. Hyponatremia and seizures presenting in the first two years of life. Pediatr Emerg Care 1985;1:190–3.
22. Moritz M, Ayus J. Preventing neurological complications from dysnatremias in children. Pediatr Nephrol 2005;20(12):1687–700.
23. Hoorn E, Geary D, Robb M, et al. Acute hyponatremia related to intravenous fluid administration in hospitalized children: an observational study. Pediatrics 2004; 113(5):1279–84.
24. Farrar H, Chande VT, Fitzpatrick DF, et al. Hyponatremia as the cause of seizures in infants: a retrospective analysis of incidence, severity, and clinical predictors. Ann Emerg Med 1995;26(1):42–8.
25. Keating J, Schears G, Dodge P. Oral water intoxication in infants. An American epidemic. Am J Dis Child 1991;145:985–90.
26. Medani C. Seizures and hypothermia due to dietary water intoxication in infants. South Med J 1987;80:421–5.
27. David R, Ellis D, Gartner J. Water intoxication in normal infants: role of antidiuretic hormone in pathogenesis. Pediatrics 1981;68(3):349–53.
28. Sharif R. Seizure from hyponatremia in infants. Early recognition and treatment. Arch Fam Med 1993;2:647–52.
29. Sarnaik A, Meert K, Hackbarth R, et al. Management of hyponatremic seizures in children with hypertonic saline: a safe and effective strategy. Crit Care Med 1991; 19(6):758–62.
30. Halberthal M, Halperin M, Bohn M. Lesson of the week: acute hyponatremia children admitted to hospital: retrospective analysis of factors contributing to its development and resolution. BMJ 2001;322(7289):780–2.
31. Vanapruks V, Prapaitrakul K. Water intoxication and hyponatremic convulsions in neonates. Arch Dis Child 1989;64:734–5.
32. Lauriat S, Berl T. The hyponatremic patient: practical focus on therapy. J Am Soc Nephrol 1997;8(10):1599–607.

33. Ayus J, Krothapalli R, Arieff A. Treatment of symptomatic hyponatremia and its relation to brain damage. A prospective study. N Engl J Med 1987;317(19): 1190–5.
34. Verbalis J. Adaptation to acute and chronic hyponatremia: implications for symptomatology, diagnosis, and therapy. Semin Nephrol 1998;18(1):3–19.
35. Fraser C, Arieff A. Epidemiology, pathophysiology, and management of hyponatremic encephalopathy. Am J Med 1997;102(1):67–77.
36. Arcara K, Tschudy M. Johns Hopkins Hospital. The Harriet Lane handbook. 19th edition. Philadelphia: Elsevier Mosby; 2012.
37. Thomas T, Smith J, White P, et al. Transient neonatal hypocalcemia: presentation and outcomes. Pediatrics 2012;129:e1461.
38. Pearce J. Congenital adrenal hyperplasia: a potential diagnosis for the neonate in shock. Aust Crit Care 1995;8(1):16–9.
39. Speiser P, White P. Congenital adrenal hyperplasia. N Engl J Med 2003;394: 776–88.
40. Pass K, Neto E. Update: newborn screening for endocrinopathies. Endocrinol Metab Clin North Am 2009;38(4):827–37.
41. Witchel S, Azziz R. Congenital adrenal hyperplasia. J Pediatr Adolesc Gynecol 2011;24(3):116–26.
42. White P. Neonatal screening for congenital adrenal hyperplasia. Nat Rev Endocrinol 2009;4:490–8.
43. Pollack C. Utility of glucagons in the emergency department. J Emerg Med 1993; 11(2):195–205.
44. Seashore M, Rinaldo P. Metabolic disease of the neonate and young infant. Semin Perinatol 1993;17(5):318–29.
45. Mathias RS, Kostiner D, Packman S. Hyperammonemia in urea cycle disorders: role of the nephrologist. Am J Kidney Dis 2001;37(5):1069–80.

Current Diagnosis and Treatment of Hyperglycemic Emergencies

Brian Corwell, MD[a],*, Brandi Knight, MD[b], Laura Olivieri, MD[b], George C. Willis, MD[b]

KEYWORDS

- Diabetic ketoacidosis (DKA) • Hyperosmolar hyperglycemic state (HHS)
- Hyperglycemic crisis • Insulin therapy • Electrolyte management

KEY POINTS

- Diabetic ketoacidosis (DKA) and hyperosmolar hyperglycemic state (HHS) are 2 hyperglycemic crises frequently encountered in emergency departments.
- DKA, characterized by hyperglycemia, ketonemia, and anion gap metabolic acidosis, results from absolute or relative insulin deficiency and counterregulatory hormone excess.
- HHS, characterized by hyperglycemia, hyperosmolarity, and profound dehydration without significant ketoacidosis, results from prolonged poor glycemic control and inadequate hydration.
- The management of both DKA and HHS hinges on treatment of precipitating illnesses, fluid resuscitation, and correction of hyperglycemia, acidosis, and electrolyte abnormalities.

INTRODUCTION

Hyperglycemia is a common occurrence in emergency department patients. As the number of new cases of diabetes mellitus increases worldwide, emergency providers are frequently faced with hyperglycemic patients and challenges surrounding their care. DKA and HHS are the most feared and life-threatening hyperglycemic emergencies in diabetes. Both of these diseases are associated with uncontrolled diabetes mellitus and may lead to significant neurologic morbidity and death. Early diagnosis and management in an emergency department is paramount to improve patient outcomes. The mainstays of treatment in both DKA and HHS are aggressive rehydration, insulin therapy, electrolyte management, and discovery and treatment of any underlying precipitating events.

[a] CAQ Sports Medicine, Department of Emergency Medicine, University of Maryland School of Medicine, 110 South Paca Street, 6th Floor, Suite 200, Baltimore, MD 21201, USA; [b] Department of Emergency Medicine, University of Maryland School of Medicine, 110 South Paca Street, 6th Floor, Suite 200, Baltimore, MD 21201, USA
* Corresponding author.
E-mail address: bcorwell@som.umaryland.edu

Emerg Med Clin N Am 32 (2014) 437–452
http://dx.doi.org/10.1016/j.emc.2014.01.004
0733-8627/14/$ – see front matter © 2014 Elsevier Inc. All rights reserved.
emed.theclinics.com

EPIDEMIOLOGY

The prevalence and financial burden of diabetes are tremendous and rising. Approximately 10% of the US population lives with diabetes, and approximately 2 million Americans are diagnosed with diabetes yearly.[1] It is projected that by the year 2050, up to 1 in 3 American adults will be diabetic.[2] An estimated 10% of health care dollars are spent treating diabetes and its complications, and 20% of health care dollars are spent caring for diabetics overall; in 2012, the direct medical costs of treating diabetes totaled $176 billion.[3]

The incidence of DKA has been estimated in older studies to range from 4 to 8 episodes per 1000 patient admissions for diabetes.[4] In 2009, DKA accounted for approximately 140,000 hospitalizations.[5] In the United States, DKA accounts for more than $1 billion in hospital costs per year.[6] The incidence of DKA is much higher among young children and persons of lower socioeconomic status. There is often low family income, poor parental support and patient education levels, and less health insurance coverage with decreased access to care, all contributing to poor compliance and high rates of recurrent DKA.[7]

The incidence of HHS is more difficult to quantify because there have been no population-based studies, but it has been estimated to account for approximately 1% of diabetic admissions.[8] This number is likely an underestimation. The mortality in HHS is much higher, however, ranging from 10% to 20%, compared with 1% to 5% in DKA.[8,9]

PATHOPHYSIOLOGY

DKA and HHS are both characterized by hyperglycemia, which stems from insulin resistance or deficiency of insulin secretion from the pancreas. In DKA, the driving force is insulin insufficiency and a subsequent increase in insulin counterregulatory hormones (ICRHs), which prevents the body from metabolizing carbohydrates.[10,11] Insulin normally stimulates the transference of glucose from the bloodstream into tissues of the body, where it is needed for energy, glycogen storage, and lipogenesis. Insulin also inhibits hepatic gluconeogenesis, preventing further glucose production by the body.[12] When insulin is absent, hepatic gluconeogenesis continues, yet glucose cannot move into the cells and instead builds up in the bloodstream. This elevated glucose leads to osmotic diuresis and dehydration.

In DKA, metabolism shifts from normal carbohydrate metabolism to a state of fasting fat metabolism. There is an increase in the aforementioned ICRHs: glucagon, catecholamines, cortisol, and growth hormones.[13] These stress hormones stimulate lipolysis, which leads to free fatty acid oxidation into the ketone bodies, acetone, acetoacetate, and β-3-hydroxybutyrate, the last being the primary contributor to the resultant metabolic acidosis.[8] The body can initially buffer mild ketonemia, and this results in a mild anion gap with a normal blood pH. Once ketonemia reaches excess of the body's limits, however, it begins to spill into urine and causes an anion gap acidosis with a drop in pH and bicarbonate levels.[8] Respiratory compensation ensues with rapid deep breathing, called Kussmaul respirations. Ketonemia further leads to nausea and vomiting, often worsening dehydration.[8] The course of DKA is usually a quick progression, often occurring in hours to days.

DKA occurs more frequently in type 1 diabetes mellitus; however, it can also occur in non–insulin-dependent (type 2) diabetes mellitus. It is growing increasingly common in type 2 diabetes mellitus, which is thought due to an acute halt of insulin secretion by temporary pancreatic beta islet cell dysfunction and temporary insulin resistance. The condition often resolves after treatment of the acute DKA episode, and patients may later resume their home oral hypoglycemic agent, not requiring long-term insulin therapy.[14]

Type 2 diabetics are more likely to develop HHS when in a hyperglycemic state. In HHS, there is enough pancreatic production of insulin to prevent the initiation of lipolysis required to generate ketosis and acidemia.[13] There is significantly higher hyperglycemia, however, with associated osmotic diuresis and worsened dehydration compared with DKA. HHS often has a longer and more protracted course, over days to weeks prior to presentation.

In either condition, fluid deficits are significant. Fluid losses in DKA average between 10% and 15% body weight, or approximately 100 mL/kg, for a net loss of between 5 and 7 L.[8,15,16] In HHS, fluid losses average between 20% and 25% body weight, or approximately 100 and 200 mL/kg, for a net loss of between 8 and 12 L.[8,16,17] There are total body losses of important electrolytes through the urine, such as sodium, chloride, and potassium. Initial laboratory measurements may appear falsely elevated secondary to volume contraction.[13]

Causes

Lack of exogenous insulin (noncompliance or undertreatment) and infection are the most common precipitants of DKA and HHS.[8,13] There are many possible triggers, however, for hyperglycemic crisis (**Box 1** lists of the most common precipitating causes for hyperglycemic crisis). Mortality, especially in HHS, is frequently due to an underlying cause rather than the complications of the condition itself; therefore, a thorough investigation for the cause should always be performed.

Differential Diagnosis

There are many disease states that may mimic the presentation of hyperglycemic crisis. DKA can be mimicked by any of the causes of anion gap metabolic acidosis. Similarly, the differential diagnosis for HHS is extensive because it can mimic many other causes of altered mental status. Other causes for confusion, acidosis, and ketosis should be sought out during initial work-up. **Box 2** outlines a list of differential diagnoses. Unfortunately, one of these alternative diagnoses can also be a precipitating event leading to the development of either hyperglycemic crisis. Therefore, it is important to keep a broad differential in acutely ill patients and realize that there may be many other concomitant conditions.

Clinical Presentation

Patients with DKA often present with nonspecific complaints, such as fatigue or classic symptoms of hyperglycemia: polyuria, polydipsia, and weight loss.[10] They commonly present with generalized abdominal pain, nausea, and vomiting, which are due to ketosis or possible decreased mesenteric perfusion secondary to dehydration.[10] Patients with DKA may present with decreased mental status, which may be due to respiratory fatigue, acidosis, or an inciting cause, such as sepsis or cerebrovascular accident (CVA). It is also important to garner a history of any possible inciting events, such as chest pain for an acute myocardial infarction (MI) or neurologic deficits for an acute cerebrovascular event. Any information in review of symptoms to suggest an infectious source, missed medication doses, new medications, or illicit drug use is a vital aspect of history taking.

Similarly, patients with HHS also complain of symptoms of hyperglycemia. The most common presenting symptom for patients with HHS is neurologic deficit. The mainstay of the diagnosis of HHS is the presence of neurologic deficits due to the profound

Box 1
Precipitating factors for hyperglycemic crisis
Medication noncompliance
Infection
Urinary tract infection
Pneumonia
Dental abscess
Skin infections
Sepsis/septic shock
Cardiovascular incidents
MI
CVA
Abdominal inflammation
Appendicitis
Pancreatitis
Trauma
Pregnancy
Ingestions
Cocaine
Alcohol abuse
Medications
Sympathomimetics
Atypical antipsychotics
Corticosteroids
Thiazide diuretics

dehydration and hyperosmolarity. It can be as simple as limb weakness or sensory deficits or as complicated as seizures or coma.

On physical examination, patients often present with vital sign abnormalities, such as tachycardia or hypotension, due to volume loss or infection. Patients in DKA may exhibit Kussmaul respirations. The breath may have a classic fruity odor in DKA patients due to acetone exhalation in ketosis,[10] which is absent in HHS. Both DKA and HHS likely show fatigue or lethargy and signs of dehydration with dry mucous membranes and poor skin turgor.

The rest of the physical examination should focus on searching for possible inciting causes. Abdominal examination is a key portion of the assessment to evaluate for additional pathology; however, palpation may reveal diffuse tenderness in DKA patients.[10] Efforts should be made to discern any localized tenderness necessitating further evaluation. Additional history should elicit a search for other physical examination findings to suggest an inciting event, such as pulmonary examination for possible pneumonia and dental, ear, and full skin examination to evaluate for hidden causes of infection, such as oral abscess, otitis media, cellulitis, abscess, or decubitus ulcers.

Box 2
Differential diagnosis in hyperglycemic crisis
Alcoholic ketoacidosis
Wernicke encephalopathy
Seizure/postictal state
Opiate overdose
Salicylate toxicity
Methanol
Toxic alcohol ingestion
Paraldehyde ingestion
Isoniazid
Lactic acidosis
Appendicitis
Pancreatitis
Pneumonia
MI
CVA
Renal failure

Diagnostic Evaluation

The diagnostic criteria for DKA and HHS are outlined in **Table 1**. The blood glucose for DKA rarely reaches the elevations seen in HHS, which are frequently greater than 600 mg/dL. Also, the presence of a neurologic deficit is necessary for the diagnosis of HHS. Calculating the serum osmolarity reveals all hyperglycemic patients to also be hyperosmolar. The hyperosmolarity leading to neurologic sequelae requires, however, much more aggressive treatment than simple hyperglycemia.

Initial evaluation should include bedside finger-stick glucose or a chemistry panel, including serum glucose, electrolytes, and serum urea nitrogen (SUN) and creatinine. Preliminary electrolyte evaluation may reveal false hypernatremia or hyperkalemia due

Table 1
Diagnostic criteria for DKA and HHS

	Mild DKA	Moderate DKA	Severe DKA	HHS
Plasma glucose (mg/dL)	>250	>250	>250	>600
pH	7.25–7.3	7.0–7.24	<7.0	>7.3
Serum bicarbonate (mEq/L)	15–18	10–15	<10	>18
Ketones (urine or serum)	Positive	Positive	Positive	Minimal or negative
Anion gap	>10	>12	>12	Variable
Osmolality (mOsm/kg)	Variable	Variable	Variable	>320
Mental status	Alert	Alert/drowsy	Stupor/coma	Stupor/coma

Data from Kitabchi AE, Umpierrez GE, Miles JM, et al. Hyperglycemic crises in adult patients with diabetes. Diabetes Care 2009;32(7):1335–43.

to volume depletion, when in reality hyperglycemic osmotic diuresis causes hyponatremia and hypokalemia.[13] Hyperkalemia occurs when potassium shifts out of cells in exchange for hydrogen ions in an attempt to compensate for acidosis. This may cause the measured potassium to appear artificially normal or elevated when total body potassium levels are depleted due to urinary and gastrointestinal losses.[18]

Despite the official definition of DKA involving serum glucose of greater than 250 mg/dL, there are reported cases of euglycemic DKA with normal to low serum glucose levels of less than 200 mg/dL, also called pseudonormoglycemic DKA. Cases are rare, occurring in 0.8% to 1.1% of DKA episodes.[19] This condition has been seen in pregnancy; in states of fasting or low caloric intake, starvation, persistent vomiting, depression, or extreme hyperlipidemia; and in those with glycogen storage disorders.[18–20] Physiology of true euglycemic DKA (not secondary to insulin administration) is thought to be due to relative insulin deficiency with increased urinary loss of glucose from increased ICRHs or decreased rate of hepatic gluconeogenesis during fasting.[21]

DKA causes an elevated anion gap metabolic acidosis due to ketogenesis, notably from the ketone body β-hydroxybutyrate, followed by acetoacetate.[8] The anion gap is calculated using the measured sodium and not the corrected sodium. **Box 3** contains a list of commonly used calculation. A venous blood gas level should be obtained for serial evaluations of pH. Studies show good correlation between arterial blood gas and venous blood gas measurement and no benefit to arterial versus venous testing in the diagnosis and treatment of DKA in an emergency department.[22] Other sources of anion gap metabolic acidosis may be assessed based on clinical suspicion, such as lactate level for differentiating lactic acidosis, salicylate level, acetaminophen level, SUN, and toxic alcohols.

Serum ketones or β-hydroxybutyrate should be obtained. Urine testing detects only acetoacetate levels meaning that a patient's urine may initially show no or low ketones. Therefore, serum β-hydroxybutyrate is more sensitive compared with urine ketones.[23] Point-of-care bedside β-hydroxybutyrate testing is available as well. These tests have been found as accurate as laboratory methods, which can shorten time to diagnosis of DKA.[7,24,25] Bedside testing may replace serial blood gas measurements in the future.[26] Another quick bedside test is end-tidal capnography. In one study, capnography values greater than 24.5 mm Hg were suggestive of the absence of DKA in hyperglycemic emergency department patients.[27]

HHS has an absence of the major laboratory findings in DKA. There are no anion gap acidosis and no ketones present, unless an alternative cause of these laboratory abnormalities is present concurrently with HHS. The serum osmolarity, however, is elevated. Therefore, serum osmolarity should also be obtained.

Glucose-induced hyponatremia is another side effect of hyperglycemic crisis. Corrected serum sodium in hyperglycemia is routinely calculated with the correction factor of 1.6.[28] Hillier and colleagues,[29] in 1999, however, found more accurate

---

Box 3
Calculations in DKA and HHS

- Anion gap: [Na (mEq/L) − [Cl (mEq/L) + HCO_3 (mEq/L)]
- Serum osmolality: [2 × measured Na (mEq/L)] + [glucose (mg/dL)/18] + [SUN (mg/dL)/2.8]
- Corrected serum sodium
  - Measured Na (mEq/L) + 0.016 × [glucose(mg/dL) − 100] for glucose <400 mg/dL
  - Measured Na (mEq/L) + 0.024 × [glucose (mg/dL) − 100] for glucose >400 mg/dL

mean correction factor of 2.4, particularly in glucose levels greater than 400. The standard correction factor of 1.6 may still remain accurate for blood glucose up to 400 mg/dL.

TREATMENT

Successful treatment of DKA and HHS involves the correction of hypovolemia, hyperglycemia, ketoacid production, and electrolyte abnormalities and treating any precipitating illnesses. The fluid, electrolyte, and insulin regimens for initial emergency department resuscitation of DKA and HHS share many commonalities.

Fluid Resuscitation

Fluid replacement therapy should be initiated immediately after diagnosis, because further delay while awaiting initial electrolyte results could lead to further deterioration of hemodynamic status. As discussed previously, the osmotic diuresis from hyperglycemia results in significant volume depletion.

Fluid resuscitation serves several functions. Initial resuscitation helps restore depleted intravascular volume, achieve normal tonicity, and decrease the level of ICRHs. Additionally, fluid resuscitation increases tissue/organ perfusion decreasing lactate formation, improves renal perfusion promoting renal excretion of glucose and ketone bodies, and decreases plasma osmolarity by decreasing serum glucose concentration.[6] Mean plasma glucose concentrations have been noted to drop by approximately 25 to 70 mg/dL/h on average, solely in response to saline in the absence of insulin.[12,14] This rate of decrease may be even more pronounced in HHS. The main function in HHS treatment is to restore intravascular volume and decrease plasma osmolarity.

The fluid of choice for initial resuscitation is 0.9% normal saline (NS). Other concentrations of saline are not useful initially. Fluids should be infused as quickly as possible in patients who are in shock. In adult patients without signs of overt shock or heart failure, 1 L of NS may be administered in the first 30 to 60 minutes with a goal of 15 to 20 mL/kg/h over the first 2 hours. Another 2 L of fluid may be given over the following 2 to 6 hours, and an additional 2 L may be given over the following 6 to 12 hours. A good rule of thumb for the subsequent rate of fluid administration is between 250 and 500 mL/h because faster rates have not been shown to be beneficial.[8,30–32] This resuscitation strategy repletes approximately 50% of the fluid losses in the first 12 hours. Similarly, in HHS, due to the larger fluid deficits, the goal is to correct one-half of the fluid deficit in the first 8 to 12 hours. The remaining fluid requirement is addressed in the following 12 to 36 hours during admission.

After initial fluid resuscitation, the subsequent type of fluid replacement should be individualized based on the corrected serum sodium. If hyponatremia is present, continued fluid hydration with 0.9% NS is recommended. If the corrected serum sodium is normal or elevated, consider transitioning using 0.45% NS (half NS). Additionally, the need for concurrent potassium administration may prompt the use of half NS. Addition of potassium to NS results in an overall hypertonic solution, thereby worsening serum osmolarity. In HHS, continued fluid administration with 0.9% NS is also recommended. Maintenance of proper circulating intravascular volume takes precedence over correcting serum osmolarity. The initial resuscitative fluid should be NS even when patients may be initially hypernatremic, because this still corrects the hyperosmolarity due to NS being hypo-osmotic to patients. NS is hyperosmolar relative to the serum when the serum osmolarity is greater than 308 mOsm/L.

Correction of hypernatremia can proceed once initial volume depletion has been corrected with half NS.

In both DKA and HHS, when the plasma glucose level falls to between 250 and 300 mg/dL, dextrose-containing fluids should be initiated. Further reduction in serum glucose below this range is unnecessary. The plasma glucose level tends to fall more rapidly than the plasma ketone level and resultant closure of the anion gap. There is no difference in capillary blood pH or level of bicarbonate when using 5% or 10% glucose solutions, although use of 10% glucose results in a greater level of hyperglycemia[33]; 5% dextrose in half NS at an initial rate of 150 to 250 mL/h is a reasonable first choice. If the serum glucose continues to fall, increasing the concentration to 10% dextrose is recommended.

Insulin

Volume therapy should always precede insulin therapy. Insulin does not need to be started at the time of diagnosis and should never be started until electrolyte results are available to prevent potentially lethal complications.

DKA cannot be reversed without insulin. Insulin therapy also addresses the core physiologic derangements of DKA. Insulin lowers the serum glucose primarily by inhibiting gluconeogenesis rather than enhancing peripheral utilization.[34] Insulin inhibits lipolysis, ketogenesis, and glucagon secretion, thereby decreasing the production of ketoacids. Insulin allows glucose to be used as the substrate for cellular energy production. This causes a steady fall in serum glucose, a decreasing anion gap, and an improvement in serum pH. In HHS, insulin serves primarily to lower the serum glucose and, subsequently, the serum osmolarity.

Continuous intravenous (IV) infusion of regular insulin is the treatment of choice. Traditional insulin regimens list 0.1 U/kg IV bolus and then 0.1 U/kg/h IV continuous infusion. This bolus dosing, or priming, bolus dose, however, prior to continuous infusion has not proved significantly different from just starting a continuous infusion.[8,35] Insulin infused at a rate of 0.14 U/kg/h achieved similar treatment endpoints as the bolus regimen.[36] Therefore, initial insulin infusion can be started with either an IV bolus (0.1 U/kg) followed by a continuous hourly infusion (0.1 U/kg/h) or with a continuous infusion alone (0.14 U/kg/h). This treatment approach mirrors normal physiology and, in combination with fluid therapy, produces a linear, predictable clearance of elevated serum glucose and ketones.

In the first 2 hours of therapy, IV administration results in a more significant decline in serum ketones and glucose compared with other routes.[37] Furthermore, this approach helps to avoid traditional complications (hypoglycemia/hypokalemia) that are more likely with large volume bolus dosing. Advantages of IV insulin administration include ease of titration, short half-life, and physician comfort.

There may be a role for subcutaneous or IV rapid-acting insulin analogs, however, such as glulisine, aspart, and lispro. Initial subcutaneous and intramuscular insulin administration has unpredictable or inadequate absorption in ill DKA/HHS patients who are likely vasoconstricted and volume depleted.[12] Subcutaneous regular insulin has a prolonged half-life and a delayed onset of action. This regimen also raises the possibility of creating an insulin deposit in tissues, which, once adequate perfusion is achieved, is released as a bolus causing a sudden fall in serum glucose. In mild, uncomplicated DKA patients, however, several small studies have demonstrated safety, efficacy, and cost effectiveness (30%–39% reduction) with this approach as well as similar amounts of insulin used, time to resolution of ketoacidosis, rates of hypoglycemia, and total hospital length of stay compared with traditional continuous insulin infusions.[38–43] Cost savings were derived from avoiding the added costs of care stemming from ICU admission. The method calls for intermittent boluses of 0.1 U/kg of subcutaneous or intramuscular insulin every 1 to 2 hours with frequent monitoring of glucose, electrolytes, and acid-base status. Care should be taken to safely implement this approach because it anticipates that hospital nursing protocols allow for frequent glucose monitoring that is inherently necessary for safe implementation and may not be applicable to most standard hospital floor care. This does represent an important area of investigation as a way to improve emergency department flow during times of hospital crowding and scarce ICU beds.

Secondary insulin resistance is suggested when the serum glucose does not decrease in an expected manner (glucose drop of 50–75 mg/dL in the first hour).[37] In these cases, the insulin infusion can be doubled every hour until a steady decline in serum glucose occurs (beginning with 0.2 U/kg/h). When the fluids are changed to dextrose-containing fluids, the insulin infusion can be reduced to half (0.02–0.05 U/kg/h), with a goal of keeping the serum glucose between 150 and 200 mg/dL until the anion gap has resolved.[44] Alternatively, at this point, the insulin drip may be discontinued and subcutaneous administration of rapid acting insulin may be started (0.1 U/kg) and repeated every 2 hours.[8,45] Subcutaneous insulin can also be started in an emergency department once ketosis has cleared and the patient's overall condition is improved. There may be a role for long-acting insulin analogs during this transition.[46]

Discontinuation of the insulin infusion can be tricky. Because of the short half-life of insulin, abrupt cessation of the insulin supply restarts ketogenesis, rebounding patients into hyperglycemia and metabolic acidosis, and DKA recurs. Appropriate patients for discontinuation of the infusion must have serum glucose below 200 to 250 mg/dL in DKA and between 250 and 300 mg/dL in HHS. Also, DKA patients must have a normal anion gap, venous pH greater than 7.30, and a serum bicarbonate greater than or equal to 18 mEq/L. A long-acting insulin agent, such as glargine, should be administered subcutaneously approximately 30 minutes before a meal and 60 to 120 minutes before discontinuing the continuous insulin infusion. This overlap allows for maintenance of steady serum insulin concentrations and for the insulin to be given at a physiologically appropriate time, preventing both a worsening hyperglycemia and a rebound into DKA. Patients who are unable to eat should continue to receive both IV insulin and fluid replacement. DKA and HHS patients with previously known diabetes can be restarted on their previous insulin regimens. Insulin-naive patients can be started on a subcutaneous multidose insulin regimen (0.5–0.8 U/kg/d).

Potassium

Potassium is the major electrolyte of importance in discussing management of DKA and HHS. Potassium replacement is always necessary, although the timing of repletion differs. Repletion is guided by initial electrolyte measurements and presence of adequate urine output. The average potassium deficit is 3 to 5 mEq/Kg in DKA and 4 to 6 mEq/Kg in HHS, although it may be as high as 10 mEq/kg.[8] The initial potassium level is commonly normal or high despite large total-body deficits.[47,48] This apparent contradiction is due to hyperosmolarity, insulin deficiency, and, to a lesser extent, the intracellular exchange of potassium for hydrogen ions in the setting of severe acidosis. Therefore, initial hypokalemia reflects a very large total-body potassium deficit and clinicians should anticipate very large repletion requirements during the hospital course.

Table 2 contains a potassium repletion guide. Insulin therapy should be held if the initial serum potassium is low (less than 3.3–3.5 mEq/L). Once adequate renal function and urine output are confirmed, hypokalemia is treated by adding 20 to 30 mEq/h of

Table 2
Potassium repletion in DKA and HHS

Serum Potassium (mEq/L)	Repletion
>5.3	No repletion, repeat in 1 h.
4.0–5.3	Add 10 mEq/L KCl/h to IV fluids.
3.5–<4.0	Add 20 mEq/L KCl/h to IV fluids.
<3.5	Hold insulin. Add 20–60 mEq/L/h to IV fluids, place on continuous cardiac monitor.

Data from McNaughton CD, Self WH, Slovis C. Diabetes in the emergency department: acute care of diabetes patients. Clin Diabetes 2011;29(2):51–9.

KCL to 0.45% NS in the IV fluids until the serum potassium is between 3.3 and 3.5 mEq/L.[8,44] In cases of initial hyperkalemia, potassium repletion is normally not necessary during the first several hours of therapy. If the initial potassium level is normal (3.3–5.0 mEq/L), 20 to 30 mEq KCL can be added to each subsequent liter of fluid with a goal of keeping serum potassium in a physiologic normal range (4–5 mEq/L). Total body potassium depletion is usually greater in HHS than in DKA, with an average requirement of 20–30 mEq/h. Furthermore, because there is no underlying acidosis in HHS, the intracellular shift of potassium is accelerated in response to treatment.

Frequent re-evaluation of serum electrolytes is recommended due to the rapid electrolyte shifts that occur during therapy and guides subsequent replacement. In the setting of renal impairment and/or oliguria, potassium replacement must be decreased and should only occur when either the serum potassium is less than 4 mEq/L or an ECG shows signs of hypokalemia. In the setting of profound hypokalemia (<3 mEq/L), due to limitations in the rate of potassium repletion through a peripheral line, peripheral infusion through 2 peripheral lines should be considered. Simultaneous oral potassium replacement has good absorption and is a recommended additional option in the absence of ileus or vomiting.

Bicarbonate

The use of bicarbonate has been long debated, although currently it is not recommended in the treatment of most cases of DKA and has no role in the treatment of HHS.[8,49] Bicarbonate therapy does not alter patient outcomes nor does it increase the rate at which the pH is corrected. Potential risks of bicarbonate use include hypokalemia, rebound metabolic alkalosis, and potential delay in improvement of both hyperosmolarity and ketosis. Furthermore, in patients with DKA with an initial pH less than 7.0, IV bicarbonate therapy did not decrease time to resolution of acidosis or time to hospital discharge.[50] Bicarbonate administration has also been implicated as an increased risk factor for cerebral edema in children.[7,51] Because of the potential adverse cardiovascular effects, the American Diabetes Association guidelines suggest using bicarbonate when the serum pH is less than 6.9 and may likely only apply when patients also have concomitant cardiogenic shock, respiratory failure, or renal failure.[8] Even this recommendation is controversial, however, and there is little supportive evidence.

Phosphate

Hypophosphatemia is common in DKA and HHS. As with potassium, initial phosphate concentration may be normal or elevated due to movement of phosphate out of the cells and dehydration. Furthermore, serum levels fall with institution of insulin therapy. Levels of hypophosphatemia in DKA and HHS are self-limited, however, and are not associated with marked whole-body phosphate depletion. Furthermore, studies on phosphate repletion in DKA have not demonstrated any benefit on morbidity/mortality or on typical clinical outcome measures for DKA, such as duration of ketoacidosis.[52,53] Therefore, there is no indication for the routine repletion of phosphate for most patients in DKA or HHS.

COMPLICATIONS

Many complications of treatment are evident only later during an ICU stay yet may result from early inappropriate management. Most complications in DKA and HHS are due to either the predisposing or associated condition or the treatment of the hyperglycemia itself. The most common complications are hypoglycemia and hypokalemia. Less common, yet significant, complications include cerebral edema, volume overload, and acute respiratory distress syndrome (ARDS). Emergency providers must be knowledgeable regarding the full course of treatment to avoid such complications.

Cerebral Edema

Cerebral edema is a rare but well-known complication during the resuscitation of patients with DKA although more commonly reported in pediatric patients. Cerebral edema has an approximate incidence of only 1%; however, this is the most common cause of mortality in children with diabetes.[51,54] The mortality rate is between 20% and 40%[8]; 95%, of cases of cerebral edema occurred in patients less than 20 years of age, and one-third of those were in children under 5 years old.[10,55]

The pathophysiology is poorly understood.[8] Risk factors may include pH less than 7.1, Pco_2 less than 20 mm Hg, greater than 50 mL/kg of fluid administered within the first 4 hours of treatment, high SUN at presentation, initiation of insulin before initial rehydration bolus, treatment with bicarbonate, and failure of serum sodium to rise as glucose decreases.[51,56] Symptoms can include headache and vomiting and progress to decreased arousal and altered mental status.[51] They may also include Cushing triad, hypertension, bradycardia, and irregular respirations—signs of increased intracranial pressure.[57] Severe cases may progress to decorticate or decerebrate posturing and, finally, herniation and death.[51] Cerebral edema can develop within 4 to 12 hours of initiating treatment.[10]

Treatment involves decreasing intracranial pressure by shifting fluid back out of the central nervous sytem. Therapy should not be delayed to obtain imaging. Initial treatment includes reducing IV fluids and elevating the head of the bed. Mannitol is recommended as soon as possible with dosing of 0.5 to 1 g/kg over 20 minutes.[10,54] This may be repeated if there is no clinical improvement in 30 to 120 minutes[58]; 3% hypertonic saline may also be given at 5 to 10 mL/kg over 30 minutes.[57,59] Be sure to monitor for rising serum sodium, because a falling level is associated with cerebral edema.[56] The best therapy is always prevention.

Pulmonary Edema

Fluid resuscitation in DKA and HHS requires large volumes of IV fluids that may be detrimental, especially to those with underlying cardiac disease or renal insufficiency.[10] Cardiogenic pulmonary edema can occur when the amount of fluid administered overwhelms the capabilities of the heart to pump or the kidneys to excrete it. Careful monitoring of fluid input and urine output should be performed in addition to slow fluid infusion, frequent pulmonary auscultation, and continued pulse oximetry monitoring in those with known disease. Treatment may require diuretics and oxygen administration with severe cases necessitating either noninvasive positive pressure ventilation or intubation.

Even those without known cardiac disease may develop noncardiogenic pulmonary edema from fluid shifts secondary to excessive or rapid volume repletion.[10,18] ARDS is a rare but potentially fatal complication in DKA that may also present with rales and pulmonary edema.[10,18] It is defined as acute-onset respiratory failure, bilateral infiltrates on chest x-ray, hypoxemia (Pao_2/Fio_2 ratio <200 mm Hg), and no evidence of cardiogenic edema.[60,61] ARDS is thought to develop from the chemical stress of DKA, which can lead to epithelial and endothelial cell damage with neutrophil infiltration and increased vascular permeability with resultant alveolar edema.[60] Patients with ARDS also require slow and lower volume fluid resuscitation and often necessitate mechanical ventilation.[10,60]

DISPOSITION

Most patients with a diagnosis of DKA or HHS require admission to a hospital for treatment, observation, and resolution of the underlying cause or modification to an appropriate medication regimen.

All patients benefit from frequent clinical and laboratory reassessment while in an emergency department for adequate urine output, electrolyte correction, and the absence of fluid overload. Emergency practitioners should anticipate that the fluid, metabolic, and electrolyte deficits be gradually corrected over a period of 18 to 24 hours. Finger-stick glucose should be monitored every hour to prevent hypoglycemia. Basic metabolic panel testing should be obtained every 1 to 2 hours to assess the potassium levels and the anion gap, because they provides a good estimate of the serum ketoacid (anion) levels. Normalization (closure) of the anion gap reflects disappearance of serum ketoacids and correction of the ketoacidosis. Criteria for resolution of DKA include a serum glucose less than 200 mg/dL and at least 2 of the following criteria: normalization of the anion gap, a venous pH greater than 7.3, and a serum bicarbonate level greater than or equal to 15 mEq/L.[30] Ketonemia and ketonuria may persist for 24 to 36 hours due to slower elimination time. In HHS, treatment endpoints indicating resolution include a normalization of serum osmolarity and a corresponding restoration of baseline mental status.

Many of those patients in DKA or HHS should be placed in an ICU or step-down unit to accommodate the requirements of hourly finger-stick glucose and frequent laboratory assessments. Patients who present with sepsis, hypoxia, altered mental status, hypotension, or persistent tachycardia despite fluid resuscitation and those with significant laboratory derangements, such as acidosis or severe electrolyte abnormalities, warrant a higher level of care.[13] Acute comorbidities, such MI or CVA, may also dictate disposition to a cardiac care unit or neurologic unit. Pediatric patients should be admitted to an ICU setting for frequent monitoring and neurologic checks due to increased risk associated with cerebral edema.

Hyperglycemic crisis itself can often be resolved in an emergency department. This is something not often performed in emergency departments. Because of the scarcity of ICU beds, emergency department overcrowding, and longer emergency department stays, however, it is becoming more of a reality to correct patients in emergency departments and lower their level of care. Average time to the resolution of anion gap acidosis is 3 hours.[10] Many patients are stable enough for general floor admission pending improved volume status after resuscitation, closed anion gap, discontinuation of the insulin infusion, and ability to tolerate fluids by mouth. They may be admitted to continue subcutaneous insulin, monitor minor electrolyte abnormalities, and determine proper medication dosing for later discharge.

Some select patients may be discharged home from an emergency department after an episode of mild DKA with a known cause, such as missed insulin doses, with resolution of hyperglycemia, acidosis, electrolyte abnormalities, normalization of vital signs, and ability to tolerate oral hydration.[13] These patients must have a pre-determined insulin regimen with available supplies and medication, a reliable way of checking their blood sugar, and close outpatient follow-up for re-evaluation.

SUMMARY

Diabetes is an increasingly prevalent chronic illness and, along with DKA and HHS, is associated with significant morbidity, mortality, and cost. Both DKA and HHS are complicated hyperglycemic states characterized by dehydration and electrolyte disturbances. The treatment of both conditions must be tailored to individual patients and relies on aggressive fluid resuscitation, strictly monitored insulin replacement, and electrolyte management, while correcting the underlying causes and monitoring for complications.

ACKNOWLEDGMENTS

Thanks to Morgan Walker, MSN, for her assistance in article editing.

REFERENCES

1. Centers for Disease Control and Prevention (CDC). National diabetes fact sheet 2011. United States Department of Health and Human Services; 2011. Available at: http://www.cdc.gov/diabetes/pubs/estimates11.htm. Accessed August 17, 2013.
2. Boyle JP, Thompson TJ, Gregg EW, et al. Projection of the year 2050 burden of diabetes in the US adult population: dynamic modeling of incidence, mortality, and prediabetes prevalence. Popul Health Metr 2010;8:29.
3. American Diabetes Association. Economic costs of diabetes in the U.S. in 2012. Diabetes Care 2013;36(4):1033–46.
4. Johnson DD, Palumbo PJ, Chu CP. Diabetic ketoacidosis in a community-based population. Mayo Clin Proc 1980;55(2):83–8.
5. CfDCaP (CDC). Number (in thousands) of hospital discharges with diabetic Ketoacidosis as first-listed diagnosis, United States, 1988–2009. 2012. Available at: http://www.cdc.gov/diabetes/statistics/dkafirst/fig1.htm. Accessed September 1, 2013.
6. Kitabchi AE, Umpierrez GE, Murphy MB. Diabetic ketoacidosis and hyperglycemic hypersmolar state. In: DeFronzo RA, Ferrannini E, Keen H, et al, editors. International textbook of diabetes mellitus. 3rd edition. Chichester (United Kingdom): John Wiley & Sons; 2004. p. 1101.
7. Rewers A. Current controversies in treatment and prevention of diabetic ketoacidosis. Adv Pediatr 2010;57(1):247–67.
8. Kitabchi AE, Umpierrez GE, Miles JM, et al. Hyperglycemic crises in adult patients with diabetes. Diabetes Care 2009;32(7):1335–43.
9. American Diabetes Association. Hyperglycemic crises in patients with diabetes mellitus. Diabetes Care 2001;24(11):1988–96.
10. Charfen MA, Fernandez-Frackelton M. Diabetic ketoacidosis. Emerg Med Clin North Am 2005;23(3):609–28, vii.

11. McNaughton CD, Self WH, Slovis C. Diabetes in the emergency department: acute care of diabetes patients. Clin Diabetes 2011;29(2):51–9.

12. American Diabetes Association. Standards of medical care in diabetes–2011. Diabetes Care 2011;34(Suppl 1):S11–61.

13. Van Ness-Otunnu R, Hack JB. Hyperglycemic crisis. J Emerg Med 2013;45(5): 797–805.

14. Umpierrez GE, Khajavi M, Kitabchi AE. Review: diabetic ketoacidosis and hyperglycemic hyperosmolar nonketotic syndrome. Am J Med Sci 1996;311(5):225–33.

15. Expert Committee on the Diagnosis and Clasification of Diabetes Mellitus. American diabetes association: clinical practice recommendations 2002. Diabetes Care 2002;25(Suppl 1):S1–147.

16. American Diabetes Association. Hyperglycemic crises in patients with diabetes mellitus. Diabetes Care 2002;25(Suppl 1):s100–8.

17. Trence DL, Hirsch IB. Hyperglycemic crises in diabetes mellitus type 2. Endocrinol Metab Clin North Am 2001;30(4):817–31.

18. Kitabchi AE, Nyenwe EA. Hyperglycemic crises in diabetes mellitus: diabetic ketoacidosis and hyperglycemic hyperosmolar state. Endocrinol Metab Clin North Am 2006;35(4):725–51, viii.

19. Usman A, Sulaiman SA, Khan AH. Euglycemia; a hideout for diabetic ketoacidosis. J Pharmaceut Sci Innovat 2012;1(3):44–5.

20. Burge MR, Hardy KJ, Schade DS. Short-term fasting is a mechanism for the development of euglycemic ketoacidosis during periods of insulin deficiency. J Clin Endocrinol Metab 1993;76(5):1192–8.

21. De P, Child DF. Euglycaemic diabetic ketoacidosis – is it on the rise? Practical Diabetes Int 2001;18(7):239–40.

22. Ma OJ, Rush MD, Godfrey MM, et al. Arterial blood gas results rarely influence emergency physician management of patients with suspected diabetic ketoacidosis. Acad Emerg Med 2003;10(8):836–41.

23. Laffel L. Ketone bodies: a review of physiology, pathophysiology and application of monitoring to diabetes. Diabetes Metab Res Rev 1999;15(6):412–26.

24. Rewers A, McFann K, Chase HP. Bedside monitoring of blood beta-hydroxybutyrate levels in the management of diabetic ketoacidosis in children. Diabetes Technol Ther 2006;8(6):671–6.

25. Sheikh-Ali M, Karon BS, Basu A, et al. Can serum beta-hydroxybutyrate be used to diagnose diabetic ketoacidosis? Diabetes Care 2008;31(4):643–7.

26. Muir AB, Quisling RG, Yang MC, et al. The direct measurement of 3-beta-hydroxybutyrate enhances the management of diabetic ketoacidosis in children and reduces time and costs of treatment. Diabetes Nutr Metab 2003; 16(5–6):312–6.

27. Soleimanpour H, Taghizadieh A, Niafar M, et al. Predictive value of capnography for suspected diabetic ketoacidosis in the emergency department. WestJ Emerg Med 2013;14(6):590–4.

28. Katz MA. Hyperglycemia-induced hyponatremia–calculation of expected serum sodium depression. N Engl J Med 1973;289(16):843–4.

29. Hillier TA, Abbott RD, Barrett EJ. Hyponatremia: evaluating the correction factor for hyperglycemia. Am J Med 1999;106(4):399–403.

30. Nyenwe EA, Kitabchi AE. Evidence-based management of hyperglycemic emergencies in diabetes mellitus. Diabetes Res Clin Pract 2011;94(3):340–51.

31. Adrogue HJ, Barrero J, Eknoyan G. Salutary effects of modest fluid replacement in the treatment of adults with diabetic ketoacidosis. Use in patients without extreme volume deficit. JAMA 1989;262(15):2108–13.

32. Caputo DG, Villarejo F, Valle GB, et al. Hydration in diabetic ketoacidosis. What is the effect of the infusion rate? Medicina 1997;57(1):15–20.
33. Krentz AJ, Hale PJ, Singh BM, et al. The effect of glucose and insulin infusion on the fall of ketone bodies during treatment of diabetic ketoacidosis. Diabet Med 1989;6(1):31–6.
34. Luzi L, Barrett EJ, Groop LC, et al. Metabolic effects of low-dose insulin therapy on glucose metabolism in diabetic ketoacidosis. Diabetes 1988;37(11):1470–7.
35. Goyal N, Miller JB, Sankey SS, et al. Utility of initial bolus insulin in the treatment of diabetic ketoacidosis. J Emerg Med 2010;38(4):422–7.
36. Kitabchi AE, Murphy MB, Spencer J, et al. Is a priming dose of insulin necessary in a low-dose insulin protocol for the treatment of diabetic ketoacidosis? Diabetes Care 2008;31(11):2081–5.
37. Kitabchi AE, Umpierrez GE, Fisher JN, et al. Thirty years of personal experience in hyperglycemic crises: diabetic ketoacidosis and hyperglycemic hyperosmolar state. J Clin Endocrinol Metab 2008;93(5):1541–52.
38. Barski L, Kezerle L, Zeller L, et al. New approaches to the use of insulin in patients with diabetic ketoacidosis. Eur J Intern Med 2013;24(3):213–6.
39. Umpierrez GE, Cuervo R, Karabell A, et al. Treatment of diabetic ketoacidosis with subcutaneous insulin aspart. Diabetes Care 2004;27(8):1873–8.
40. Umpierrez GE, Latif K, Stoever J, et al. Efficacy of subcutaneous insulin lispro versus continuous intravenous regular insulin for the treatment of patients with diabetic ketoacidosis. Am J Med 2004;117(5):291–6.
41. Della Manna T, Steinmetz L, Campos PR, et al. Subcutaneous use of a fast-acting insulin analog: an alternative treatment for pediatric patients with diabetic ketoacidosis. Diabetes Care 2005;28(8):1856–61.
42. Mazer M, Chen E. Is subcutaneous administration of rapid-acting insulin as effective as intravenous insulin for treating diabetic ketoacidosis? Ann Emerg Med 2009;53(2):259–63.
43. Ersoz HO, Ukinc K, Kose M, et al. Subcutaneous lispro and intravenous regular insulin treatments are equally effective and safe for the treatment of mild and moderate diabetic ketoacidosis in adult patients. Int J Clin Pract 2006;60(4):429–33.
44. Kitabchi AE, Umpierrez GE, Murphy MB, et al. Management of hyperglycemic crises in patients with diabetes. Diabetes Care 2001;24(1):131–53.
45. Umpierrez GE, Jones S, Smiley D, et al. Insulin analogs versus human insulin in the treatment of patients with diabetic ketoacidosis: a randomized controlled trial. Diabetes Care 2009;32(7):1164–9.
46. Savage MW, Dhatariya KK, Kilvert A, et al. Joint British Diabetes Societies guideline for the management of diabetic ketoacidosis. Diabet Med 2011; 28(5):508–15.
47. Adrogue HJ, Lederer ED, Suki WN, et al. Determinants of plasma potassium levels in diabetic ketoacidosis. Medicine 1986;65(3):163–72.
48. Martin HE, Smith K, Wilson ML. The fluid and electrolyte therapy of severe diabetic acidosis and ketosis; a study of twenty-nine episodes (twenty-six patients). Am J Med 1958;24(3):376–89.
49. Chua HR, Schneider A, Bellomo R. Bicarbonate in diabetic ketoacidosis - a systematic review. Ann Intensive Care 2011;1(1):23.
50. Duhon B, Attridge RL, Franco-Martinez AC, et al. Intravenous sodium bicarbonate therapy in severely acidotic diabetic ketoacidosis. Ann Pharmacother 2013; 47(7–8):970–5.
51. Glaser NS, Wootton-Gorges SL, Marcin JP, et al. Mechanism of cerebral edema in children with diabetic ketoacidosis. J Pediatr 2004;145(2):164–71.

52. Wilson HK, Keuer SP, Lea AS, et al. Phosphate therapy in diabetic ketoacidosis. Arch Intern Med 1982;142(3):517–20.
53. Fisher JN, Kitabchi AE. A randomized study of phosphate therapy in the treatment of diabetic ketoacidosis. J Clin Endocrinol Metab 1983;57(1):177–80.
54. Edge JA, Ford-Adams ME, Dunger DB. Causes of death in children with insulin dependent diabetes 1990-96. Arch Dis Child 1999;81(4):318–23.
55. Rosenbloom AL. Intracerebral crises during treatment of diabetic ketoacidosis. Diabetes Care 1990;13(1):22–33.
56. Mahoney CP, Vlcek BW, DelAguila M, et al. Risk factors for cerebral edema in children with diabetic keotacidosis. The Pediatric Emergency Medicine Collaborative Research Committee of the American Academy of Pediatrics. N Engl J Med 2001;344:264–9.
57. Olivieri L, Chasm R. Diabetic ketoacidosis in the pediatric emergency department. Emerg Med Clin North Am 2013;31(3):755–73.
58. Shabbir N, Oberfield SE, Corrales R, et al. Recovery from symptomatic brain swelling in diabetic ketoacidosis. Clin Pediatr 1992;31(9):570–3.
59. Curtis JR, Bohn D, Daneman D. Use of hypertonic saline in the treatment of cerebral edema in diabetic ketoacidosis (DKA). Pediatr Diabetes 2001;2(4):191–4.
60. Fanelli V, Vlachou A, Ghannadian S, et al. Acute respiratory distress syndrome: new definition, current and future therapeutic options. J Thorac Dis 2013;5(3):326–34.
61. Ferguson ND, Fan E, Camporota L, et al. The Berlin definition of ARDS: an expanded rationale, justification, and supplementary material. Intensive Care Med 2012;38(10):1573–82.

Approach to Metabolic Alkalosis

Jennifer T. Soifer, MD*, Hyung T. Kim, MD

KEYWORDS

- Metabolic alkalosis • Chloride depletion • Mineralocorticoid excess syndrome
- Apparent mineralocorticoid excess syndrome

KEY POINTS

- Metabolic alkalosis is a common disorder amongst patients presenting to the emergency department.
- Patients often present without any symptoms but can develop neurologic and respiratory symptoms as their alkalosis worsens.
- The mainstay of treatment is supportive care; however, once a specific cause is identified, it should be addressed to correct the alkalosis and any electrolyte abnormalities.

INTRODUCTION

Metabolic alkalosis is defined as increased arterial pH greater than 7.42 or an increase in serum bicarbonate to greater than 30 mmol/L. It is the result of an increase in bicarbonate production, a decrease in bicarbonate excretion, or a loss of hydrogen ions. In a person with normal renal function, the regulatory response of the kidney leads to a decrease in bicarbonate by excreting the excess alkali. Metabolic alkalosis can be sustained only when renal regulation is disrupted.[1,2]

Metabolic alkalosis is common, accounting for half of all acid-base disorders in hospitalized patients.[3] Although most of the patients can tolerate mild metabolic alkalosis, severe alkalosis can have significant adverse effects on cellular function and can lead to increased mortality.[4] Patients with mild to moderate metabolic alkalosis, with serum bicarbonate levels less than 40 mmol/L, are typically asymptomatic. However, mortality approaches 45% when patients develop arterial pH of 7.55% and 80% when the pH is greater than 7.65.[5]

CLINICAL PRESENTATION

The workup of any patient in the emergency department should always begin by obtaining a history. Any history of excessive vomiting or diarrhea, recently added or

Department of Emergency Medicine, Keck School of Medicine, University of Southern California, 1200 North State Street, Los Angeles, CA 90033, USA
* Corresponding author.
E-mail address: jtsoifer@yahoo.com

Emerg Med Clin N Am 32 (2014) 453–463
http://dx.doi.org/10.1016/j.emc.2014.01.005
0733-8627/14/$ – see front matter © 2014 Elsevier Inc. All rights reserved.

emed.theclinics.com

increased dosages of diuretics, recent history of surgery that required nasogastric tube insertion, or a history of family members with excessive thirst and urination as children or fatigue and muscle wasting as adults may lead the clinician to a diagnosis of metabolic alkalosis.

Patients with mild to moderate metabolic alkalosis, with serum bicarbonate levels less than 40 mmol/L, are typically asymptomatic. When symptoms do occur, they are usually a consequence of an electrolyte abnormality rather than the alkalosis itself. For instance, in patients with ischemic heart disease, hypokalemia increases the risks of developing cardiac arrhythmias. Other symptoms include paresthesias, muscular cramping, and tetany, which are again likely caused by electrolyte abnormalities associated with the alkalosis. As bicarbonate levels increase to 45 mmol/L, the physiologic compensation is to correct the alkalosis by hypoventilation, leading to hypoxemia, especially in patients with chronic obstructive pulmonary disease. Once bicarbonate levels increase higher than 50 mmol/L, patients may develop seizures, altered mental status, and coma. Therefore, identifying the cause of this acid-base disorder and initiating specific treatment is important.

DIAGNOSIS

The diagnosis of metabolic alkalosis is sometimes a clinical one, but it is often found incidentally of laboratory work. On a routine serum chemistry panel, a bicarbonate level higher than 30 mmol/L in association with hypokalemia is pathognomonic for metabolic alkalosis. Once the diagnosis of metabolic alkalosis has been established, it is important to fully characterize the disorder by obtaining an arterial or venous blood gas to obtain a pH and $Paco_2$ measurement (partial pressure of carbon dioxide, arterial), especially if the alkalosis is severe with bicarbonate levels greater than 40 mmol/L. As the serum bicarbonate level increases, there is an increase in $Paco_2$ which is caused by compensatory hypoventilation.

Another useful tool in the diagnosis of metabolic alkalosis is the measurement of the urine chloride concentration. Urine chloride concentration of less than 10 mmol/L is usually observed in chloride-responsive metabolic alkalosis, whereas a concentration greater than 30 mmol/L is usually seen in non–chloride-responsive metabolic disorders such as mineralocorticoid excess or apparent excess syndromes. Patients with metabolic alkalosis associated with severe hypokalemia, volume depletion caused by diuretic use, Bartter and Gitelman syndromes, or alkali ingestion can have a urine chloride concentration in an indeterminate range between 10 and 30 mmol/L. There is little usefulness of urine chloride concentration alone as a diagnostic tool if the result is in this range.[1,6]

CAUSE AND MANAGEMENT

There are several possible causes of metabolic alkalosis in patients. The most common causes are listed in **Box 1**. The major decision point in making the diagnosis is based on volume status and blood pressure. An algorithmic approach to the workup and management of metabolic alkalosis is detailed in **Fig. 1**. Patients with evidence of volume depletion who are either normotensive or hypotensive are more likely to have metabolic alkalosis caused by chloride depletion. If the cause is clear, such as a history of vomiting, nasogastric suction, or diuretic use, the appropriate management is to treat the underlying disorder. If the cause is unclear, a trial of chloride repletion often helps elucidate the cause. Metabolic alkalosis that is easily corrected is usually caused by a simple chloride depletion disorder. If it is not easily corrected, then a hereditary chloride wasting disorder such as Gitelman syndrome or Bartter syndrome

Box 1
Common causes of metabolic alkalosis
Chloride depletion syndrome
Gastrointestinal losses
Vomiting
Nasogastric suction
Congenital chloridorrhea
Villous adenomas
High-volume ileostomy losses
Renal losses
Diuretic administration
Impairment of Chloride-linked sodium transport
Bartter syndrome
Gitelman syndrome
Mineralocorticoid excess
Primary hyperaldosteronism
Glucocorticoid-remediable aldosteronism
Secondary hyperaldosteronism (high renin syndrome)
Renal artery stenosis
Accelerated hypertension
Renin-secreting tumor
Apparent mineralocorticosteroid excess
Liddle syndrome
11β-Hydroxysteroid dehydrogenase deficiency
Fludrocortisone administration
Other causes
Alkali intake or administration
Milk alkali syndrome
Severe potassium depletion

should be considered. In the hypertensive patient with metabolic alkalosis, mineralo-corticoid excess or apparent excess syndromes should be considered, which can be examined by measuring serum aldosterone and renin levels.[7,8]

The causes of metabolic alkalosis can be divided into the following groups based on pathophysiology: chloride depletion syndromes, mineralocorticoid excess syndromes, apparent mineralocorticoid excess syndromes, alkali administration, and other causes.

Chloride Depletion Alkalosis

Chloride depletion is the most common cause of metabolic alkalosis. Traditionally, metabolic alkalosis has been described in the literature as either contraction alkalosis or noncontraction alkalosis, but it has become clear that it is truly chloride depletion or

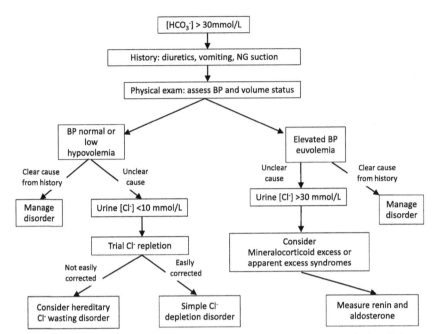

Fig. 1. An algorithmic approach to the workup and management of metabolic alkalosis. BP, blood pressure; NG, nasogastric.

non–chloride depletion alkalosis. Studies have shown that chloride repletion in the absence of volume administration can correct alkalosis. In contrast, volume expansion in the absence of chloride administration does not. On its own, potassium depletion causes a small increase in serum bicarbonate concentration. However, when this increase occurs in conjunction with chloride depletion, the resultant alkalosis is 4 times as great.[9] Chloride depletion alkalosis is associated with hyponatremia and hypokalemia as a result of gastrointestinal or renal losses.[10]

Gastrointestinal losses

Chloride absorption takes place throughout the gastrointestinal tract. Approximately 7 to 8 L of fluids and electrolytes are excreted and absorbed daily. Chloride is secreted as hydrochloric acid in the stomach. Hydrochloric acid activates pepsinogen into pepsin, which functions in numerous antibacterial and nutrient absorption roles. Hydrochloric acid also removes iron from food and aids in its conversion to the ferrous form. Chloride is secreted into the intestine through 3 channels, which depend on osmotic gradients.

Vomiting or nasogastric suction Gastric fluid is a chloride ion-rich solution, which is balanced by sodium, potassium, and hydrogen ions. Vomiting or nasogastric suction causes major chloride losses, which are coupled with losses of hydrogen ions as well. This loss of hydrogen ions leads to an increase in serum bicarbonate at levels often several times greater than 45 mmol/L.[11] Subsequently, this leads to a decrease in serum potassium as potassium ions enter the cell to replace the hydrogen ions. Thus, suctioning leads to a metabolic alkalosis, which is associated with hypochloremia and hypokalemia. This alkalosis persists until both chloride and potassium are repleted.[8]

Congenital chloridorrhea Congenital chloridorrhea is a disorder caused by a genetic mutation, which leads to an absence of intestinal bicarbonate/chloride exchange in the intestine. Consequently, chloride is not absorbed and bicarbonate is not excreted, resulting in large-volume watery diarrhea, which contains mostly sodium, chloride, and potassium. Management of fluid and electrolyte losses in these patients is difficult, such that they have sustained metabolic alkalosis throughout their lives and are chronically hypovolemic.[11]

Villous adenoma of the colon Most patients with villous adenoma are asymptomatic. However, patients with villous adenoma with McKittrick-Wheelock syndrome can present with severe dehydration and hypovolemic shock as a result of chronic diarrhea, with daily fluid losses up to 4 L. Large amounts of sodium and chloride ions are lost as a result of copious diarrhea caused by these rare tumors.[12] Although little is known about the mechanism of the tumor, the secretory complication is a known cause of metabolic alkalosis.[12]

High-output ileostomy drainage Patients with ileostomy are susceptible to electrolyte disturbances as a result of obligatory large volume and electrolyte loss. When the drainage increases unexpectedly, patients can develop severe metabolic acidosis or alkalosis. Although most patients develop metabolic acidosis as a result of highly concentrated HCO_3 ileostomy fluids, few patients develop metabolic alkalosis. The mechanism is not clear, but these patients produce abnormally high concentrated chloride ion in ileostomy fluids, which leads to severe metabolic alkalosis.[13] Because these patients are extremely sensitive to electrolyte and acid-base balance, it is important to treat the underlying cause for increased ileostomy output and replenish extracellular fluids and electrolytes.

Renal losses
Excretion of chloride primarily occurs in the kidney. **Fig. 2** shows where the chloride transporters are. The proximal convoluted tubule is the site for most of the sodium, chloride, and bicarbonate reabsorption. The site of aldosterone action for the reabsorption of sodium and chloride and secretion of potassium and hydrogen ions occurs in the distal tubule. The collecting duct plays an important role in acid-base transport via hydrogen ion–adenosine triphosphatase (ATPase) and chloride/bicarbonate exchangers. Chloride is also secreted into the lumen and absorbed into the interstitium of the kidney through the sodium-potassium-chloride and chloride-bicarbonate cotransporters. Net loss of chloride causes a net gain of bicarbonate through the cotransporters, adding to the alkalosis.[14]

Diuretic administration Diuretics that inhibit chloride transport proteins in the kidney are the most common cause of metabolic alkalosis. Loop diuretics inhibit the sodium-potassium-chloride cotransporter in the thick ascending limb of the loop of Henle. Thiazide diuretics inhibit the sodium-potassium cotransporter in the distal convoluted tubule. Inhibition of these cotransporter proteins impairs chloride reabsorption, resulting in chloride excretion. It also leads to potassium excretion by increasing sodium delivery to the collecting duct. The alkalosis is typically mild ($[HCO_3^-]$ <36 mmol/L).[1]

Impairment of chloride-linked sodium transport Bartter and Gitelman syndromes are characterized by hypochloremic metabolic alkalosis, hypokalemia, and normal to low blood pressure. Bartter syndrome is caused by one of several mutations that inactivate or impair the function of the sodium-potassium-chloride transporter in the thick ascending limb of the loop of Henle. The pathophysiologic process of metabolic alkalosis is the same as that induced by loop diuretics. In the classic presentation

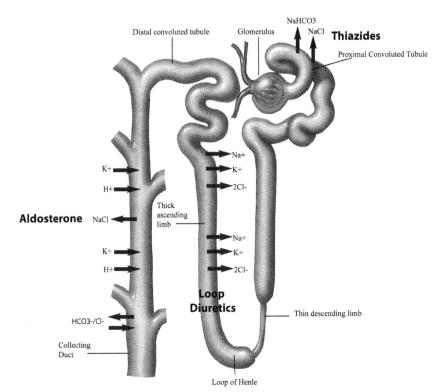

Fig. 2. The nephron with locations of ion channels and sites of action of diuretics. Netter illustration from www.netterimages.com. © Elsevier Inc. All rights reserved.

of Bartter syndrome, the symptoms of polyuria, polydipsia, dehydration, vomiting, and growth retardation begin in the first 2 years of life.

Gitelman syndrome is a mild, but not asymptomatic, syndrome. Gitelman syndrome is caused by a mutation in the sodium-chloride cotransporter in the distal tubule. The pathophysiologic process of metabolic alkalosis is the same as that induced by thiazide diuretics. Routine laboratory tests show hypochloremic, hypokalemic metabolic alkalosis combined with hypocalciuria. Patients can present as adults with the following symptoms: muscle weakness, muscle cramps, polyuria, polydipsia, hypotension, dizziness, salt craving, and joint pain. Approximately 40% of patients with Gitelman syndrome have QT interval prolongation on electrocardiography.[15]

Treatment The first step in treating patients with chloride depletion metabolic alkalosis is to diagnose and correct the underlying cause. Replacing the chloride losses results in a correction of the alkalosis. In patients with nasogastric suction or vomiting, hypovolemia poses an additional challenge to chloride loss. Administration of intravenous normal saline replaces the chloride and provides volume repletion. If nasogastric suctioning cannot be terminated, hydrogen and chloride losses can be minimized by administration of an H_2 blocker or a proton pump inhibitor.[1]

On the other hand, if a patient develops metabolic alkalosis while in a volume-overloaded state (cirrhosis or congestive heart failure), to replenishing chloride with potassium chloride must be considered. Hypokalemia plays an integral role in development and maintenance of metabolic alkalosis and should be replaced appropriately with potassium chloride either orally or intravenously.

The carbonic anhydrase inhibitors (acetazolamide) can be used to enhance bicarbonate excretion and subsequently lower serum bicarbonate levels.[16,17] The carbonic anhydrase inhibitors can be particularly useful when hyperkalemia coexists with the need to diurese in the setting of metabolic alkalosis. They can decrease the serum level of bicarbonate within 12 to 24 hours, but careful monitoring of potassium is indicated.[18]

Rarely, rapid reversal with hydrochloric acid infusion is indicated in severe metabolic alkalosis with pH greater than 7.55 or in patients who have altered mental status or cardiac arrhythmia. Hydrochloric acid infusion is indicated in a patient who cannot tolerate intravenous saline or potassium chloride administration because of volume overload status or renal failure.[19,20] The infusion must be given in a central line, because it can lead to sloughing of perivascular tissue. Close monitoring of potassium and other electrolytes is necessary, because shifts can occur. Dialysis can also be used for severe metabolic alkalosis but should be reserved for patients who have advanced renal failure and are unable to tolerate other traditional therapy.[21]

Mineralocorticoid Excess Syndromes

Metabolic alkalosis in the setting of excess or apparent excess of mineralocorticoids occurs as a result of stimulation of the collecting duct ion transport. Aldosterone stimulates sodium reabsorption in the collecting duct of the kidney by activating the mineralocorticoid receptor of sodium-potassium-ATPase pumps and hydrogen ion secretion through activating the mineralocorticoid receptor of hydrogen ion-ATPase pumps. It also stimulates extracellular reuptake of potassium, resulting in significant hypokalemia (<3 mmol/L) and mild alkalosis. Aldosterone secretion is increased in states of hypochloremia caused by concomitant volume depletion.[7] The excess sodium reabsorption also leads to increased potassium losses, renal ammonium excretion, and serum bicarbonate levels.[8]

Primary hyperaldosteronism results from either unilateral or bilateral aldosterone-secreting adrenal adenomas or from hyperplasia of the zona glomerulosa, the aldosterone-forming area of the adrenal glands. The characteristics of the disorder include early-onset hypertension that is refractory to multiple medications. Half of these patients also have hypokalemia and metabolic alkalosis.

Glucocorticoid-remediable aldosteronism is an autosomal-dominant mutation in which aldosterone secretion is stimulated by adrenocorticotropic hormone (ACTH) rather than angiotensin. This situation causes sustained increased aldosterone levels. Patients present with features of primary hyperaldosteronism, including hypertension and hypokalemia. Affected individuals have early-onset hypertension, which is usually refractory to treatment. There is also a high incidence of hemorrhagic stroke at a young age (<40 years), often caused by ruptured intracranial aneurysms.

Secondary hyperaldosteronism, also known as high renin syndrome, is another cause of metabolic alkalosis. Renin is secreted in response to a decrease in blood volume or a reduction in sodium to increase plasma volume and increase blood pressure. Conditions such as renal artery stenosis can trigger release of rennin, which results in increased levels of aldosterone. The result of this condition is retention of sodium and extracellular water.

The causes for secondary hyperaldosteronism can be divided into 2 categories: hypertensive state secondary to a renin-producing tumor or increased renin production as a result of poor renal perfusion. Constant edematous states such as cirrhosis and nephrotic syndrome result in a deficit in effective extracellular fluid and blood volume, resulting in activation of renin-angiotensin-aldosterone cascade.[22] This situation increases absorption of sodium ions and excretion of hydrogen ions via the apical proton pump. Aldosterone also activates the chloride-bicarbonate exchanger, which adds bicarbonate into the systemic circulation.

Treatment

The treatment of primary hyperaldosteronism includes either laparoscopic adrenalectomy or administering mineralocorticoid receptor antagonists (spironolactone and eplerenone), depending if the patient is a surgical candidate or has bilateral aldosterone secretion.[23] Glucocorticoid-remediable aldosteronism is treated with glucocorticoid administration to suppress the secretion of ACTH, thereby decreasing the secretion of aldosterone.[24] The treatment of secondary hyperaldosteronism begins with identifying and addressing the underlying cause. Surgical interventions are indicated in rennin-producing tumors.

Apparent Mineralocorticosteroid Excess Syndromes

Clinically, apparent mineralocorticosteroid excess syndromes cause metabolic alkalosis, which is impossible to differentiate from hyperaldosteronism. Liddle syndrome, also known as pseudohyperaldosteronism, is an autosomal-dominant genetic mutation that prevents downregulation of the sodium ion channel.[25] This situation causes continuous sodium reabsorption, hypertension, and hypokalemic alkalosis. However, renin and aldosterone levels in these patients are very low. Typical presentation is that of a child or adolescent with hypertension, and at times, with renal failure, who may have siblings with the same symptoms.

11β-Hydroxysteroid dehydrogenase is an enzyme that is adjacent to the mineralocorticoid receptor in the collecting duct, which rapidly converts cortisol to cortisone, decreasing the binding of cortisol to the receptor. 11β-Hydroxysteroid dehydrogenase deficiencies, caused by a mutation of this enzyme, increase the binding of cortisol to the receptor and thus stimulate sodium reabsorption and potassium secretion independent of aldosterone. This situation produces a chloride-resistant metabolic alkalosis and hypertension in the setting of low aldosterone levels. Glycyrrhizic acid, a component of natural licorice, inhibits the activity of 11β-hydroxysteroid dehydrogenase and can cause the same clinic picture.[1]

Treatment

Metabolic alkalosis caused by apparent mineralocorticoid excess syndromes is treated by restricting a patient's sodium intake and adding potassium supplementation. Liddle syndrome and 11β-hydroxysteroid dehydrogenase deficiencies also respond to amiloride.[24]

OTHER CAUSES
Alkali Ingestion or Administration

Under normal circumstances, the kidney responds quickly to excess alkali by increasing bicarbonate excretion, and thus, metabolic alkalosis exists only transiently. However, in patients with renal failure, ingested or administered alkali cannot be excreted as efficiently, which causes a sustained increase in serum bicarbonate levels. In addition, patients with preexisting hypochloremia or hypokalemia or patients placed on a diet with little chloride who are given alkali supplementation also experience a sustained metabolic alkalosis.[26]

Alkali ingestion

Pronounced metabolic alkalosis can occur with consumption of a large amount of bicarbonate or its precursors, such as citrate or acetate. Several cases have been reported in which patients presented with severe metabolic alkalosis after ingestion of large amounts of bicarbonate to treat various ailments as a home remedy for the treatment of peptic ulcer disease and wound care or the treatment of common cold.[6,27] In addition, the administration of citrate to be used as anticoagulants in renal patients has been linked to the development of metabolic alkalosis.[28,29]

Recently, there has been an increase in the practice of ingesting of bicarbonate to improve sports performance.[30,31] It has been suggested that bicarbonate improves performance by promoting the efflux of hydrogen ions from working cells and tissues.[32] The efficacy is not clear-cut based on recent literature. However, patients may present to the emergency department after ingestion of a large amount of sodium bicarbonate before the planned event with gastrointestinal symptoms, including abdominal cramps, vomiting, and stomach bloating.[33] Routine workup of these patients may show alkalosis. Most patients recover without any sequelae with supportive therapy.

Milk alkali syndrome

This syndrome was described in the early 20th century, when ingestion of milk and large amounts of alkali (sodium bicarbonate, magnesium bicarbonate, and bismuth subcarbonate) was used to treat peptic ulcer disease. It consists of hypercalcemia, renal failure, and metabolic alkalosis.[34] However, with the introduction of other H_2 blockers and proton pump inhibitors as the treatment modality of peptic ulcer disease, the occurrence of milk alkali syndrome has reduced significantly. Recently, a similar condition called the calcium alkali syndrome has emerged, with ingestion of a large amount of calcium carbonate to increase calcium uptake to prevent osteoporosis and over-the-counter treatment of dyspepsia. Similar to the traditional milk alkali syndrome, patients present with hypercalcemia, acute renal failure, and metabolic alkalosis. However, serum phosphorus levels can be normal to low in calcium alkali syndrome in contrast to the traditional milk alkali syndrome, in which phosphorus is high because of the large load from milk and cream.[35]

The initial treatment consists of fluid resuscitation with normal saline to improve calcium and bicarbonate excretion. It is also important to educate patients on appropriate dosing of the calcium containing medications.

Profound hypokalemia

Hypokalemia is often found in patients with metabolic alkalosis. In patients deficient in potassium, as the serum potassium decreases, potassium ions are transported from the intracellular space out to extracellular space in exchange with a hydrogen ion to maintain electric equilibrium. The movements of hydrogen ion contribute to the development of alkalosis. Hypokalemia also activates aldosterone to stimulate potassium/hydrogen ion exchange enzymes to further enhance hydrogen ion secretion.[4] Because potassium is closely linked to the development and maintenance of metabolic alkalosis, it is crucial to monitor the potassium status of these patients.

Posthypercapnic alkalosis

The kidney compensates for chronic respiratory acidosis by increasing bicarbonate reabsorption and accelerating excretion of chloride. When hypercapnia is corrected rapidly by means of mechanical ventilation, increased plasma bicarbonate levels persist in the setting of hypochloremia.[17] Presence of posthypercapnic alkalosis in the intensive care unit setting may be associated with ventilator dependence and increase stay in the intensive care unit.[36] The treatment consists of correcting the chloride deficit and expanding the volume.

SUMMARY

Metabolic alkalosis is a common disorder amongst patients presenting to the emergency department. Patients often present without any symptoms but can develop neurologic and respiratory symptoms as their alkalosis worsens. The cause of metabolic alkalosis can be divided into 4 main groups: chloride depletion syndromes, which include gastrointestinal and renal losses; mineralocorticoid excess syndromes; apparent mineralocorticoid syndromes; and excess alkali administration. The cause of this acid-base disturbance is identified by obtaining a history from the patient, then assessing the blood pressure and volume status. The mainstay of treatment is supportive care; however, once a specific cause is identified, it should be addressed correct the alkalosis and any electrolyte abnormalities.

REFERENCES

1. Gennari FJ. Metabolic alkalosis. In: Feehally J, Floege J, Johnson RJ, editors. Comprehensive clinical nephrology. 3rd edition. New York: Mosby; 2007. p. 167–75.
2. DuBose TD. Acidosis and alkalosis. In: Longo DL, Fauci AS, Kasper DL, editors. Harrison's principles of internal medicine. 18th edition. New York: McGraw-Hill; 2012. p. 363–73.
3. Hodgkin JE, Soeprono FF, Chan DM. Incidence of metabolic alkalemia in hospitalized patients. Crit Care Med 1980;8:725–32.
4. Peixito AJ, Alpern RJ. Treatment of severe metabolic alkalosis in a patient with congestive heart failure. Am J Kidney Dis 2013;61(5):822–7.
5. Anderson LE, Henrich WL. Alkalemia associated morbidity and mortality in medical and surgical patients. South Med J 1987;80:729–33.
6. Yi JH, Han SW, Song JS, et al. Metabolic alkalosis from unsuspected ingestion: use of urine pH and anion gap. Am J Kidney Dis 2012;59(4):577–81.
7. Gennari FJ, Hussain-Khan S, Segal A. An unusual case of metabolic alkalosis: a window into the pathophysiology and diagnosis of this common acid-base disturbance. Am J Kidney Dis 2010;55(6):1130–5.
8. Gennari FJ. Pathophysiology of metabolic alkalosis: a new classification based on the centrality of stimulated collecting duct ion transport. Am J Kidney Dis 2011;58(4):626–36.
9. Schaefer T, Wolford R. Disorders of potassium. Emerg Med Clin North Am 2005; 23:723–47.
10. Luke RG, Galla JH. It is chloride depletion alkalosis, not contraction alkalosis. J Am Soc Nephrol 2012;23(2):204–7.
11. Gennari FJ, Weise WJ. Acid-base disturbances in gastrointestinal disease. Clin J Am Soc Nephrol 2008;3:1861–8.
12. Miles LF, Wakeman CJ, Farmer KC. Giant villous adenoma presenting as McKittrick-Wheelock syndrome and pseudo-obstruction. Med J Aust 2010; 192(4):225–7.
13. Weise WJ, Serrano FA, Fought J, et al. Acute electrolyte and acid-base disorders in patients with ileostomies: a case series. Am J Kidney Dis 2008;52(3):494–500.
14. Berend K, van Hulsteijn LH, Gans RO. Chloride: the queen of electrolytes? Eur J Intern Med 2012;23:203–11.
15. Naesens M, Steels P, Verberckmoes R, et al. Bartter's and Gitelman's syndromes: from gene to clinic. Nephron Physiol 2004;96:65–78.
16. Kassamali R, Sica DA. Acetazolamide: a forgotten diuretic agent. Cardiol Rev 2011;19(6):276–8.

17. Mazur JE, Devlin JW, Peters MJ, et al. Single versus multiple doses of acetazolamide for metabolic alkalosis in critically ill medical patients: a randomized, double-blind trial. Crit Care Med 1999;27(7):1257–61.
18. Galla JH. Metabolic alkalosis. J Am Soc Nephrol 2000;11:269–375.
19. Brimioulle S, Berre J, Dufaye P, et al. Hydrochloric acid infusion for treatment of metabolic alkalosis associated with respiratory acidosis. Crit Care Med 1989;17(3):232–6.
20. Korkmaz A, Yildirim E, Aras N, et al. Hydrochloric acid for treating metabolic alkalosis. Jpn J Surg 1989;19(5):519–23.
21. Lu H, Gennari FJ. Severe metabolic alkalosis in a hemodialysis patient. Am J Kidney Dis 2011;58(1):144–9.
22. Bansal S, Lindenfeld J, Schrier RW. Sodium retention in heart failure and cirrhosis: potential role of natriuretic doses of mineralocorticoid antagonist? Circ Heart Fail 2009;2(4):370–6.
23. Weiner D, Wingo C. Endocrine causes of hypertension–aldosterone. In: Feehally J, Floege J, Johnson RJ, editors. Comprehensive clinical nephrology. 3rd edition. New York: Mosby; 2007. p. 469–76.
24. Gross P, Hedushka P. Inherited disorders of sodium and water handling. In: Feehally J, Floege J, Johnson RJ, editors. Comprehensive clinical nephrology. 3rd edition. New York: Mosby; 2007. p. 573–83.
25. Shimkets RA, Warnock DG, Bositis CM, et al. Liddle's syndrome: heritable human hypertension caused by mutations in the p subunit of the epithelial sodium channel. Cell 1994;79:407–14.
26. Gennari FJ. Acid-base disorders in end stage renal disease: part II. Semin Dial 1991;3:161–5.
27. John RS, Simoes S, Reddi AS. A patient with foot ulcer and severe metabolic alkalosis. Am J Emerg Med 2012;30(1):260.e5–8.
28. Kindgen-Milles D, Amman J, Kleinekofort W, et al. Treatment of metabolic alkalosis during continuous renal replacement therapy with regional citrate anticoagulation. Int J Artif Organs 2008;31(4):363–6.
29. Tolwani A, Wille KM. Advances in continuous renal replacement therapy: citrate anticoagulation update. Blood Purif 2012;34(2):88–93.
30. Van Montfoort MC, Van Dieren L, Hopkins WG, et al. Effects of ingestion of bicarbonate, citrate, lactate, and chloride on sprint running. Med Sci Sports Exerc 2004;36(7):1239–43.
31. Carr AJ, Hopkins WG, Gore CJ. Effects of acute alkalosis and acidosis on performance: a meta-analysis. Sports Med 2011;41(10):801–14.
32. Peart DJ, Siegler JC, Vince RV. Practical recommendations for coaches and athletes: a meta-analysis of sodium bicarbonate use for athletic performance. J Strength Cond Res 2012;26(7):1975–83.
33. Cameron SL, McLay-Cooke RT, Brown RC, et al. Increased blood pH but not performance with sodium bicarbonate supplementation in elite rugby union players. Int J Sport Nutr Exerc Metab 2010;20(4):307–21.
34. Medarov BI. Milk-alkali syndrome. Mayo Clin Proc 2009;84(3):261–7.
35. Arroyo M, Fenves A, Emmett M. The calcium alkali syndrome. Proc (Bayl Univ Med Cent) 2013;26(2):179–81.
36. Banga A, Khilnani GC. Post-hypercapnic alkalosis is associated with ventilator dependence and increased ICU stay. COPD 2009;6(6):437–40.

The Clinical Manifestations, Diagnosis, and Treatment of Adrenal Emergencies

Veronica Tucci, MD, JD*, Telematé Sokari, MD

KEYWORDS

- Adrenal emergencies • Primary adrenal insufficiency (Addison disease)
- Secondary adrenal insufficiency • Tertiary adrenal insufficiency • Adrenal crisis
- Pheochromocytomas

KEY POINTS

- Adrenal insufficiency occurs because of a disruption in the hypothalamic-pituitary-adrenal axis. The resultant hormonal deficiencies cause a myriad of nonspecific symptoms, complicating the clinical picture and delaying diagnosis.
- The hallmark of adrenal crisis is hypotension and shock refractory to fluid resuscitation and vasopressors. Adrenal crisis is a life-threatening condition and treatment should not be delayed for confirmatory testing.
- Hydrocortisone is the drug of choice for treating cases of adrenal crisis or insufficiency because of its glucocorticoid and mineralocorticoid effects.
- Pheochromocytoma is a rare, catecholamine-secreting tumor of the adrenal medulla, which may precipitate life-threatening hypertension and lead to multiorgan system failure.

INTRODUCTION

With his perfectly tanned, boyish good looks, athleticism, intelligence, and wit, John F. Kennedy (JFK) was the picture of vitality. Even 50 years after his assassination, his presidential administration, still referred to as Camelot, embodies the hopes, dreams, and exuberant idealism of many Americans. Yet beneath the facade, JFK was plagued by the myriad of health problems seen in patients with adrenal insufficiency and those on chronic steroids. JFK's medical records reveal that he was diagnosed with adrenal insufficiency in 1947 and hypothyroidism in 1955. Experts now believe that JFK suffered from autoimmune polyendocrine syndrome type 2. Unlike the participants of more recent political campaigns, JFK's health issues remained largely hidden from the public domain. Decades later, we know that JFK's physicians prescribed him

Section of Emergency Medicine, Emergency Center, Ben Taub General Hospital, Baylor College of Medicine, 1 Baylor Plaza, 1504 Taub Loop, Houston, TX 77030, USA
* Corresponding author.
E-mail address: vtuccimd@gmail.com

Emerg Med Clin N Am 32 (2014) 465–484
http://dx.doi.org/10.1016/j.emc.2014.01.006   emed.theclinics.com
0733-8627/14/$ – see front matter © 2014 Elsevier Inc. All rights reserved.

numerous medications but the extent to which his illness impacted his presidential decision-making and the course of American history remains largely unknown.[1,2]

Emergency medicine physicians should be able to identify and treat patients whose clinical presentations including key historical, physical examination, and laboratory findings are consistent with diagnoses of primary, secondary, and tertiary adrenal insufficiency, adrenal crisis, and pheochromocytoma. Failure to make a timely diagnosis leads to increased morbidity and mortality. As great mimickers, adrenal emergencies often present with a constellation of nonspecific signs and symptoms that can lead even the most diligent emergency physician astray. As discussed in this article, the emergency physician must include adrenal emergencies in the differential diagnosis when encountering such clinical pictures.

EMERGENCIES OF THE ADRENAL CORTEX
Primary Adrenal Insufficiency (Addison Disease)

Epidemiology
In the United States, the prevalence of Addison disease is 40 to 60 cases per 1 million population. Internationally, the occurrence is equally rare. The reported prevalence in countries where data are available is 39 cases per 1 million population in Great Britain, 60 cases per 1 million population in Denmark, and 144 cases per million in Norway.[3,4] It is more common in women and diagnosis peaks during the fourth to sixth decades of life. In the United States, roughly 80% of cases are caused by autoimmune disorders.[5] These autoimmune disorders can occur as an isolated process or as part of an autoimmune polyendocrine syndrome known as the polyglandular autoimmune syndrome types I and II. Type I polyglandular autoimmune syndrome is associated with candidiasis, hypoparathyroidism, and adrenal failure. Type II polyglandular autoimmune syndrome consists of Addison disease plus either an autoimmune thyroid disease or type 1 diabetes mellitus associated with hypogonadism, pernicious anemia, celiac disease, or primary biliary cirrhosis.[6] Causes of Addison disease are shown in **Table 1**.

Anatomy and physiology
The adrenal glands are encapsulated, retroperitoneal organs comprised of an outer cortex and an inner medullary zone. The cortex is subdivided into three zones: the zona fasiculata and zona reticularis, which secrete glucocorticoids and androgens, and the zona glomerulosa, which produces mineralocorticoids.[7] The most clinically important glucorticoid produced by the adrenal cortex is cortisol. Aldosterone and dehydroepiandrosterone acetate (DHEA) are the most clinically important mineralocorticoid and androgen, respectively. Aldosterone functions in the setting of hypovolemia and regulates blood pressure by acting on the distal tubules and collecting ducts of the nephron to cause the conservation of sodium, secretion of potassium, which leads to increased water retention and blood pressure. DHEA acts as a metabolic intermediate in the biosynthesis of the androgen and estrogen sex steroids.[7] **Table 2** reviews the actions of the adrenal hormones and the target systems they affect. The inner medullary zone produces catecholamines including epinephrine and norepinephrine. Adrenal function and secretion of hormones is maintained by the body until approximately 80% to 90% of the glands are destroyed.

Released during periods of stress including trauma and infection, cortisol is vital to the body's response and impacts immune function; vascular tone; and lipid, protein, and carbohydrate metabolism. Its release is regulated by the hypothalamic-pituitary-adrenal (HPA) axis (**Fig. 1**). Signals from the body (eg, cytokine release, tissue injury, pain, hypotension, hypoglycemia, hypoxemia) are sensed by the central nervous

Table 1
Causes of primary adrenal insufficiency

Disorders in the Adrenal Gland	Examples
Autoimmune (80% of cases)	Polyglandular autoimmune syndrome type I and II, isolated adrenal insufficiency
Adrenal hemorrhage or thrombosis	Coagulation disorders Overwhelming sepsis (Waterhouse-Friderichsen syndrome) Necrosis caused by meningococcal sepsis
Associated endocrinopathies	Hypoparathyroidism Hepatitis Type 1 diabetes mellitus Hypogonadism Hypothyroidism
Drugs	Ketoconazole Suramin Aminogluthimide Etomidate (in children)
Infections	Disseminated tuberculosis Cytomegalovirus Histoplasmosis Cryptococcus Toxoplasmosis HIV Candidiasis
Infiltrative disorders	Amyloidosis Sarcoidosis Hemochromatosis Metastatic disease
Surgery and trauma	Bilateral adrenalectomy Adrenal trauma
Genetic diseases	Congenital adrenal hyperplasia Neonatal and X-linked adrenoleukodystrophy Familial glucocorticoid deficiency

Table 2
Key actions of adrenal hormones

Target System	Action
Cardiovascular	Increases contractility and the vascular response to vasoconstrictors
Endocrine	Inhibits insulin secretion, promotes peripheral insulin resistance Increases epinephrine synthesis
Inflammatory	Causes demargination of granulocytes, suppresses adhesion Reduces circulating eosinophils and lymphocytes Decreases production of inflammatory cytokines
Metabolism	Stimulates gluconeogenesis Promotes lipolysis Induces muscle protein catabolism Increases plasma glucose during stress
Renal	Increases the glomerular filtration rate; pharmacologic doses act at mineralocorticoid receptors

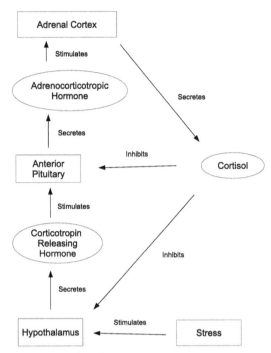

Fig. 1. Hypothalamic-pituitary-adrenal axis.

system and transmitted to the hypothalamus. The hypothalamus integrates these signals and increases or decreases the release of corticotropin-releasing hormone (CRH). CRH circulates to the anterior pituitary gland, where it stimulates the release of adrenal corticotropin hormone (ACTH), which in turn circulates to the adrenal cortex where it stimulates the release of cortisol.

Figs. 1 and **2** illustrate the feedback loop of cortisol and the HPA axis and aldosterone and the renin-angiotensin system. Cortisol levels have a negative and positive feedback effect on the hypothalamus and the anterior pituitary.

Aldosterone acts at the renal tubules to maintain Na+, K+, and water balance by way of the renin-angiotensin system, which is illustrated by **Fig. 2**. The renin-angiotensin system regulates aldosterone production.[7]

Clinical presentation

Patients with Addison disease generally have chronic, vague, and nonspecific complaints. As a result, they may be misdiagnosed with various psychiatric and gastrointestinal diseases.[8,9] Indeed, one study found that up to 20% of patients had symptoms for more than 5 years before they were diagnosed.[8] A recent analysis in Poland found that 54% of patients were only diagnosed after presenting with adrenal crisis.[10] Fulminant presentations may also occur with adrenal hemorrhage. The type and severity of clinical symptoms depends largely on the extent of the patient's hormonal deficiency, the rate at which the deficiency developed, and the underlying cause of the patient's condition.

Signs and symptoms of chronic primary adrenal insufficiency (PAI) and their frequencies are listed in **Box 1**. **Box 2** reports laboratory findings associated with PAI and the frequency for each laboratory result.

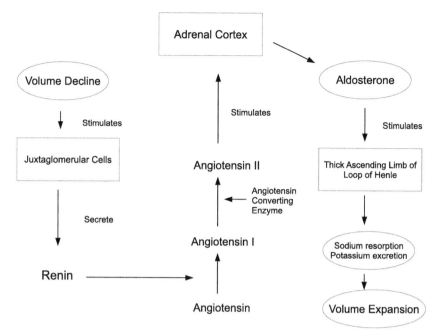

Fig. 2. Effect of volume decline on adrenal cortex and renin-angiotensin-aldosterone system.

Secondary Adrenal Insufficiency

Epidemiology

Secondary adrenal insufficiency (SAI) occurs when the integrity of the HPA axis is lost (see **Fig. 1**) because of pituitary disease. The causes of SAI are listed in **Table 3** but in each instance, secretion of ACTH is diminished and cortisol production is reduced. The lack of ACTH stimulation can eventually result in adrenal atrophy. Aldosterone release, sex hormone release, and catecholamine synthesis are usually normal.[14]

Anatomy and physiology

The pituitary gland, also known as the hypophysis, is a pea-sized gland that sits in a protective bony enclosure called the sella turcica. It is divided into the anterior pituitary, which produces several hormones, and the posterior pituitary, which secretes vasopressin, also known as antidiuretic hormone, and oxytocin.

Clinical presentation

SAI is a chronic disease process and patients may present with many of the same signs and symptoms as PAI. Fulminant presentations may be caused by pituitary hemorrhage or necrosis.

Clinical signs and symptoms of SAI are summarized in **Box 3**. There are some notable clinical and laboratory differences between PAI, SAI, and tertiary adrenal insufficiency (TAI; see **Boxes 1** and **3**, **Table 5**). Patients with Addison disease typically have hyperpigmented skin, particularly of sun-exposed areas, axillae, palmar creases, and mucous membranes. The cause of hyperpigmentation in Addison disease is believed to reflect increased stimulation of melanocyte receptors by ACTH.[15] Patients with SAI, however, do not manifest this finding because the anterior pituitary produces only low levels of ACTH. In addition, in Addison disease, the mineralocorticoid

Box 1
Clinical signs and symptoms of primary adrenal insufficiency

Weight loss, 25%–100%

Hyperpigmentation, 76%–94%

Vitiligo, 10%–20%

Hypotension (systolic blood pressure <110 mm Hg), 88%–94%

Shock, 5%

Auricular calcification, 5%

Amenorrhea, 25%

Infertility and premature ovarian insufficiency, 6%

Constitutional symptoms including weakness, fatigue, 100%

Anorexia, 100%

Nausea, 25%–86%

Vomiting, 25%–75%

Constipation, 33%

Abdominal pain, 31%

Diarrhea, 16%

Salt craving, 16%

Postural dizziness and syncope, 12%–20%

Musculoskeletal complaints including myalgias and arthralgias, 6%–37%

Psychiatric complaints including depression, apathy, psychosis, and pseudodementia

Data from Refs.[10–13]

Box 2
Laboratory abnormalities seen with primary adrenal insufficiency

Hyponatremia, 57%–88%

Hyperkalemia, 64%–85%

Hypercalcemia, 6%–33%

Azotemia, 55%

Mild hypoglycemia, 67%

Hypochloremia and acidosis

Anemia, 40%

Eosinophilia, 17%

Vitamin B_{12} deficiency, 10%

Type 1 diabetes, 12%

Data from Taub YR, Wolford RW. Adrenal insufficiency and other adrenal oncologic emergencies. Emerg Med Clin North Am 2009;27:273; and Erichsen MM, Husebye ES, Michelsen TM, et al. Sexuality and fertility in women with Addison's disease. J Clin Endocrinol Metab 2010;95(9):4354–60.

Table 3
Causes of secondary adrenal insufficiency

Reason for Dysfunction of HPA Axis	Examples
Sudden cessation of prolonged glucocorticoid therapy (most common)	Chronic use of steroid inhibits ACTH production
Brain tumors	Pituitary tumor Local invasion (craniopharyngioma)
Medications (eg, megesterol, medroxyprogesterone, opioids)	Progestin binds to glucocorticoid receptor resulting in some glucocorticoid activity leading to decreased response to ACTH Opioids impacts diurnal release of cortisol, diminishes response to exogenous ACTH
Pituitary irradiation Pituitary surgery Head trauma involving the pituitary gland	Disrupts ACTH production capacity in HPA axis
Pituitary necrosis or bleeding	Postpartum pituitary necrosis (Sheehan syndrome)
Infiltrative disorders of the pituitary or hypothalamus	Sarcoidosis Amyloidosis Hemosiderosis Hemochromatosis Histiocytosis X Metastatic cancer Lymphoma
Infectious diseases	Tuberculosis Meningitis Fungus HIV

Box 3
Clinical signs and symptoms of secondary adrenal insufficiency

Weight gain

Thin axillary and/or pubic hair

Decreased libido

Infertility, amenorrhea

Auricular calcification

Constitutional symptoms including weakness, fatigue, weight gain, cold intolerance

Anorexia

Headache and visual disturbance

Gastrointestinal complaints including abdominal pain, nausea, vomiting, diarrhea, constipation

Musculoskeletal complaints including myalgias and arthralgias

Psychiatric complaints including depression, apathy, psychosis, and pseudodementia deficiency often produces significant salt craving, and evidence in laboratory analysis, including hyperkalemia and hyponatremia.[15] Because mineralocorticoids are not primarily affected by ACTH, patients with SAI are not hypokalemic, hypernatremic (aldosterone functioning), or hyponatremic (because of water retention). Pathology of the anterior pituitary gland produces clinical manifestations of adrenal insufficiency in addition to the effects that are seen with deficiencies of the other hormones produced by the anterior pituitary.

Tertiary Adrenal Insufficiency

Epidemiology
TAI occurs secondary to hypothalamic disease. CRH secretion is diminished, leading to minimal ACTH and cortisol production. As with SAI, the lack of ACTH stimulation can lead to adrenal atrophy. Aldosterone release, sex hormone release, and catecholamine synthesis are usually normal.[14]

The most common cause of TAI is long-term, high-dose glucocorticoid therapy (eg, prednisone, hydrocortisone, and dexamethasone) for autoimmune and inflammatory conditions. Exogenous steroid administration suppresses CRH synthesis and secretion, which also leads to decreased ACTH production. Adrenal atrophy is the result of this long-term therapy with levels of ACTH being suppressed. Recovery of the HPA axis may take a few months to 1 year after cessation of long-term glucocorticoid therapy. A summary of causes of TAI is listed in **Table 4**.

Anatomy and physiology
The hypothalamus is located below the thalamus, just above the brainstem and is roughly the size of an almond. One of the most important functions of the hypothalamus is to link the nervous system to the endocrine system by the pituitary gland. It synthesizes and secretes certain neurohormones, often called hypothalamic-releasing hormones, and these in turn stimulate or inhibit the secretion of pituitary hormones (see **Fig. 1**).

Table 4
Causes of tertiary adrenal insufficiency

Reason for Dysfunction of HPA Axis	Examples
Exogenous high-dose glucocorticoid use	Chronic use of steroid inhibits CRH, ACTH production
Brain tumors	Hypothalamic tumor
Isolated CRH deficiency (rare)	Idiopathic
Cushing syndrome cure	Removal of pituitary tumor or other tumor that secretes ACTH or cortisol
Infiltrative disorders of the pituitary or hypothalamus	Sarcoidosis Amyloidosis Hemosiderosis Hemochromatosis Histiocytosis X Metastatic cancer Lymphoma
Infectious diseases	Tuberculosis Meningitis Fungus HIV

Clinical presentation
TAI is a chronic disease process and patients may present with many of the same signs and symptoms as PAI and SAI.

Differentiating PAI, SAI, and TAI
It can be difficult for practitioners to tease out differences in clinical presentation between PAI, SAI, and TAI. The key differences in signs and symptoms and noteworthy laboratory findings are listed in **Table 5**.

Differential Diagnosis
The differential diagnoses of neoplasia, acute appendicitis, cardiac dysrhythmias, subarachnoid hemorrhage, and acute coronary syndrome must be considered in patients with this disease. The nonspecific constellation of signs and symptoms, such as headache, visual changes, fatigue, generalized weakness, weight loss, abdominal pain, nausea and vomiting, syncope, and postural dizziness, often makes chronic adrenal insufficiency an elusive diagnosis for practitioners.

Table 5
Differences in clinical presentation and laboratory findings between primary, secondary, and tertiary adrenal insufficiency

	Primary Adrenal Insufficiency	Secondary Adrenal Insufficiency	Tertiary Adrenal Insufficiency
Signs and Symptoms			
Cushingoid features including abdominal striae and central obesity, humpback	Absent	May be present (if caused by long-term glucocorticoid use)	May be present (if caused by long-term glucocorticoid use)
Volume depletion and hypotension	Marked	Absent or mild (caused by decreased vascular tone)	Absent or mild (caused by decreased vascular tone)
Axillary hair loss, decreased libido, amenorrhea	Present	Present	Present
Hyperpigmentation	Present	Absent	Absent
Laboratory Findings			
Aldosterone deficiency	Present	Absent	Absent
Serum potassium level	Hyperkalemia	Normal or hypokalemia	Normal or hypokalemia
Serum sodium level	Hyponatremia (caused by salt wasting)	Hypernatremia (aldosterone functioning) or hyponatremia (caused by water retention)	Hypernatremia (aldosterone functioning) or hyponatremia (caused by water retention)
Serum chloride	Hypochloremia	Normal	Normal
Blood-urea-nitrogen	Mildly elevated	Normal	Normal
Serum glucose	Mild hypoglycemia	Marked hypoglycemia	Marked hypoglycemia

Adrenal Crisis

Epidemiology

Most cases of adrenal crisis occur in a person with Addison disease caused by mineralocorticoid deficiency but can be seen in patients with SAI or TAI and who are under severe physiologic stress, such as sepsis, trauma, burns, surgery, and myocardial infarction. Severe physiologic stress rapidly depletes the patient's already limited cortisol reserves, making the patient unable to mount an adequate stress response.

Hahner and colleagues[16] investigated the frequency, precipitating conditions, and risk factors for adrenal crisis in patients with chronic adrenal insufficiency. They found that 47% and 35% experienced at least one crisis in patients with PAI and SAI, respectively. Precipitating factors were fever (24% in PAI, 15% in SAI), gastrointestinal illness (33% in PAI, 22% in SAI), surgery (7% in PAI, 16% in SAI), and strenuous activity. Risk factors for adrenal crisis included nonendocrine comorbidities for PAI and female gender and diabetes insipidus for patients with SAI.

Clinical presentation The hallmark of adrenal crisis is hypotension and shock refractory to fluid resuscitation and vasopressors. As with adrenal insufficiency, patients have nonspecific symptoms including abdominal pain, nausea, vomiting, fever, lethargy, malaise, weakness, and confusion. The frequency of clinical signs and symptoms are listed in **Box 4**.

Emergency Department Management of Adrenal Insufficiencies and Adrenal Crisis

Treatment before diagnostic testing

Emergency physicians should begin empiric treatment of patients with suspected adrenal crisis before receiving the results of any confirmatory laboratory testing. **Table 6** serves as a treatment guide for adrenal crisis.

Hydrocortisone is the drug of choice for cases of adrenal crisis or insufficiency (provides both glucocorticoid and mineralocorticoid effects).[17,18] Although not necessary in the acute phase, fludrocortisone, 0.1 mg, is often part of a daily maintenance regimen. Although still controversial, DHEA may also be considered because of its reported improvement in patient quality of life.[19]

A thorough search for a precipitating cause should be undertaken. Empiric antibiotics may be given based on the patient's clinical presentation. Reversal of coagulopathy, if present, should be attempted with fresh frozen plasma. Patients with primary failure of the HPA axis may have concurrent clinical hypothyroidism and require

---

Box 4
Clinical signs and symptoms of adrenal crisis

Hypotension and shock, 90%

Fever, 66%

Abdominal rebound tenderness or rigidity, 22%

Anorexia, nausea, and vomiting, 47%

Abdominal pain, flank pain, back pain, lower chest pain, 86%

Neuropsychiatric complaints (confusion, disorientation), 42%

Data from Rao RH, Vagnucci AH, Amico JA. Bilateral massive adrenal hemorrhage: early recognition and treatment. Ann Intern Med 1989;110(3):227–35.

Table 6
Treatment guide for adrenal crisis

Treatment	Adult	Pediatric
Fluids	5% dextrose in normal saline or normal saline boluses may be used	Shock and hypotension is addressed with standard fluid resuscitation measures: 20 mL/kg normal saline boluses up to a maximum of 60 mL/kg over 1 h
Vasopressors	May be necessary if shock is refractory	May be necessary if shock is refractory
Steroids	Hydrocortisone, 100 mg bolus Followed by daily doses of 100 mg divided two to three times per day	Hydrocortisone Infants and toddlers to age 3: 25 mg IV Children ages 3–12: 50 mg IV Adolescents older than 12: 100 mg IV
Glucose	D50 may be used as necessary	Infants and children to age 12: 2.5 mL/kg of 10% dextrose Adolescents older than 12: 1 mL/kg of 25% dextrose

thyroxine supplementation. Hyperkalemia must be addressed in adult patients but is generally well tolerated in pediatric populations and resolves with normal saline infusions.[18]

Guillamondegui and colleagues,[20] in their retrospective review, found that compared to their untreated counterparts, trauma patients promptly identified and treated for acute adrenal insufficiency had an almost 50% reduction in mortality, spent less time in the intensive care unit and on ventilators and had shorter overall hospital stays.

Table 7 provides a summary of current maintenance recommendations for patients with chronic adrenal insufficiency.

Confirmatory diagnostic testing
Patients with all forms of adrenal insufficiency exhibit a deficiency of cortisol. In the outpatient setting, patients are generally screened with an early morning plasma cortisol level.[21] Readings lower than 3 µg/dL confirm adrenal insufficiency and values higher than 13 to 15 µg/dL make the diagnosis highly unlikely.[22]

The second step is to establish whether the cortisol deficiency is caused by ACTH or CRH deficiency. Adrenal function testing begins with the administration of 250 µg of synthetic ACTH (Cosyntropin). A rise in serum cortisol to greater than 8 µg/dL within 30 minutes is considered a normal response. Such a finding excludes PAI but does not evaluate the HPA axis–related causes of SAI. To differentiate between PAI and

Table 7
Management of chronic adrenal insufficiency

Treatment	Primary	Secondary
Glucocorticoid	20–25 mg hydrocortisone per 24 h divided in two to three doses	15–20 mg hydrocortisone per 24 h divided in two to three doses
Mineralocorticoid	0.1 mg per day	Not required
Androgen	May consider DHEA 25–50 mg and using transdermal testosterone	Not required

Data from Marik PE, Zaloga GP. Adrenal insufficiency during septic shock. Crit Care Med 2003;31(1):141–5; and Arlt W. The approach to the adult with newly diagnosed adrenal insufficiency. J Clin Endocrinol Metab 2009;94(4):1059–67.

SAI, basal corticotropin (ACTH) levels must be obtained. Levels are high in primary adrenal disorders (>100 pg/mL) and low or normal in SAI.

Early morning cortisol testing followed by ACTH stimulation testing in the emergency department is impractical and alternative testing algorithms have been sought. For critically ill patients, random serum cortisol levels above 34 μg/dL generally exclude a diagnosis of adrenal insufficiency and levels below 15 μg/dL in a patient with severe sepsis or shock suggest adrenal crisis.[23] Care must be taken in interpreting cortisol measurements in critically ill patients because those with hypoproteinemia may have low serum cortisol but normal free cortisol levels.[24]

Laboratory testing and imaging should also seek to establish whether the patient's adrenal insufficiency is caused by a treatable condition, such as infection. Computed tomography (CT) of the abdomen may reveal calcifications (associated with tuberculosis), adrenal hemorrhages, or metastatic infiltration. In cases of SAI, a head CT scan may show destruction of the pituitary gland (ie, empty sella syndrome).

In summary, serum cortisol levels are low in PAI, SAI, and TAI. ACTH levels are high in PAI, whereas they are low or normal in SAI and TAI. The ACTH stimulation test has no effect on cortisol in PAI but restores normal cortisol production in SAI and TAI. There is absent or minimal ACTH response to the CRH stimulation test in SAI but an exaggerated ACTH release in TAI.

Disposition

All patients with adrenal crisis should be admitted to an intensive care unit for resuscitation, and electrolyte and hemodynamic monitoring. Inpatient teams should continue to search for the inciting event that precipitated the patient's crisis (eg, infections, acute coronary syndrome). Patients with the more classically indolent and chronic presentations of PAI or SAI may be managed on an outpatient basis.

EMERGENCIES OF THE ADRENAL MEDULLA
Pheochromocytomas

Epidemiology

Pheochromocytomas are neuroendocrine tumors that secrete excess catecholamines and may cause life-threatening hypertensive crises. Pheochromocytomas account for only 0.05% to 0.2% of hypertensive individuals. Pheochromocytomas occur in people of all races but are less commonly diagnosed in blacks. Pheochromocytomas may occur in persons of any age, but the peak incidence is from the third to the fifth decades of life. An estimated 500 to 1600 cases occur with an annual prevalence between 1:2500 and 1:6500.[25] The true incidence of pheochromocytoma in the United States is difficult to determine because of the number of patients with asymptomatic cases found incidentally at autopsy. Indeed, one retrospective study from the Mayo Clinic revealed that in 50% of cases of pheochromocytoma, the diagnosis was made at autopsy.[26]

Traditional teachings regarding pheochromocytoma include the Rule of 10s (**Box 5**). The tumor is malignant in 10% of cases. However, surgical removal is often curative. Approximately 10% of pheochromocytomas are discovered incidentally.[27] Approximately 10% occur in children. Fifty percent of pheochromocytomas in children are solitary intra-adrenal lesions, 25% are present bilaterally, and 25% are extra-adrenal.

Pheochromocytomas occur in certain familial syndromes and are inherited in an autosomal-dominant manner. These include multiple endocrine neoplasia, neurofibromatosis (von Recklinghausen disease), and von Hippel-Lindau disease.

Box 5 **Rule of 10s**
10% Bilateral
10% Malignant (higher in familial cases)
10% Extra-adrenal (most commonly in the sympathetic chain in the thorax, abdomen, and pelvis)
10% Familial (now estimated to be as high as 24%)

Anatomy and physiology

The inner zone of the adrenal gland is the medulla. It consists of chromaffin cells that produce mainly the catecholamines norepinephrine, epinephrine, and a small amount of dopamine. The catecholamines are secreted in response to stimulation by sympathetic preganglionic neurons and receptors for catecholamines are widely distributed throughout the body. The physiologic effects of catecholamines are well known and include increased heart rate and blood pressure, blood vessel constriction in the skin and gastrointestinal tract, smooth muscle (bronchiole and capillary) dilation, and increased metabolism. Pheochromocytomas can occur anywhere along the sympathetic chain, although 85% to 90% are discovered within the adrenal gland.

Clinical presentation

Pheochromocytoma classically presents with paroxysmal "spells" wherein the afflicted patient experiences headaches, palpitations, diaphoresis, and severe hypertension. These spells may occur monthly, weekly, daily, or multiple times per day, and the duration may vary from seconds to hours. Typically, they worsen with time, occurring more frequently and becoming more severe with tumor progression.

The clinical symptoms and signs and their frequencies (when available) of pheochromocytoma are listed in **Boxes 6** and **7**, respectively. The most common sign of pheochromocytoma, found in upward of 95% of patients, is hypertension.[28] Approximately 50% of patients have sustained hypertension, 45% present with the "classic picture" of paroxysmal hypertension, and the remainder is normotensive.[29] One recent review noted, however, that approximately 30% of patients with pheochromocytoma or paraganglioma are normotensive or have orthostatic hypotension.[30]

Box 6 **Clinical symptoms of pheochromocytoma**
Headache, 82%
Palpitations, 48%
Diaphoresis
Anxiety, 35%
Dizziness, 18%
Abdominal pain, flank pain
Myalgias, arthralgias
Data from Anderson NE, Chung K, Willoughby E, et al. Neurologic manifestations of phaeochromocytomas and secretory paragangliomas: a reappraisal. J Neurol Neurosurg Psychiatry 2013;84(4):452–7.

> **Box 7**
> **Clinical signs of pheochromocytoma**
>
> Weight loss
>
> Pallor
>
> Fever
>
> Hypertensive crisis
>
> Paroxysmal hypertension
>
> Malignant hypertension
>
> Orthostatic hypotension
>
> Frank shock
>
> Diaphoresis
>
> Tachycardia and arrhythmias
>
> Acute coronary syndrome
>
> Cardiomyopathy
>
> Acute heart failure
>
> Myocarditis
>
> Dissecting aortic aneurysm
>
> Acute respiratory distress syndrome
>
> Hypertensive retinopathy
>
> Seizure, 7%
>
> Hemiplegia
>
> Tremors, 15%
>
> Melena
>
> Hematochezia
>
> Café au lait spots
>
> Neurofibromas
>
> Hematuria
>
> Pain
>
> Pallor
>
> Paresthesias
>
> Rales
>
> Pulmonary edema
>
> *Data from* Anderson NE, Chung K, Willoughby E, et al. Neurologic manifestations of phaeochromocytomas and secretory paragangliomas: a reappraisal. J Neurol Neurosurg Psychiatry 2013;84(4):452–7.

Cerebrovascular accidents are frequently responsible for neurologic symptoms in patients with pheochromocytoma.[31,32] Intracranial and subarachnoid hemorrhages have been reported during paroxysmal attacks of hypertension and may be seen in connection with seizures. Patients may also present with generalized seizures secondary to cerebral ischemia and vasospasm.[33]

Adrenal tumor hemorrhages or necrosis can present as severe abdominal pain, nausea, and vomiting. The destruction of the adrenal medulla by either process may result in the excretion of vast quantities of catecholamines and precipitate a hypertensive crisis, cardiovascular collapse, and shock.[34] Moreover, emergency surgery or angiographic embolization by interventional radiology may be required to stop associated arterial bleeding with hemorrhage. Emergency surgery may also be indicated if a catecholamine surge induces vasoconstriction or spasms of the mesenteric arteries resulting in bowel ischemia.

Pheochromocytoma multisystem crisis is the most severe presentation of a pheochromocytoma that an emergency physician may encounter in practice. Patients with this condition may present with temperatures exceeding 40°C, encephalopathy, hypertension or hypotension, and multisystem organ failure. Mortality rates can exceed 85%.[35] Treatment with imipramine, metoclopramide, and glucocorticoids including dexamethasone have been reported to precipitate acute crises.[36–41]

Pheochromocytoma in pregnancy also warrants special consideration. Up to 65% of practitioners fail to diagnose pheochromocytoma in their pregnant patients before delivery despite the high maternal and fetal morbidity and mortality rates (40.3% and 56%, respectively).[42]

Hypertension complicates an estimated 8% of pregnancies and is classically divided into four categories: (1) chronic/essential hypertension, (2) preeclampsia, (3) preeclampsia complicated by chronic hypertension, and (4) transient hypertension of pregnancy.[43–45] Diagnosis of pheochromocytoma during pregnancy is complicated by the similarities in its clinical presentation with preeclampsia. The key differences are hypertension is generally not seen until 20 weeks after gestation in preeclampsia but may be seen at anytime during the pregnancy with pheochromocytoma. Edema and proteinuria are present in preeclampsia but are usually absent in pheochromocytoma.

Differential diagnosis

Also known as the great mimicker, patients with pheochromocytoma may present to the emergency department with a wide range of signs and symptoms, as seen in **Boxes 6** and **7**. Screening for pheochromocytoma should be done in children and young adults without any other explanation for hypertension and in older adults that are hypertensive and refractory to any medication regimens.

Surgical and Medical Management of Pheochromocytoma

Treatment of hypertension associated with pheochromocytoma depends in part on the clinical severity. Surgery is the only curative measure.

The indications for emergency surgery in the context of pheochromocytoma multisystem crisis are controversial with some advocates stating that emergent surgical resection may be the only means to halt disease progression, and others that medical stabilization followed by elective or urgent surgery is the best course of action.[46] Scholten and colleagues[47] conducted a retrospective cohort study enrolling 137 patients with pheochromocytoma, including 25 who presented in crisis. None of the crisis patients underwent emergent surgery and those who received urgent surgery had a higher rate of complications and longer intensive care unit stays and overall hospital admission compared with patients who received elective surgery. Their literature review found that emergency resection of pheochromocytoma resulted in higher intraoperative and postoperative surgical morbidity and mortality. They concluded that pheochromocytoma crisis should be treated with medical stabilization and elective or urgent surgery rather than emergency surgery.

Despite the controversies surrounding emergent versus urgent versus elective operative resection, pharmacotherapy is essential to preoperative and perioperative management. Pharmacotherapy is the mainstay of treatment of inoperable metastatic disease.

There is no consensus with respect to the ideal preoperative medical management. α-Blockers, calcium channel blockers, β-blockers, and angiotensin-receptor blockers have all been used by practitioners. Local practice patterns and drug shortages can complicate pharmacologic choices.[48]

The most common preoperative drug regimen used in the United States is phenoxybenzamine, 10 mg taken twice daily for 10 to 14 days. Shorter courses have also been used successfully and there is no universally recommended treatment duration.[49] The dose is titrated to symptom resolution by an irreversible, noncompetitive, α-adrenergic blockade. α-Blockers are typically started to control blood pressure and prevent a hypertensive crisis triggered by the high levels of circulating catecholamines that stimulate α-receptors and cause vasoconstriction.

β-Blockers are often included in preoperative regimens to treat the tachyarrhythmias that occur with α-blockade. However, β-blockade should not be used as a lone therapy and should not be started before initiation of the α-blockade because unopposed β-blockade potentiates the α-agonist effects of epinephrine and may precipitate a hypertensive crisis. Both noncardioselective β-blockers, such as propranolol or nadolol, and cardioselective agents, such as atenolol and metoprolol, may be used. The use of labetolol and carvedilol is controversial. Although both agents have α- and β-antagonist activity at a ratio of approximately 1:7, their use has been associated with paradoxic episodes of hypertension thought to be secondary to incomplete α-blockade.

Calcium channel blockers have also successfully been used preoperatively particularly in patients who are unable to tolerate the side effects of α-blockade.

A tyrosine analog, metyrosine, is sometimes used as an adjunct to α-blockade to inhibit catecholamine synthesis by inhibiting tyrosine hydroxylase.[50] This therapy may be beneficial to patients with refractory hypertension despite α-blockade and those patients with a high tumor burden or biochemically active tumors.[51,52]

There are also no consensus guidelines for intraoperative management of pheochromocytomas and this condition often presents significant challenges to our anesthesia colleagues because of the rapid hemodynamic shifts often seen in such cases. Tumor manipulation during surgery can result in bursts of catecholamine activity and hypertensive spikes. So called background infusions of nitroprusside or nitroglycerin can be used to prevent and address such spikes. Similarly, nicardipine has been used to prevent and treat hypertensive spikes.[53] Treatment with magnesium sulfate boluses (20–40 mg/kg) and infusions (1–2 mg/h) has also gained popularity in the

Table 8
Sensitivity and specificity of laboratory testing in pheochromocytomas

Diagnostic Test	Sensitivity and Specificity
Plasma metanephrine testing	96% sensitivity, 85% specificity
24-h urinary collection for catecholamines and metanephrines	87.5% sensitivity, 99.7% specificity

Data from Waguespack SG, Rich T, Grubbs E, et al. A current review of the etiology, diagnosis, and treatment of pediatric pheochromocytoma and paraganglioma. J Clin Endocrinol Metab 2010;95(5):2023–37; and Sheps SG, Jiang NS, Klee GG, et al. Recent developments in the diagnosis and treatment of pheochromocytoma. Mayo Clin Proc 1990;65(1):88–95.

Table 9
Sensitivity and specificity of imaging modalities in pheochromocytomas

Test	Sensitivity (%)	Specificity (%)
Abdominal CT scan	93	95
Magnetic resonance imaging	86–100	93
I-MIBG scintigraphy	90	100

Data from Luster M, Karges W, Zeich K, et al. Clinical value of (18)F-fluorodihydroxyphenylalanine positron emission tomography/computed tomography ((18)F-DOPA PET/CT) for detecting pheochromocytoma. Eur J Nucl Med Mol Imaging 2010;37(3):484–93; and Ilias I, Pacak K. Diagnosis, localization and treatment of pheochromocytoma in MEN 2 syndrome. Endocr Regul 2009;43(2):89–93.

last 15 years because of magnesium's anti-arrhythmic properties and its ability to decrease catecholamine stores and cause arteriolar vasodilation.[54–62]

Confirmatory Diagnostic Testing

Biochemical tests including 24-hour collection of urinary metanephrines and vanillylmandelic acid and plasma metanephrines are used to confirm a diagnose of pheochromocytoma. The sensitivity and specificity of these tests are listed in **Table 8**.

CT, magnetic resonance imaging, and scintigraphy scans are generally reserved to assist with planning operative course and are not part of the emergency department evaluation. The sensitivity and specificity of each imaging modality for diagnosing pheochromocytoma are provided in **Table 9**.

Disposition

Postoperatively, patients should be monitored closely for 24 hours in an intensive or immediate care unit. Hypotension and hypoglycemia are the most common postoperative complications.

Incidentalomas

Patients presenting to the emergency department increasingly receive CT scans of their chest, abdomen, or pelvis to evaluate for a myriad of complaints. Incidental adrenal masses are found in up to 4% of these scans.[63] Patients being discharged from the emergency department should be directed to follow up with their primary care provider in a timely manner to ascertain whether these masses are benign, nonfunctioning, hormonally active, malignant, or metastatic.

REFERENCES

1. PBS News Hour. President Kennedy's health secrets. Available at: http://www.pbs.org/newshour/bb/health/july-dec02/jfk_11-18.html. Accessed October 10, 2013.
2. Maugh TH III. John F. Kennedy's Addison's disease was probably caused by rare autoimmune disease: a navy doctor's report sheds light on the late president's medical records. Available at: http://articles.latimes.com/2009/sep/05/science/sci-jfk-addisons5. Accessed October 10, 2013.
3. Griffing GT, Odeke S, Nagelberg SB, et al. Addison disease. In Medscape. 2012. Available at: http://emedicine.medscape.com/article/116467-overview#a0199. Accessed August 30, 2013.

4. Erichsen MM, Løvås K, Skinningsrud B, et al. Clinical, immunological, and genetic features of autoimmune primary adrenal insufficiency: observations from a Norwegian registry. J Clin Endocrinol Metab 2009;94(12):4882–90.

5. Oelkers W. Adrenal insufficiency. N Engl J Med 1996;335:1206.

6. Tintinalli J, Stapczynski J, Ma OJ, et al. Tintinalli's emergency medicine: a comprehensive study guide. 7th edition. New York: The McGraw-Hill Companies, Inc; 2011. p. 1453.

7. Adams JG, Barton ED, Collings J, et al. Emergency medicine: clinical essentials. 2nd edition. Philadelphia: Saunders; 2013. p. 3098–9.

8. Bleicken B, Hahner S, Ventz M, et al. Delayed diagnosis of adrenal insufficiency is common: a cross-sectional study in 216 patients. Am J Med Sci 2010;339(6): 525–31.

9. Bender SL, Sherry NA, Masia R. Case records of the Massachusetts General Hospital: case 16–2013. A 12-year-old girl with irritability, hypersomnia, and somatic symptoms. N Engl J Med 2013;368:2015–24.

10. Papierska L, Rabijewski M. Delay in diagnosis of adrenal insufficiency is a frequent cause of adrenal crisis. Int J Endocrinol 2013;2013:482370.

11. Ross IL, Levitt NS. Addison's disease symptoms: a cross sectional study in urban South Africa. PLoS One 2013;8(1):e53526.

12. Taub YR, Wolford RW. Adrenal insufficiency and other adrenal oncologic emergencies. Emerg Med Clin North Am 2009;27:273.

13. Erichsen MM, Husebye ES, Michelsen TM, et al. Sexuality and fertility in women with Addison's disease. J Clin Endocrinol Metab 2010;95(9):4354–60.

14. Zaloga GP, Marik P. Hypothalamic-pituitary-adrenal insufficiency. Crit Care Clin 2001;17:27.

15. Kong MF, Jeffcoate W. Eighty-six cases of Addison's disease. Clin Endocrinol 1994;41:757–61.

16. Hahner S, Loeffler M, Bleicken B, et al. Epidemiology of adrenal crisis in chronic adrenal insufficiency: the need for new prevention strategies. Eur J Endocrinol 2010;162(3):597–602.

17. Hahner S, Allolio B. Therapeutic management of adrenal insufficiency. Best Pract Res Clin Endocrinol Metab 2009;23(2):167–79.

18. Baren J, Rothrock S. Pediatric emergency medicine. Philadelphia: Saunders; 2007.

19. Coles AJ, Thompson S, Cox AL, et al. Dehydroepiandrosterone replacement in patients with Addison's disease has a bimodal effect on regulatory (CD4+CD25hi and CD4+FoxP3+) T cells. Eur J Immunol 2005;35(12):3694–703.

20. Guillamondegui OD, Gunter OL, Patel S, et al. Acute adrenal insufficiency may affect outcome in the trauma patient. Am Surg 2009;75(4):287–90.

21. Bouillon R. Acute adrenal insufficiency. Endocrinol Metab Clin North Am 2006; 35:767.

22. Satre TJ, Kovach F. Clinical inquiries. What's the most practical way to rule out adrenal insufficiency? J Fam Pract 2009;58(5):281a-b.

23. Cooper MS, Stewart PM. Corticosteroid insufficiency in acutely ill patients. N Engl J Med 2003;348(8):727–34.

24. Hamrahian AH, Oseni TS, Arafah BM. Measurements of serum free cortisol in critically ill patients. N Engl J Med 2004;350(16):1629–38.

25. Chen H, Sippel RS, O'Dorisio MS, et al. The North American Neuroendocrine Tumor Society consensus guideline for the diagnosis and management of neuroendocrine tumors: pheochromocytoma, paraganglioma, and medullary thyroid cancer. Pancreas 2010;39(6):775–83.

26. Beard CM, Sheps SG, Kurland LT, et al. Occurrence of pheochromocytoma in Rochester, Minnesota, 1950 through 1979. Mayo Clin Proc 1983;58(12):802–4.
27. Young WF Jr. Clinical practice. The incidentally discovered adrenal mass. N Engl J Med 2007;356(6):601–10.
28. Manger WM. The protean manifestations of pheochromocytoma. Horm Metab Res 2009;41(9):658–63.
29. Calhoun DA, Jones D, Textor S, et al. Resistant hypertension: diagnosis, evaluation, and treatment: a scientific statement from the American Heart Association Professional Education Committee of the Council for High Blood Pressure Research. Hypertension 2008;51(6):1403–19.
30. Mazza A, Armigliato M, Marzola MC, et al. Anti-hypertensive treatment in pheochromocytoma and paraganglioma: current management and therapeutic features. Endocrine 2013 [Epub ahead of print]. Available at: http://link.springer.com/article/10.1007%2Fs12020-013-0007-y. Accessed October 10, 2013.
31. Dagartzikas MI, Sprague K, Carter G, et al. Cerebrovascular event, dilated cardiomyopathy, and pheochromocytoma. Pediatr Emerg Care 2002;18:33–5.
32. Fox JM, Manninen PH. The anaesthetic management of a patient with a phaeochromocytoma and acute stroke. Can J Anaesth 1991;38:775–9.
33. Leiba A, Bar-Dayan Y, Leker RR, et al. Seizures as a presenting symptom of phaeochromocytoma in a young soldier. J Hum Hypertens 2003;17:73–5.
34. Hendrickson RJ, Katzman PJ, Queiroz R, et al. Management of massive retroperitoneal hemorrhage from an adrenal tumor. Endocr J 2001;48:691–6.
35. Browers FM, Lenders JW, Eisenhofer G, et al. Pheochromocytoma as an endocrine emergency. Rev Endocr Metab Disord 2003;4:121–8.
36. Ferguson KL. Imipramine-provoked paradoxical pheochromocytoma crisis: a case of cardiogenic shock. Am J Emerg Med 1994;12:190–2.
37. Brown K, Ratner M, Stoll M. Pheochromocytoma unmasked by imipramine in an 8 year old girl. Pediatr Emerg Care 2003;1(9):174–7.
38. Maxwell PH, Buckley C, Gleadle JM, et al. Nasty shock after an anti-emetic. Nephrol Dial Transplant 2001;16:1069–72.
39. Leow MK, Loh KC. Accidental provocation of phaeochromocytoma: the forgotten hazard of metoclopramide? Singapore Med J 2005;46:557–60.
40. Takagi S, Miyazaki S, Fujii T, et al. Dexamethasone-induced cardiogenic shock rescued by percutaneous cardiopulmonary support (PCPS) in a patient with pheochromocytoma. Jpn Circ J 2000;64:785–8.
41. Rosas AL, Kasperlik-Zaluska AA, Papierska L, et al. Pheochromocytoma crisis induced by glucocorticoids: a report of four cases and review of the literature. Eur J Endocrinol 2008;158(3):423–9.
42. Oishi S, Sato T. Pheochromocytoma in pregnancy: a review of the Japanese literature. Endocr J 1994;41:219–25.
43. Ndayambagye E, Nakalembe M, Kaye D. Factors associated with persistent hypertension after puerperium among women with preeclampsia/eclampsia in Mulago hospital, Uganda. BMC Pregnancy Childbirth 2010;10:12.
44. Lalitha R, Opio CK. A missed diagnosis or a masquerading disease: back to the basics. Pan Afr Med J 2013;15:29.
45. Anderson NE, Chung K, Willoughby E, et al. Neurological manifestations of phaeochromocytomas and secretory paragangliomas: a reappraisal. J Neurol Neurosurg Psychiatry 2013;84(4):452–7.
46. Uchida N, Ishiguro K, Suda T, et al. Pheochromocytoma multisystem crisis successfully treated by emergency surgery: report of a case. Surg Today 2010;40(10):990–6.

47. Scholten A, Cisco RM, Vriens MR, et al. Pheochromocytoma crisis is not a surgical emergency. J Clin Endocrinol Metab 2013;98(2):581–91.
48. Wong C, Yu R. Preoperative preparation for pheochromocytoma resection: physician survey and clinical practice. Exp Clin Endocrinol Diabetes 2010; 118(7):400–4.
49. Russell WJ, Metcalfe IR, Tonkin AL, et al. The preoperative management of phaeochromocytoma. Anaesth Intensive Care 1998;26(2):196–200.
50. Steinsapir J, Carr AA, Prisant LM, et al. Metyrosine and pheochromocytoma. Arch Intern Med 1997;157(8):901–6.
51. Bogdonoff DL. Pheochromocytoma: specialist cases that all must be prepared to treat? J Cardiothorac Vasc Anesth 2002;16(3):267–9.
52. Perry RR, Keiser HR, Norton JA, et al. Surgical management of pheochromocytoma with the use of metyrosine. Ann Surg 1990;212(5):621–8.
53. Lentschener C, Gaujoux S, Thillois JM, et al. Increased arterial pressure is not predictive of haemodynamic instability in patients undergoing adrenalectomy for phaeochromocytoma. Acta Anaesthesiol Scand 2009;53(4):522–7.
54. Van Braeckel P, Carlier S, Steelant PJ, et al. Perioperative management of phaeochromocytoma. Acta Anaesthesiol Belg 2009;60(1):55–66.
55. James MF, Cronjé L. Pheochromocytoma crisis: the use of magnesium sulfate. Anesth Analg 2004;99(3):680–6.
56. James MF. Use of magnesium sulphate in the anaesthetic management of phaeochromocytoma: a review of 17 anaesthetics. Br J Anaesth 1989;62(6): 616–23.
57. Bullough A, Karadia S, Watters M. Phaeochromocytoma: an unusual cause of hypertension in pregnancy. Anaesthesia 2001;56(1):43–6.
58. Morton A. Magnesium sulphate for phaeochromocytoma crisis. Emerg Med Australas 2007;19(5):482.
59. Waguespack SG, Rich T, Grubbs E, et al. A current review of the etiology, diagnosis, and treatment of pediatric pheochromocytoma and paraganglioma. J Clin Endocrinol Metab 2010;95(5):2023–37.
60. Sheps SG, Jiang NS, Klee GG, et al. Recent developments in the diagnosis and treatment of pheochromocytoma. Mayo Clin Proc 1990;65(1):88–95.
61. Luster M, Karges W, Zeich K, et al. Clinical value of (18)F-fluorodihydroxyphenylalanine positron emission tomography/computed tomography ((18)F-DOPA PET/CT) for detecting pheochromocytoma. Eur J Nucl Med Mol Imaging 2010;37(3):484–93.
62. Ilias I, Pacak K. Diagnosis, localization and treatment of pheochromocytoma in MEN 2 syndrome. Endocr Regul 2009;43(2):89–93.
63. Bovio S, Cataldi A, Reimondo G, et al. Prevalence of adrenal incidentaloma in a contemporary computerized tomography series. J Endocrinol Invest 2006; 29(4):298–302.

Index

Note: Page numbers of article titles are in **boldface** type.

Emerg Med Clin N Am 32 (2014) 485–493
http://dx.doi.org/10.1016/S0733-8627(14)00018-2
0733-8627/14/$ – see front matter © 2014 Elsevier Inc. All rights reserved.

Moving?

Make sure your subscription moves with you!

To notify us of your new address, find your **Clinics Account Number** (located on your mailing label above your name), and contact customer service at:

Email: journalscustomerservice-usa@elsevier.com

800-654-2452 (subscribers in the U.S. & Canada)
314-447-8871 (subscribers outside of the U.S. & Canada)

Fax number: 314-447-8029

**Elsevier Health Sciences Division
Subscription Customer Service
3251 Riverport Lane
Maryland Heights, MO 63043**

*To ensure uninterrupted delivery of your subscription, please notify us at least 4 weeks in advance of move.

Printed and bound by CPI Group (UK) Ltd, Croydon, CR0 4YY

03/10/2024

01040489-0005